Challenges in Diagnosis and Treatment of Infertility

Challenges in Diagnosis and Treatment of Infertility

Guest Editor

Konstantinos A. Zikopoulos

MDPI

Basel • Beijing • Wuhan • Barcelona • Belgrade • Novi Sad • Cluj • Manchester

Guest Editor
Konstantinos A. Zikopoulos
Department of Obstetrics and
Gynaecology
University of Ioannina
Ioannina
Greece

Editorial Office
MDPI AG
Grosspeteranlage 5
4052 Basel, Switzerland

This is a reprint of the Special Issue, published open access by the journal *Journal of Clinical Medicine* (ISSN 2077-0383), freely accessible at: https://www.mdpi.com/journal/jcm/special_issues/233D25OURQ.

For citation purposes, cite each article independently as indicated on the article page online and as indicated below:

Lastname, A.A.; Lastname, B.B. Article Title. *Journal Name* **Year**, *Volume Number*, Page Range.

ISBN 978-3-7258-4365-7 (Hbk)
ISBN 978-3-7258-4366-4 (PDF)
https://doi.org/10.3390/books978-3-7258-4366-4

Contents

Journal of
Clinical Medicine

MDPI

Article

High-Risk Outcomes in In Vitro Fertilization Pregnancies for Women of a Very Advanced Maternal Age: Insights from a Multi-Hospital Study in Greece

Themistoklis Loukopoulos [1,*], Athanasios Zikopoulos [2], Efstratios Kolibianakis [3], Anastasia Vatopoulou [1], Fani Gkrozou [1], Sotirios Sotiriou [4], Athanasios Zachariou [5] and Charikleia Skentou [1]

1 Department of Obstetrics and Gynecology, Medical School of Ioannina, University General Hospital, 45110 Ioannina, Greece
2 Obstetrics and Gynecology, Royal Devon and Exeter Hospital Barrack Rd, Exeter EX 25 DW, UK
3 3rd Department of Obstetrics and Gynecology, Aristotle University of Thessaloniki, 54128 Thessaloniki, Greece
4 Department of Embryology, Faculty of Medicine, University of Thessaly, 38221 Larissa, Greece
5 Department of Urology, Medical School of Ioannina, University General Hospital, 45110 Ioannina, Greece; zahariou@otenet.gr
* Correspondence: themistoklis.loukopoulos@gmail.com

Abstract: Background: In vitro fertilization (IVF) has transformed infertility treatment, yet it is associated with increased risks of adverse perinatal outcomes, particularly in women of advanced maternal age. This study aimed to investigate the prevalence of complications such as preeclampsia (PE), gestational diabetes mellitus (GDM), preterm labor (PTL), low birth weight (LBW), and placental abnormalities (PA) among women over 50 undergoing assisted reproductive technology (ART) in Greece, where the eligibility age limit has been recently raised to 54 years. **Methods:** We conducted a retrospective analysis of pregnancy outcomes in women over 50 compared to those under 50, utilizing medical records mainly from University Hospital of Ioannina but also from other public hospitals and private clinics in Greece. **Results:** Our findings indicate that women over 50 face an increased risk of developing preeclampsia (PE) by 4.61 times, GDM by 1.69 times, PTL by 1.82 times, LBW by 1.67 times, and PA by 3.92 times. **Conclusions:** These results underscore the need for heightened awareness and the monitoring of pregnancy complications in this demographic, informing clinical strategies to improve maternal and neonatal outcomes.

Keywords: assisted reproduction; in vitro fertilization; aging; preeclampsia; gestational diabetes; preterm labor; low birth weight; placenta abnormalities

1. Introduction

The development of in vitro fertilization (IVF) has revolutionized the management of infertility, offering an effective therapeutic option for individuals across diverse age groups. Greece attracts over 1000 women annually, owing to its notable IVF success rates, progressive legislative framework, and access to advanced medical infrastructure equipped with cutting-edge technologies. These factors have positioned Greece as a prominent hub for reproductive tourism, facilitating access to assisted reproductive technologies (ART) for international patients [1].

The recent expansion of age restrictions for IVF eligibility in Greece has led to an increase in the number of women over 50 seeking treatment. Similar trends are being observed globally, driven by socioeconomic factors that contribute to an increasing desire among women to conceive at an advanced maternal age. However, advanced maternal age (AMA) remains consistently associated with an elevated risk of adverse pregnancy outcomes. It is important to note that the significantly higher reliance on egg donation among women of advanced maternal age (AMA) distinguishes these pregnancies from those of younger women. This distinction complicates the assessment of age-related risks, as adverse outcomes in older women undergoing IVF may result not only from advanced maternal age itself but also from the specific consequences of utilizing donor eggs.

Complications frequently associated with pregnancies in AMA women include placental abnormalities, low birth weight, preterm labor, preeclampsia, and gestational diabetes mellitus (GDM). Recent studies have provided further insights into these risks. For example, Sugai et al. (2023) conducted a systematic review and meta-analysis focusing on pregnancies in women over 45 years of age, reporting a significantly higher incidence of adverse outcomes such as preeclampsia and GDM [2]. Similarly, Thilaganathan investigated the cardiovascular-placental axis in the context of preeclampsia, identifying mechanisms that impair physiological adaptations during pregnancy in older mothers [3].

In addition, Sacha et al. evaluated live births from both fresh and frozen embryo transfers, emphasizing the critical influence of placental health on IVF pregnancy outcomes [4]. Their findings indicate that pregnancies following frozen embryo transfers exhibit more anatomical and vascular placental pathology compared to those from fresh transfers, despite similar maternal outcomes. Furthermore, Masoudian et al. (2023) identified a concerning correlation between oocyte donation pregnancies and the heightened incidence of preeclampsia and gestational hypertension, underscoring the unique risks associated with donor egg pregnancies [5].

This retrospective study aimed to compare the prevalence of pregnancy complications—specifically preterm labor (PTL) [6], low birth weight (LBW), placental abnormalities (PA), gestational diabetes mellitus (GDM), and preeclampsia (PE)—among women over 50 undergoing IVF in Greece with those under 50 [7]. By identifying these disparities, we seek to enhance awareness of the risks associated with advanced maternal age (AMA) in assisted reproductive technology (ART) pregnancies and to inform clinical strategies aimed at improving maternal and neonatal outcomes.

2. Materials and Methods

This retrospective cohort study was conducted at the University Hospital of Ioannina and other public hospitals and private clinics across Greece from 2014 to 2024.

2.1. Participant Selection

Women who underwent successful in vitro fertilization (IVF) procedures and delivered at the University Hospital of Ioannina during the study period were identified through computerized hospital discharge records. Additionally, data were collected from women over 50 years of age who received IVF treatment at other public hospitals and private clinics throughout Greece. A total of 383 participants were selected based on the following inclusion criteria: women who had undergone a standardized IVF procedure that included both oocyte donation and autologous cycles. Specifically, women over the age of 50 were more likely to receive donor oocytes due to their menopausal status, as they had not undergone ovarian stimulation.

2.2. IVF Procedures

Women who underwent ovarian stimulation received a gonadotropin-based protocol, with dosages tailored to individual ovarian responses. Ovarian response was monitored through regular ultrasound examinations and serum hormone level assessments (estradiol, progesterone, and LH), allowing for adjustments in medication as necessary. Oocyte retrieval was performed using transvaginal ultrasound-guided aspiration.

Endometrial preparation was conducted for both frozen and donor cycles, which included the administration of estrogen and progesterone to promote endometrial development necessary for successful implantation.

Of the 383 participants, 296 women were categorized as the "Below 50 Years" group, while 87 women were designated as the "Above 50 Years" group. In the "Below 50 Years" group, 73 women (24.7%) utilized donor eggs, and 156 women (52.7%) underwent a stimulation protocol; 177 women (59.7%) received endometrial preparation. In contrast, the "Above 50 Years" group had 81 women (93.1%) using donor eggs, and all received endometrial preparation.

2.3. Outcomes and Data Collection

A retrospective analysis was performed to compare the incidence of pre-eclampsia, gestational diabetes mellitus, preterm labor, low birth weight, and placental abnormalities (including placenta previa, placenta accreta, and placental abruption) between the two groups. Twin pregnancies were documented, with 107 women (36%) in the "Below 50 Years" group experiencing twin pregnancies, although two cases resulted in singleton deliveries due to fetal demise at 14 and 21 weeks of gestation, respectively. In the "Above 50 Years" group, twin pregnancies were observed in 38 out of 87 women (43.6%).

2.4. Prenatal Care and Delivery

Prenatal care and ultrasound examinations were conducted by physicians certified by the Fetal Medicine Foundation (FMF). All deliveries were performed in tertiary care hospitals exclusively via cesarean section. Women identified as being at moderate or high risk for preeclampsia were prescribed 150 mg of aspirin daily, in accordance with the latest guidelines from the European Society of Hypertension.

3. Statistical Analysis

All categorical outcomes, along with the age group classifications, were summarized using frequencies and percentages. The statistical relationships between each outcome and the age groups were evaluated using Pearson's Chi-Square test, following verification of its underlying assumptions. Odds ratios (ORs) with corresponding 95% confidence intervals (CIs) were calculated to quantify the strength of these associations. Data analysis was performed using SPSS software (version 26.0), with a significance threshold set at $p < 0.05$ for all tests.

4. Results

The sample comprised 383 women, 22.7% of whom were aged between 50 and 54 years (above 50 years group). Recorded adverse outcomes included preeclampsia, gestational diabetes, preterm labor, low birth weight, and placenta abnormalities. The analysis revealed statistically significant differences between age groups for all examined adverse outcomes, except for a low birth weight.

The adverse outcomes in two groups are displayed in Table 1.

The odds of preeclampsia were 4.61 times higher in the above 50 years group compared to the below 50 years group (95% CI: 2.31–9.19; $p < 0.001$). Similarly, the odds of GDM were 1.69 times higher in the above 50 years group (95% CI: 1.01–2.82; $p = 0.043$).

For preterm labor, the odds were 1.82 times higher in the above 50 years group (95% CI: 1.01–3.27; $p = 0.043$). The odds regarding low birth weight were 1.67 but not significantly different to 1 with a 95% CI: (0.90–3.09; $p = 0.101$). Lastly, the odds of placenta abnormalities were 3.92 times higher (95% CI: 2.22–6.91; $p < 0.001$).

These statistical differences are illustrated in Figure 1.

Table 1. Adverse outcomes in the two age groups.

	Age					
	Below 50 Years		**Above 50 Years**			
	$n = 296$	%	$n = 97$	%	OR (95% CI)	p
Preeclampsia	18	6.10%	20	23.00%	4.61 (2.31–9.19))	<0.001
Gestational diabetes	73	24.70%	31	35.60%	1.69 (1.01–2.82)	0.043
Preterm labor	44	14.90%	21	24.10%	1.82 (1.01–3.27)	0.043
Low birth weight	40	13.50%	18	20.70%	1.67 (0.90–3.09)	0.101
Placenta abnormalities	35	11.80%	30	34.50%	3.92 (2.22–6.91)	<0.001

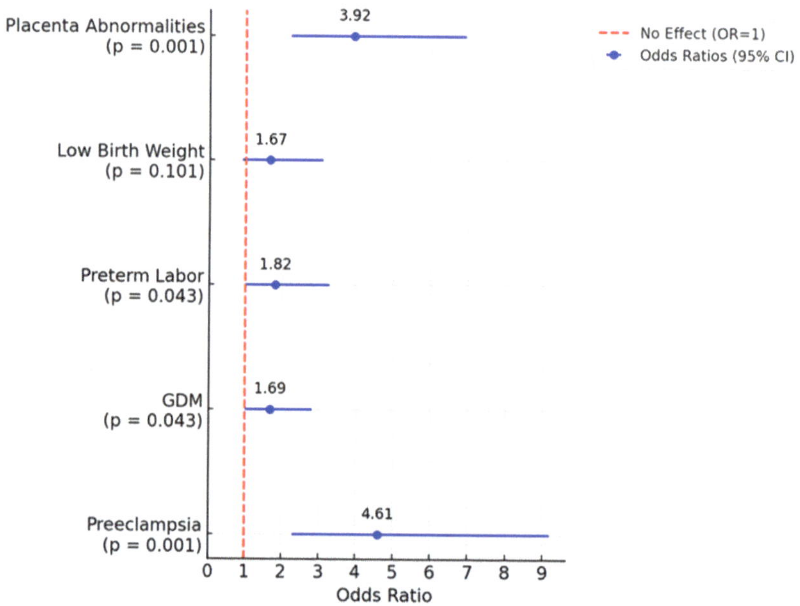

Figure 1. Forest plot comparing pregnancy complications between women aged above 50-year-old and those below 50-year-old.

5. Discussion

This retrospective cohort study aimed to evaluate the association between maternal age and the incidence of common pregnancy complications in pregnancies achieved through in vitro fertilization (IVF). The findings demonstrated a significant increase in the prevalence of major complications among women aged over 50 years compared to those under 50 years. These complications included preeclampsia, gestational diabetes mellitus, preterm labor, and placental abnormalities.

5.1. Preeclampsia

The existing literature indicates that pregnancies conceived via in vitro fertilization (IVF) have a higher risk of developing preeclampsia (PE) compared to spontaneous pregnancies [8–11]. In the present study, the incidence of preeclampsia among women under 50 years of age (6.1%) aligns with previous findings. However, the incidence observed in women over 50 years of age (23%) was markedly higher than the rates reported in earlier studies.

The exact etiology of preeclampsia (PE) remains incompletely understood; however, improper placentation is widely recognized as a critical factor in its pathogenesis [11–13]. This process involves deficient trophoblast invasion, inadequate placental implantation, insufficient spiral artery remodeling, and placental hypoperfusion [14,15]. Additional factors potentially contributing to PE include immunological dysfunction, inflammation, and genetic predispositions. The role of in vitro fertilization (IVF) and associated risk factors in the development of PE remains a subject of debate.

A retrospective population analysis identified multiple pregnancies as a primary contributor to the increased prevalence of PE in assisted reproductive technologies (ARTs) [16]. This finding may partially explain the significant differences observed in our study, where twin pregnancies were more frequent among older women (43.6%) compared to younger women (36%). Another interesting finding in our study concerns endometrial preparation. While many women under 50 years old received stimulation, not all of them received endometrial preparation. In contrast, every woman in the "Above 50 Years" group received endometrial preparation as a part of their treatment, which is essential due to their menopausal status. This difference in estrogen and progesterone administration could help explain why we observed a higher incidence of preeclampsia (PE) in the older group.

While prior studies have reported an elevated risk of PE in overweight or obese women, no significant differences in body mass index (BMI) were identified between the age groups in our study [17,18].

Despite the multifactorial etiology of preeclampsia (PE), poor trophoblastic invasion and improper placentation—often linked to endometrial dysplasia during ovarian stimulation therapy—are considered key triggers for its onset [16]. In IVF pregnancies, the embryo is transferred to the uterine cavity via the cervix, and the hormonal alterations associated with IVF can disrupt the establishment of the maternal–fetal interface, potentially resulting in defective placental function [9].

A recent systematic review and meta-analysis identified advanced maternal age as an independent risk factor for PE, along with other complications such as gestational diabetes, stillbirth, intrauterine growth restriction, and placenta previa [19]. These complications may be associated with poor placentation and the progressive decline in uterine vascular endothelial function that occurs with aging [20–22]. The findings of our retrospective study align with these observations, further substantiating the evidence on the relationship between advanced maternal age, IVF, and adverse pregnancy outcomes.

5.2. Gestational Diabetes Mellitus

Gestational diabetes mellitus (GDM) is the most prevalent metabolic disorder during pregnancy, characterized by insulin resistance and an insufficient compensatory function of pancreatic islet β cells [23]. The higher incidence of GDM in women of advanced maternal age is thought to be linked to age-related dysregulation of lipid metabolism and increased oxidative stress [24]. Emerging evidence suggests that GDM has a multifactorial etiology, influenced by both genetic and environmental factors. Notably, interactions between maternal age, body mass index (BMI), and ethnicity play a significant role in the development of GDM [20].

Assisted reproductive technology (ART) is associated with an increased risk of gestational diabetes mellitus (GDM), with studies reporting a 1.59-fold higher risk in ART-conceived pregnancies compared to spontaneously conceived pregnancies [25]. This risk is particularly pronounced in women undergoing in vitro fertilization (IVF) compared to those utilizing intracytoplasmic sperm injection (ICSI) [23]. Additionally, maternal age has been shown to have a significant positive correlation with the risk of GDM, with a 7.90% increase in risk for each additional year of maternal age [26,27]. Our findings are consistent with the existing literature, demonstrating a higher incidence of GDM in older women (24.7% in the younger group vs. 35.6% in women over 50 years old).

5.3. Preterm Labor

The World Health Organization (WHO) defines preterm labor (PTL) as any birth occurring before 37 weeks (259 days) of gestation, irrespective of whether the pregnancy involves a single or multiple gestation [28]. PTL is a leading contributor to increased fetal and neonatal mortality and morbidity, even in high-income countries [29]. While the precise etiology of PTL remains unknown, it is believed to result from either early idiopathic activation or pathological deviations from the processes of normal labor.

Current understanding suggests that PTL is a multifactorial condition initiated by various triggers, including infection or inflammation, uterine–placental ischemia or hemorrhage, uterine overdistension, stress, and immune-mediated mechanisms [30].

The association between preterm labor (PTL) and advanced maternal age (AMA) remains a subject of ongoing investigation [31]. Multiple studies have reported a link between AMA and an elevated risk of PTL, even after adjusting for confounding factors such as body mass index (BMI), education level, parity, pre-existing health conditions, and the method of conception [31]. In our study, women of very advanced maternal age exhibited a 1.82-fold increased likelihood of experiencing PTL compared to younger women. Although this association did not reach statistical significance, it indicates a potential trend consistent with the existing literature.

Interestingly, the older cohort in our study also showed higher rates of preeclampsia and gestational diabetes mellitus, both of which are well-documented risk factors for PTL [31–33]. Therefore, the observed increased risk of PTL in this group may be partially attributable to these underlying complications.

5.4. Low Birth Weight

Low birth weight (LBW) is defined by the World Health Organization (WHO) as a birth weight of less than 2500 g (up to and including 2499 g), irrespective of gestational age. It is further categorized into very low birth weight (VLBW) for infants weighing less than 1500 g and extremely low birth weight (ELBW) for those under 1000 g [34]. LBW is typically associated with preterm delivery, intrauterine growth restriction (IUGR), or a combination of both factors [35]. In contrast, "small for gestational age" (SGA) specifically refers to newborns with a birth weight below the 10th percentile for their gestational age [34]. This study focused exclusively on infants with birth weights below 2500 g.

The literature suggests that LBW risk parallels the risk of preterm labor (PTL), with both increasing with maternal age [36]. In our analysis, women over 50 years of age demonstrated a 1.67-fold higher likelihood of delivering LBW infants compared to younger women. However, this association did not reach statistical significance. The observed elevated risk of LBW is likely attributable to the higher incidence of preterm labor among older women in our study.

A well-established link exists between fetal growth restriction (FGR) and placental trophoblast aging [37]. Placentas affected by FGR often exhibit inadequate vascularization, reduced vascular branching, and diminished capillary density. Additionally, these placentas display increased rates of apoptosis, decreased cellular proliferation, and an elevated presence of syncytial nuclear aggregates (SNAs) [38]. While physiological placental aging is a normal process, abnormal or premature placental senescence can disrupt key functions, particularly nutrient and oxygen exchange, thereby contributing to adverse pregnancy outcomes [39].

Recent research indicates that advanced maternal age is associated with reduced expression of the anti-aging protein α-Klotho in placental trophoblasts. This reduction accelerates premature senescence and diminishes placental functionality, potentially leading to placental malformations and poor perinatal outcomes, such as FGR and low birth weight (LBW) [40].

5.5. Placental Abnormalities

Advanced maternal age has been strongly associated with compromised placental function, often attributed to reduced uterine blood flow, uteroplacental hypoperfusion, and increased prevalence of extensive placental infarctions. These factors contribute to a heightened risk of hemorrhagic conditions and placental abnormalities, which are more common in older women [41].

In our study, we investigated three categories of placental abnormalities: placenta previa, placenta accreta, and placental abruption [42]. According to the existing literature, the risks of these complications are elevated in pregnancies conceived through in vitro fertilization (IVF) compared to spontaneous conceptions, with reported prevalence rates of 4.8% for placenta previa, 4.7% for placenta accreta, and 1% for placental abruption. The absolute risk of these complications further increases with maternal age [42].

The results of our cohort were consistent among women under 50 years old, since the incidence of combined placental abnormalities in this group was 11.8%. However, this rate rose markedly with age, reaching 34.5% in women over 50. This significant difference may be attributed to the higher use of donor eggs, which occurred in 24.7% of the younger group and 93.1% of the older group. IVF using donor eggs is associated with a greater risk of placental anomalies, likely due to a combination of immunological, vascular, and endometrial factors.

In donor egg pregnancies, the genetic disparity between the mother and fetus induces heightened immunological activity at the maternal–fetal interface, resembling a host-versus-graft rejection. This response is characterized by severe chronic deciduitis, extensive fibrinoid deposition, and enhanced villitis of unknown origin, all of which impair placental development and functionality [43]. Furthermore, the absence of a corpus luteum in most donor egg pregnancies above 50 years of age reduces endometrial receptivity and decidualization, creating a suboptimal environment for trophoblast invasion and vascular remodeling.

Genome-wide studies have also identified altered expression of coagulation and immunological regulatory proteins in donor egg pregnancies, which contribute to placental dysfunction and complications such as preeclampsia and fetal growth restriction [44]. These mechanisms likely explain the increased risk of placental abnormalities observed in our study, particularly among the older age group undergoing IVF with donor eggs.

5.6. Impact of Egg Donation on Outcomes Between Two Groups

Pregnancies resulting from egg donation tend to have a higher chance of developing complications—such as preeclampsia and the rest of the conditions we included in our study—as compared to spontaneous conception and in vitro fertilization (IVF) with autologous eggs.

Keukens' most current and extensive meta-analysis, published in 2022, evaluated the risk of developing preeclampsia and severe preeclampsia in pregnancies resulting from spontaneous conception, IVF with autologous eggs, or egg donation. Specifically, among the group that received egg donation and those who achieved pregnancy naturally, the likelihood of preeclampsia was approximately five times greater in the former group (OR: 5.09, 95% CI: 4.29–6.04), while the risk for severe preeclampsia was over seven times greater in the first group (OR: 7.42, 95% CI: 4.64–11.88). The increased risk associated with egg donation remained significant when compared to the IVF group using autologous eggs. In this case, the risk of both preeclampsia and severe preeclampsia was approximately three times higher in pregnancies with egg donation (OR: 2.97, 95% CI: 2.49–3.53, OR: 2.97, 95% CI: 2.15–4.11, respectively) [45].

Regarding the rates of egg donor usage in our retrospective study, among women under 50, it was 24.7%, while in participants over 50 years old, it was 93.1%. Statistical analysis showed that the likelihood of preeclampsia was 4.6 times higher in the latter group (6.10% vs. 23.00%, OR: 4.61 (2.31–9.19) $p < 0.001$). Considering the aforementioned literature, the significant difference observed in the rates of egg donation between the two groups may explain part of the markedly increased frequency of preeclampsia in the older age group of our study.

Other placental-related conditions, including placenta previa, placenta accreta, and placenta abruption, may occur more frequently in pregnancies resulting from oocyte donation. This higher risk is likely due to a variety of factors, including aberrant immunological responses at the fetal–maternal interface, abnormalities in endometrial receptivity, and underlying maternal features. These variables may contribute to placental dysfunction, resulting in a greater frequency of complications that impact placentation and overall pregnancy outcomes in this patient population [44].

Besides preeclampsia, pregnancies achieved through oocyte donation tend to have a higher chance of complications, such as preterm birth (PTB) and low birth weight (LBW), too. A systematic review and meta-analysis by Mascarenhas showed an increased risk of PTB following fresh embryo transfer in OD pregnancies compared to AO IVF pregnancies (OR 1.45, 95% CI 1.20–1.77). Similarly, the risk of LBW is higher after fresh embryo transfer in OD pregnancies than in AO IVF pregnancies (OR 1.34, 95% CI 1.12–1.60). When examining preterm birth before 32 weeks and very low birth weight, the likelihood of both outcomes remained higher in the OD group (OR 2.14, 95% CI 1.40–3.25 for early PTB and OR 1.51, 95% CI 1.17–1.95 for very low birth weight, respectively) [46].

Concerning gestational diabetes mellitus, there is a disagreement in the literature about whether it is independently influenced by oocyte donation. A meta-analysis by Moreno–Sepulveda found a significantly increased risk of GDM in singleton pregnancies resulting from oocyte donation compared to those from IVF, with an odds ratio of 1.27 (95% CI: 1.0, 1.56) [47]. In contrast, Storgaard's meta-analysis reported a non-significant pooled risk estimate (aOR: 1.33, 95 %CI: 0.71, 2.50) [48].

It is important to acknowledge the inclusion of a limited number of participants, as the age limit for in vitro fertilization (IVF) in Greece was only recently raised to 54 years. This constraint highlights the need for cautious interpretation of our findings. Nonetheless, despite this limitation, statistical analyses revealed significant differences across all examined outcomes, with the exception of low birth weight (LBW). Although the difference in low birth weight (LBW) was not statistically significant, the direction and magnitude of the observed difference were consistent with the trends seen in other adverse outcomes among older vs. younger women. This finding may reflect a lack of statistical power as a potential explanation for the absence of significance. Alternatively, other factors, such as the higher utilization of frozen embryos in this age group compared to younger women, may also contribute to this result. To enhance the applicability and robustness of our findings, future research should aim to include larger and more diverse samples of women over the age of 50.

Moreover, while the study accounted for BMI as a potential confounder, other lifestyle factors and pre-existing health conditions were not included due to data limitations. Factors such as smoking, physical activity, and socio-economic status are known to influence pregnancy outcomes and could interact with advanced maternal age (AMA) to amplify risks. Additionally, the prevalence of pre-existing conditions like hypertension or diabetes, which are more common in AMA populations, may have contributed to the observed complications. Future studies should integrate detailed data on these variables to enhance the understanding of their independent and combined effects on maternal and neonatal outcomes in this high-risk group.

Healthcare providers should engage in comprehensive pre-treatment counseling that addresses the unique risks and benefits associated with IVF in women over 50. This includes discussing potential complications, such as all age-related risks mentioned in this paper. It is essential to develop individualized treatment plans that take into account the patient's overall health and reproductive goals.

6. Conclusions

Our retrospective study provides valuable insights into the relationship between very advanced maternal age and the increased incidence of pregnancy complications following in vitro fertilization (IVF) therapy in Greece. The findings underscore the significantly higher risks faced by women over 50 years of age compared to their younger counterparts. Women in this age group were found to have a markedly increased risk of preeclampsia, gestational diabetes, preterm labor, and placental abnormalities. These results contribute to the growing body of literature exploring the complex interplay between advanced maternal age and adverse perinatal outcomes. They emphasize the importance of providing comprehensive prenatal care and informed decision-making for older women pursuing IVF therapy. Consequently, clinicians should consider the high-risk profile of women of advanced maternal age and provide appropriate counseling and close monitoring for this population. To build upon these findings, further research with larger sample sizes is essential to confirm the observed associations and investigate the underlying mechanisms driving these relationships. Such research will ultimately inform clinical practice and support interventions aimed at improving maternal and neonatal health outcomes in this high-risk group.

Author Contributions: Conceptualization, T.L., C.S. and A.Z. (Athanasios Zikopoulos); methodology, T.L. and A.Z. (Athanasios Zikopoulos); validation, C.S., F.G., A.V., A.Z. (Athanasios Zikopoulos), A.Z. (Athanasios Zachariou) and S.S.; resources, T.L. and C.S.; data curation, T.L. and A.Z. (Athanasios Zikopoulos); writing-original draft preparation, T.L.; writing-review and editing, T.L., E.K. and A.Z. (Athanasios Zikopoulos); visualization, T.L., C.S. and A.Z. (Athanasios Zikopoulos); supervision, C.S. and E.K. All authors have read and agreed to the published version of the manuscript.

Funding: This research received no external funding.

Institutional Review Board Statement: Ethical review and approval were waived for this study due to this is a retrospective analysis.

Informed Consent Statement: Patient consent was waived due to this is a retrospective analysis.

Data Availability Statement: The data presented in this study are available on request from the corresponding author.

Conflicts of Interest: The authors declare no conflicts of interest.

References

1. Athanasopoulou, P.; Giovanis, A.N.; Gdonteli, K. Health Tourism in Greece: The Fertility Center in Crete. In *Strategic Innovative Marketing and Tourism*; Kavoura, A., Borges-Tiago, T., Tiago, F., Eds.; Springer Proceedings in Business and Economics; Springer Nature: Cham, Switzerland, 2024; pp. 141–146. Available online: https://link.springer.com/10.1007/978-3-031-51038-0_16 (accessed on 28 November 2024).
2. Sugai, S.; Haino, K.; Yoshihara, K.; Nishijima, K. Pregnancy outcomes at maternal age over 45 years: A systematic review and meta-analysis. *Am. J. Obstet. Gynecol. MFM* **2023**, *5*, 100885. [CrossRef] [PubMed]
3. Thilaganathan, B. Pre-eclampsia and the cardiovascular-placental axis. *Ultrasound Obstet. Gynecol.* **2018**, *51*, 714–717. [CrossRef] [PubMed]
4. Sacha, C.R.; Harris, A.L.; James, K.; Basnet, K.; Freret, T.S.; Yeh, J.; Kaimal, A.; Souter, I.; Roberts, D.J. Placental pathology in live births conceived with in vitro fertilization after fresh and frozen embryo transfer. *Am. J. Obstet. Gynecol.* **2020**, *222*, 360.e1–360.e16. [CrossRef] [PubMed]
5. Masoudian, P.; Nasr, A.; de Nanassy, J.; Fung-Kee-Fung, K.; Bainbridge, S.A.; El Demellawy, D. Oocyte donation pregnancies and the risk of preeclampsia or gestational hypertension: A systematic review and metaanalysis. *Am. J. Obstet. Gynecol.* **2016**, *214*, 328–339. [CrossRef]
6. Glick, I.; Kadish, E.; Rottenstreich, M. Management of Pregnancy in Women of Advanced Maternal Age: Improving Outcomes for Mother and Baby. *Int. J. Women's Health* **2021**, *13*, 751–759. [CrossRef]
7. Correa-de-Araujo, R.; Yoon, S.S.S. Clinical Outcomes in High-Risk Pregnancies Due to Advanced Maternal Age. *J. Women's Health* **2021**, *30*, 160–167. [CrossRef]
8. Thomopoulos, C.; Tsioufis, C.; Michalopoulou, H.; Makris, T.; Papademetriou, V.; Stefanadis, C. Assisted reproductive technology and pregnancy-related hypertensive complications: A systematic review. *J. Hum. Hypertens.* **2013**, *27*, 148–157. [CrossRef] [PubMed]
9. Watanabe, N.; Fujiwara, T.; Suzuki, T.; Jwa, S.C.; Taniguchi, K.; Yamanobe, Y.; Kozuka, K.; Sago, H. Is in vitro fertilization associated with preeclampsia? A propensity score matched study. *BMC Pregnancy Childbirth* **2014**, *14*, 69. [CrossRef]
10. Xiong, F.; Hu, L.; Zhang, Y.; Xiao, X. Correlation of hypertensive disorders in pregnancy with procedures of in vitro fertilization and pregnancy outcomes. *Exp. Ther. Med.* **2017**, *14*, 5405–5410. [CrossRef] [PubMed]
11. Wang, S.; Chinnasamy, T.; Lifson, M.A.; Inci, F.; Demirci, U. Flexible Substrate-Based Devices for Point-of-Care Diagnostics. *Trends Biotechnol.* **2016**, *34*, 909–921. [CrossRef] [PubMed]
12. Stern, J.E.; Luke, B.; Tobias, M.; Gopal, D.; Hornstein, M.D.; Diop, H. Adverse pregnancy and birth outcomes associated with underlying diagnosis with and without assisted reproductive technology treatment. *Fertil. Steril.* **2015**, *103*, 1438–1445. [CrossRef] [PubMed]
13. Kroener, L.; Wang, E.; Pisarska, M. Predisposing Factors to Abnormal First Trimester Placentation and the Impact on Fetal Outcomes. *Semin. Reprod. Med.* **2015**, *34*, 027–035. [CrossRef] [PubMed]
14. Gui, J.; Ling, Z.; Hou, X.; Fan, Y.; Xie, K.; Shen, R. In vitro fertilization is associated with the onset and progression of preeclampsia. *Placenta* **2020**, *89*, 50–57. [CrossRef] [PubMed]
15. Ness, R.B.; Sibai, B.M. Shared and disparate components of the pathophysiologies of fetal growth restriction and preeclampsia. *Am. J. Obstet. Gynecol.* **2006**, *195*, 40–49. [CrossRef] [PubMed]
16. Wang, Y.A.; Chughtai, A.A.; Farquhar, C.M.; Pollock, W.; Lui, K.; Sullivan, E.A. Increased incidence of gestational hypertension and preeclampsia after assisted reproductive technology treatment. *Fertil. Steril.* **2016**, *105*, 920–926.e2. [CrossRef] [PubMed]
17. O'Brien, T.E.; Ray, J.G.; Chan, W.S. Maternal body mass index and the risk of preeclampsia: A systematic overview. *Epidemiology* **2003**, *14*, 368–374. [CrossRef] [PubMed]
18. Myers, J.E. What are the metabolic precursors which increase the risk of pre-eclampsia and how could these be investigated further. *Placenta* **2017**, *60*, 110–114. [CrossRef]
19. Zhao, J.; Huang, B.; Li, N.; Wang, X.; Xu, B.; Li, Y. Relationship between advanced maternal age and decline of endometrial receptivity: A systematic review and meta-analysis. *Aging* **2023**, *15*, 2460–2472. [CrossRef]
20. Cleary-Goldman, J.; Malone, F.D.; Vidaver, J.; Ball, R.H.; Nyberg, D.A.; Comstock, C.H.; Saade, G.R.; Eddleman, K.A.; Klugman, S.M.; Dugoff, L.; et al. Impact of Maternal Age on Obstetric Outcome. *Obstet. Gynecol.* **2005**, *105 Pt 1*, 983–990. [CrossRef]
21. Crawford, N.M.; Steiner, A.Z. Age-related Infertility. *Obstet. Gynecol. Clin. N. Am.* **2015**, *42*, 15–25. [CrossRef] [PubMed]
22. Ethics Committee of the American Society for Reproductive Medicine; Ethics Committee of the American Society for Reproductive Medicine. Oocyte or embryo donation to women of advanced reproductive age: An Ethics Committee opinion. *Fertil. Steril.* **2016**, *106*, e3–e7. [CrossRef] [PubMed]
23. American Diabetes Association. Diagnosis and Classification of Diabetes Mellitus. *Diabetes Care* **2013**, *36* (Suppl. S1), S67–S74.

24. Sun, M.; Luo, M.; Wang, T.; Wei, J.; Zhang, S.; Shu, J.; Zhong, T.; Liu, Y.; Chen, Q.; Zhu, P.; et al. Effect of the interaction between advanced maternal age and pre-pregnancy BMI on pre-eclampsia and GDM in Central China. *BMJ Open Diabetes Res. Care* **2023**, *11*, e003324. [CrossRef]
25. Li, M.; Chen, Y.; Wang, Y.; Wang, H.; Ding, X.; Li, G. Maternal gestational diabetes in singleton pregnancies conceived by ART may be modified by periconceptional B vitamins. *Front. Nutr.* **2022**, *9*, 1069911. [CrossRef] [PubMed]
26. Vaajala, M.; Liukkonen, R.; Ponkilainen, V.; Mattila, V.M.; Kekki, M.; Kuitunen, I. In vitro fertilization increases the odds of gestational diabetes: A nationwide register-based cohort study. *Acta Diabetol.* **2023**, *60*, 319–321. [CrossRef] [PubMed]
27. Li, Y.; Ren, X.; He, L.; Li, J.; Zhang, S.; Chen, W. Maternal age and the risk of gestational diabetes mellitus: A systematic review and meta-analysis of over 120 million participants. *Diabetes Res. Clin. Pract.* **2020**, *162*, 108044. [CrossRef]
28. WHO. WHO: Recommended definitions, terminology and format for statistical tables related to the perinatal period and use of a new certificate for cause of perinatal deaths. Modifications recommended by FIGO as amended October 14, 1976. *Acta Obstet. Gynecol. Scand.* **1977**, *56*, 247–253.
29. Esposito, G.; Mauri, P.A.; Cipriani, S.; Franchi, M.; Corrao, G.; Parazzini, F. The role of maternal age on the risk of preterm birth among singletons and multiples: A retrospective cohort study in Lombardy, Northern Italy. *BMC Pregnancy Childbirth* **2022**, *22*, 234.
30. Gondane, P.; Kumbhakarn, S.; Maity, P.; Kapat, K. Recent Advances and Challenges in the Early Diagnosis and Treatment of Preterm Labor. *Bioengineering* **2024**, *11*, 161. [CrossRef] [PubMed]
31. Ye, X.; Baker, P.N.; Tong, C. The updated understanding of advanced maternal age. *Fundam. Res.* **2023**, *4*, 1719–1728. [CrossRef] [PubMed]
32. Köck, K.; Köck, F.; Klein, K.; Bancher-Todesca, D.; Helmer, H. Diabetes mellitus and the risk of preterm birth with regard to the risk of spontaneous preterm birth. *J. Matern-Fetal Neonatal Med.* **2010**, *23*, 1004–1008. [CrossRef] [PubMed]
33. Bramham, K.; Parnell, B.; Nelson-Piercy, C.; Seed, P.T.; Poston, L.; Chappell, L.C. Chronic hypertension and pregnancy outcomes: Systematic review and meta-analysis. *BMJ* **2014**, *348*, g2301. [CrossRef]
34. World Health Organization. *International Statistical Classification of Diseases and Related Health Problems, Tenth Revision*, 2nd ed.; World Health Organization: Geneva, Switzerland, 2004.
35. Cutland, C.L.; Lackritz, E.M.; Mallett-Moore, T.; Bardají, A.; Chandrasekaran, R.; Lahariya, C.; Nisar, M.I.; Tapia, M.D.; Pathirana, J.; Kochhar, S.; et al. Low birth weight: Case definition & guidelines for data collection, analysis, and presentation of maternal immunization safety data. *Vaccine* **2017**, *35 Pt A*, 6492–6500.
36. Aradhya, S.; Tegunimataka, A.; Kravdal, Ø.; Martikainen, P.; Myrskylä, M.; Barclay, K.; Goisis, A. Maternal age and the risk of low birthweight and pre-term delivery: A pan-Nordic comparison. *Int. J. Epidemiol.* **2023**, *52*, 156–164. [CrossRef] [PubMed]
37. Toutain, J.; Prochazkova-Carlotti, M.; Cappellen, D.; Jarne, A.; Chevret, E.; Ferrer, J.; Idrissi, Y.; Pelluard, F.; Carles, D.; Maugey-Laulon, B.; et al. Reduced Placental Telomere Length during Pregnancies Complicated by Intrauterine Growth Restriction. Tian X (Cindy), editor. *PLoS ONE* **2013**, *8*, e54013. [CrossRef] [PubMed]
38. Fuchs, F.; Monet, B.; Ducruet, T.; Chaillet, N.; Audibert, F. Effect of maternal age on the risk of preterm birth: A large cohort study. *PLoS ONE* **2018**, *13*, e0191002. [CrossRef] [PubMed]
39. Sultana, Z.; Maiti, K.; Dedman, L.; Smith, R. Is there a role for placental senescence in the genesis of obstetric complications and fetal growth restriction? *Am. J. Obstet. Gynecol.* **2018**, *218*, S762–S773. [CrossRef] [PubMed]
40. Chen, Z.; Xiong, L.; Jin, H.; Yu, J.; Li, X.; Fu, H.; Wen, L.; Qi, H.; Tong, C.; Saffery, R.; et al. Advanced maternal age causes premature placental senescence and malformation via dysregulated α-Klotho expression in trophoblasts. *Aging Cell* **2021**, *20*, e13417. [CrossRef] [PubMed]
41. Martinelli, K.G.; Garcia, É.M.; Santos Neto, E.T.D.; Gama, S.G.N.D. Advanced maternal age and its association with placenta praevia and placental abruption: A meta-analysis. *Cad. Saúde Pública* **2018**, *34*, e00206116. [CrossRef] [PubMed]
42. Kong, F.; Fu, Y.; Shi, H.; Li, R.; Zhao, Y.; Wang, Y.; Qiao, J. Placental Abnormalities and Placenta-Related Complications Following In-Vitro Fertilization: Based on National Hospitalized Data in China. *Front. Endocrinol.* **2022**, *13*, 924070. [CrossRef]
43. Gundogan, F.; Bianchi, D.W.; Scherjon, S.A.; Roberts, D.J. Placental pathology in egg donor pregnancies. *Fertil. Steril.* **2010**, *93*, 397–404. [CrossRef] [PubMed]
44. Caradeux, J.; Fernández, B.; Ávila, F.; Valenzuela, A.; Mondión, M.; Figueras, F. Pregnancies through oocyte donation. A mini review of pathways involved in placental dysfunction. *Front. Med.* **2024**, *11*, 1338516. [CrossRef] [PubMed]
45. Keukens, A.; van Wely, M.; van der Meulen, C.; Mochtar, M.H. Pre-eclampsia in pregnancies resulting from oocyte donation, natural conception or IVF: A systematic review and meta-analysis. *Hum. Reprod.* **2022**, *37*, 586–599. [CrossRef]
46. Mascarenhas, M.; Sunkara, S.K.; Antonisamy, B.; Kamath, M.S. Higher risk of preterm birth and low birth weight following oocyte donation: A systematic review and meta-analysis. *Eur. J. Obstet. Gynecol. Reprod. Biol.* **2017**, *218*, 60–67. [CrossRef]

47. Moreno-Sepulveda, J.; Checa, M.A. Risk of adverse perinatal outcomes after oocyte donation: A systematic review and meta-analysis. *J. Assist. Reprod. Genet.* **2019**, *36*, 2017–2037. [CrossRef] [PubMed]
48. Storgaard, M.; Loft, A.; Bergh, C.; Wennerholm, U.B.; Söderström-Anttila, V.; Romundstad, L.B.; Aittomaki, K.; Oldereid, N.; Forman, J.; Pinborg, A. Obstetric and neonatal complications in pregnancies conceived after oocyte donation: A systematic review and meta-analysis. *BJOG Int. J. Obstet. Gynaecol.* **2017**, *124*, 561–572. [CrossRef]

Journal of
Clinical Medicine

MDPI

Article

Association of Obesity with Telomere Length in Human Sperm

Efthalia Moustakli [1,*], Athanasios Zikopoulos [2], Charikleia Skentou [3], Stefanos Dafopoulos [4], Sofoklis Stavros [5], Konstantinos Dafopoulos [6], Peter Drakakis [5], Ioannis Georgiou [1] and Athanasios Zachariou [7]

[1] Laboratory of Medical Genetics, Faculty of Medicine, School of Health Sciences, University of Ioannina, 45110 Ioannina, Greece; igeorgio@uoi.gr
[2] Obstetrics and Gynecology, Royal Devon and Exeter Hospital, Barrack Rd., Exeter EX 25 DW, UK; thanzik92@gmail.com
[3] Department of Obstetrics and Gynecology, Medical School of Ioannina, University General Hospital, 45110 Ioannina, Greece; haraskentou@gmail.com
[4] Department of Health Sciences, European University Cyprus, Nicosia 2404, Cyprus; stefanosntf2001@gmail.com
[5] Third Department of Obstetrics and Gynecology, Attikon Hospital, Medical School, National and Kapodistrian University of Athens, 12462 Athens, Greece; sfstavrou@med.uoa.gr (S.S.); pdrakakis@med.uoa.gr (P.D.)
[6] IVF Unit, Department of Obstetrics and Gynecology, Faculty of Medicine, School of Health Sciences, University of Thessaly, 41500 Larissa, Greece; kdafop@yahoo.gr
[7] Department of Urology, School of Medicine, Ioannina University, 45110 Ioannina, Greece; zahariou@otenet.gr
* Correspondence: thaleia.moustakli@gmail.com

Abstract: Background: Telomere attrition and mitochondrial dysfunction are two fundamental aspects of aging. Calorie restriction (CR) is the best strategy to postpone aging since it can enhance telomere attrition, boost antioxidant capacity, and lower the generation of reactive oxygen species (ROS). Since ROS is produced by mitochondria and can readily travel to cell nuclei, it is thought to be a crucial molecule for information transfer between mitochondria and cell nuclei. Important variables that affect the quality and functionality of sperm and may affect male reproductive health and fertility include telomere length, mitochondrial content, and the ratio of mitochondrial DNA (mtDNA) to nuclear DNA (nDNA). Telomere damage results from mitochondrial failure, whereas nuclear DNA remains unaffected. This research aims to investigate potential associations between these three variables and how they might relate to body mass index. **Methods:** Data were collected from 82 men who underwent IVF/ICSI at the University Hospital of Ioannina's IVF Unit in the Obstetrics and Gynecology Department. Evaluations included sperm morphology, sperm count, sperm motility, and participant history. To address this, male participants who were categorized into three body mass index (BMI) groups—normal, overweight, and obese—had their sperm samples tested. **Results:** For both the normal and overweight groups, our results show a negative connection between relative telomere length and BMI. As an illustration of a potential connection between mitochondrial health and telomere maintenance, a positive correlation was found for the obese group. Only the obese group's results were statistically significant ($p < 0.05$). More evidence that longer telomeres are associated with lower mitochondrial content can be found in the negative connection between telomere length and mitochondrial content in both the normal and overweight groups. However, the obese group showed a positive association. The data did not reach statistical significance for any of the three groups. These associations may affect sperm quality since telomere length and mitochondrial concentration are indicators of cellular integrity and health. Moreover, the ratio of mtDNA to nDNA was positively correlated with the relative telomere lengths of the obese group, but negatively correlated with the normal and overweight groups. In every group that was studied, the results were not statistically significant. According to this, male fertility may be negatively impacted by an imbalance in the copy number of the mitochondrial genome compared to the nuclear DNA in sperm. **Conclusions:** Essentially, the goal of our work is to determine whether mitochondria and telomere length in human sperm interact. Understanding these connections may aid in the explanation of some male infertility causes and possibly contribute to the creation of new treatment modalities for problems pertaining to reproductive health. The functional implications of these connections and their applications in therapeutic settings require further investigation.

Keywords: telomeres; telomere length; mitochondria; oxidation; body mass index; IVF/ICSI; male infertility; spermatozoa

1. Introduction

The accumulation of abnormally high amounts of fat in the body is the hallmark of obesity. The obesogenic phenotype is driven by a confluence of hormonal, genetic, and metabolic factors that impact significant aspects of energy expenditure and nutritional intake [1]. Obesity accelerates aging-related pathologies including several cancer types, cardiovascular illnesses, type 2 diabetes (T2D), and non-alcoholic fatty liver disease (NAFLD), as well as organ degeneration [2–4]. Obesity causes early cellular senescence in a number of different tissues, which contributes to these difficulties, at least in part [5]. Obese adults exhibit telomere shortening, a defining feature of cellular senescence [6–9].

Cellular senescence is an irreversible cell cycle arrest caused by various types of stress. It can be triggered by DNA damage, telomere attrition, oxidative damage, mitotic stress, mitochondrial dysfunction, endoplasmic reticulum (ER) stress, and oncogene activation [10]. A process known as the mitochondrial dysfunction-associated senescent response (MiDAS) is a response that occurs when mitochondrial ROS and sirtuins are depleted. Hayflick and Moorhead first used the term "cellular senescence" to describe how human somatic cells gradually lose their ability to proliferate [11]. Along with the loss of the capacity to replicate, this condition also exhibits a variety of important modifications in cell structure, gene expression, metabolism, epigenetics, and other areas [12]. The knowledge of how telomeres can signal senescence arrest has progressed significantly since then. These mechanisms are particularly crucial in the study of aging since it has been established that cellular senescence, which is fueled by telomere disruption, is a primary cause of aging and age-related disease [12].

Telomeres are DNA tandem repeats (TTAGGG) linked to a variety of proteins that together make up the "Shelterin" complex. At the end of linear chromosomes, there is a ribonucleoprotein called telomere repeats, which elongates the telomeric TTAGGG [13]. The core holoenzyme of this multi-subunit ribonucleoprotein enzyme only consists of catalytic telomerase reverse transcriptase (TERT) and an RNA template (TERC) [14]. Telomerase silencing occurs because TERC is widely expressed, while the TERT gene is strongly repressed in the majority of human somatic cells [15]. Hence, the factor that sets a rate limit for telomerase activity regulation is TERT. Telomeres have a 3′ overhang made up of single-stranded nucleotide repeats, as well as a lagging strand that is high in cytosine and a leading strand that is high in guanine [16]. Since continued cell division requires the maintenance of telomere length, telomerase is more active in cells that require this maintenance. Furthermore, telomerase's reverse transcriptase structure is specifically made to withstand telomere shortening. In order to maintain ongoing cell division, which delays aging, the two major components of human telomerase—TERT and TERC—serve as templates for telomere extension. Telomerase activity increases with telomere length [17].

Extra-nuclear pools of the telomerase protein TERT are known to exist. Telomere independent functions were initially used to characterize TERT's activities outside of the nucleus [18]. It is now well established that these activities are crucial for maintaining telomeres, maintaining genomic stability, and allowing interaction between the nucleus and mitochondria. TERT is released from the nucleus and imported into the mitochondria during conditions of stress, where it may have a protective role [19]. Furthermore, the TERC component is brought into the mitochondria, where it is converted to TERC-53 and subsequently released back to the cytosol, where it prevents GADPH from nuclear translocating [20,21]. Cytosolic TERC-53 is implicated in cellular senescence and organismal aging and transmits the signal of mitochondrial abnormalities to the nucleus. Genes implicated in the inflammatory response can also have their transcription increased by nuclear TERC binding directly to their promoter regions [22].

DNA breaks into single and double strands when the oxidative stress (OS) is high. Due to their higher guanine content and increased vulnerability to oxidative damage, telomeres also shorten more quickly as a result of it. The majority of somatic cells lack the telomerase enzyme, which results in a condition known as the "end-replication problem" during cell division. This is due to DNA polymerases' innate inability to completely duplicate the lagging strand with a high concentration of telomere C [23]. By allowing DNA polymerases to start DNA replication, RNA primers contribute to the synthesis of the lagging strand. However, when the final primer at the 3′ end is deleted, telomere repeats are lost, and unavoidably, the recently formed strand will be a few nucleotides shorter [23].

It has been determined that the telomere length (TL) in human spermatozoa is roughly 6–20 kb, longer than that in somatic cells [24–26]. The arrangement of telomeres in sperm cells, specifically their location near the nuclear membrane or at the nuclear periphery, may have a purpose. This purpose is theorized to facilitate the oocyte's access to these regions during fertilization, potentially influencing the growth of pronuclei. Another explanation for the differential distribution of telomeres concerning infertile males could be that poor telomere positioning makes the oocyte less accessible, which could be the cause of infertility. Telomere distribution in this case may suggest infertility, but it may also be the cause of infertility rather than just a symptom in an infertile man. Given that telomeres are histone-bound and positioned near nuclear boundaries, it is hypothesized that this may have a functional effect on the process of fertilization [27].

Telomeres, the protective caps at the ends of chromosomes, play a major role in cellular aging and senescence, in contrast to BMI, which is commonly used as a measure of general health and obesity. Mitochondrial DNA is essential for the cellular synthesis of energy and has implications for age-related disorders. The purpose of this research is to investigate any possible relationships between body mass index, mitochondrial function, and relative telomere length.

2. Materials and Methods

2.1. Participants' Characteristics and Semen Sample Collection

The current study included eighty-two (82) men who underwent IVF/ICSI at the IVF Unit of the Obstetrics and Gynecology Department of the University Hospital of Ioannina, Ioannina, Greece. Men were classified into three groups based on their BMI. Twenty-five [25] of the men recruited had normal BMI (ranging from 18 to 24.9 kg/m^2), twenty-nine [28] men were overweight (ranging from 25 to 29.9 kg/m^2), and twenty-eight [29] men were obese (class I and II) with a BMI higher than 30 kg/m^2. Each participant signed an informed consent form. The characteristics of each sperm sample were identified using Kruger's criteria.

According to Kruger's criteria, tougher sperm morphology standards may be a reliable indicator of infertility during in vitro fertilization (IVF). The sperm head needs to meet Kruger's specifications, which include having an oval form, regularity, and a smooth, continuous outline. Additionally, the acrosome must be intact. Furthermore, midpiece and tail abnormalities are not permitted. Another indication of morphological issues may be bent, numerous, or short tails as well as coiled, bowed, or sloppy midpieces. Finally, a high cytoplasmic droplet count may be a sign of sperm immaturity.

2.2. Sperm DNA Extraction and Quantification

In the fresh semen samples, sperm parameters such as sperm count, motility, morphology, and DFI using computer-aided semen analysis (CASA), were measured within an hour of ejaculation. The Sperm Class Analyzer (SCA) software SCA 6 Evolution from MICROPTIC Automatic Diagnostic Systems SL (Barcelona, Spain), an Axio Zeiss® Lab.A1 microscope, and a Basler Ace digital recording camera (Jena, Germany), were used to measure concentration and motility. The samples were then frozen at a temperature of –20 °C for storage. The Qiagen (Venlo, The Netherlands) methodology was used in the current investigation along with a matching kit, the QIAmp DNA blood Mini kit by Qiagen.

During the first stage, 100 μL of semen sample was combined with an X2 buffer, and heated for at least an hour at 56 °C in the heat block. Each sample was vortexed at regular intervals. Following this, a volume of 200 μL from each preheated semen sample was processed for sperm DNA extraction using the QIAmp DNA blood Mini kit according to the manufacturer's instructions.

Using a NanoDrop Spectrophotometer from Thermo Fisher Scientific, Waltham, MA, USA, the isolated sperm DNA was eluted in 80 μL of elution buffer and measured to determine purity and concentrations. By evaluating the A260/A80 ratio using spectroscopy for DNA analysis, the quality of the isolated DNA was evaluated. A human cell population's average telomere length can be measured directly using the Absolute Human Telomere Length Quantification qPCR Assay Kit (AHTLQ) from ScienCell Research Laboratories, San Diego, California. Recognizing and amplifying telomere sequences is the function of the telomere primer pair. Data normalization was accomplished using the single-copy reference (SCR) primer pair, which identifies and amplifies the human chromosome 17 region of 100 base pairs.

Two genes were chosen for DNA quantification, both nuclear and mitochondrial DNA. The human retinoid isomerohydrolase gene (RPE65) served as the nuclear DNA reference gene for the quantification of nDNA using the RPE primers 5′-ATAGGAAGCCAGAGAAGAGAGACT-3′ and 5′-TCTATCTCTGCGGACTTTGAGCAT-3′ (200 bp). Meanwhile, the combination of primers 5′-TAGAGGAGCCTGTTCTGTAATCG-3′ and 5′-TAAGGGCTATCGTAGTTTTCTGG-3′ (205 bp) was utilized for the mitochondrial DNA quantification, which corresponds to a section of the mitochondrially produced 12S RNA (Table 1).

Table 1. Primer sequences, amplicon base pair, and Tm.

Primer Pair	Sequence (Forward/Reverse)	Amplicon Base Pair (bp)	Tm
Nuclear region (RPE gene)	Forward 5′-ATAGGAAGCCAGAGAAGAGAGACT-3′ Reverse 5′-TCTATCTCTGCGGACTTTGAGCAT-3′	200	60 °C
Mitochondrial region	Forward 5′-TAGAGGAGCCTGTTCTGTAATCG-3′ Reverse 5′-TAAGGGCTATCGTAGTTTTCTGG-3′	205	59 °C

2.3. Real-Time Quantitive PCR (qPCR)

A quantitative polymerase chain reaction was employed to measure the absolute telomere length. Every genomic DNA sample was used in two separate qPCR procedures, one using telomere primer stock solution and the other using SCR primer stock solution. We employed the following components in each reaction: 0.5–0.5 ng/μL of genomic DNA template, 2 μL of primer stock solution (Telomere or SCR), 10 μL of 2X GoldNStart TaqGreen qPCR master mix, and 7 μL of nuclease-free water, for a total volume of 20 μL. The reaction was conducted on a Corbett Rotor-Gene 3000 Real-Time Rotary Analyzer (Corbett Research, Sydney, Australia) using the following cycling conditions: initial denaturation at 95 °C for 10 min, followed by 32 cycles of denaturing at 95 °C for 20 s, annealing at 52 °C for 20 s, and extension at 72 °C for 45 s. Following data collection, a hold at 25 °C for 1 min was performed.

2.4. Quantification Method: Comparative ΔΔCq Method Based on the AHTLQ Assay Kit

1. The difference in the number of quantification cycles of telomeres (TEL) between the target and reference genomic DNA samples is known as Cq (TEL).

$$\Delta Cq\ (TEL) = Cq\ (TEL,\ target\ sample) — Cq\ (TEL,\ reference\ sample)$$

2. For single-copy references, Cq (SCR) is the number of quantification cycles that differ between the reference and target genomic DNA samples.

$$\Delta\Delta Cq = \Delta Cq\ (TEL) - \Delta Cq\ (SCR)$$

3. The target sample's relative telomere length to the reference sample (fold) = $2^{-\Delta\Delta Cq}$.

The mitochondrial DNA content and the mtDNA to nDNA ratio were evaluated using quantitative polymerase chain reaction (qPCR). The following ingredients were added to each reaction: 0.02–0.03 μg of extracted DNA, 0.25 μL of each 10 μM forward and reverse primer, 5 μL of SYBR Green Master Mix (PowerUp SYBR Green Master Mix, Applied Biosystems, Thermo Fisher Scientific, USA), and 2.5 μL of distilled water, for a total volume of 10 μL. The following cycling conditions were used for the reaction on a Corbett Rotor-Gene 3000 Real-Time Rotary Analyzer (Corbett Research, Sydney, Australia): 50 °C for 2 min, 95 °C for 2 min, and then 40 cycles of denaturing at 95 °C for 15 s and 60 °C for 1 min. A duplicate of each sample was analyzed. The proportion of mitochondrial DNA in each sperm was measured. After calculating the ratio of mtDNA to nDNA using the ΔΔCt technique—which is described below—the relative mitochondrial DNA content per sperm sample was determined.

Selecting a control group, we used the cycle threshold Ct values for the relative quantification (also referred to as the "ΔΔCt method" as follows [28,29]:

(a) By subtracting each sample's mean nuclear Ct value from its mean mitochondrial Ct value, as shown by the formula ΔCt = mtDNA − nDNA;
(b) In this case, the control group comprised men with normal body mass index (18.5 to 24.9 kg/m^2) and normal semen characteristics, that is, the average ΔCt value;
(c) A sample's ΔΔCt is determined by deducting the control group's ΔCt from the sample's mean ΔCt. In other words, ΔΔCt = a sample's ΔCt minus the control group's ΔCt [28];
(d) The fold difference is calculated using the formula $2^{-\Delta\Delta Ct}$.

2.5. Statistical Analysis

The association between the two variables was evaluated statistically using Spearman's correlation coefficient. The statistical software SPSS 28.0 was used to analyze the data between the groups under study. The direction and correlation coefficient (r_s) between the variables shown in the graph are reported numerically in the analysis. Microsoft Excel spreadsheets were used to organize the extraction data, mtDNA copy numbers, and Ct rates to create graphs. Statistical significance was defined as $p < 0.05$.

2.6. Inclusion and Exclusion Criteria

The inclusion and exclusion criteria that were taken into consideration for the conduct of the particular study are referenced in the following table (Table 2).

Table 2. Inclusion and exclusion criteria for this study.

Inclusion Criteria	Exclusion Criteria
IVF/ICSI participants	Males without informed consent
Lifestyle (smoking, alcohol, drugs, etc.)	Urological conditions (e.g., varicocele)
	Abnormal Karyotype
	AZF deletions

3. Results

The individuals were divided into three groups according to their BMI. The mean values for the males' semen characteristics are displayed in the table below (Table 3).

Furthermore, the median values of the relative length of the telomeres for the three groups under study are reported in the graph below.

The overweight group's TL differs by almost half from that of the groups with normal and obese BMIs. However, this difference is not significant in terms of statistics ($p > 0.05$).

Following that, in each group separately, we examined the interaction regarding relative telomere length (TL). For the three groups with normal, overweight, and obese BMI, the relative length of telomeres was examined, as shown in the figures below. A substantial negative association was found between telomere length (TL) and the group of people with normal BMI (Figure 1A).

Table 3. Male participants' age, morphology, progressive motility, and sperm count, with a 95% confidence interval (CI), were among the parameters of their semen that were examined in this study. p values were determined by ANOVA. $p < 0.05$ was used to indicate statistical significance.

Semen Characteristics	Normal	Overweight	Obese	*p*-Values
No. of participants	25	29	28	
Progressive motility (%), CI 95%	47.71 ± 6.14	37.53 ± 5.61	4.2 ± 3.56	0.0062
Sperm morphology (%), CI 95%	13.48 ± 4.11	16 ± 9.04	10.16 ± 3.02	0.4073
Sperm count, million/mL, CI 95%	30.54 ± 14.84	16.98 ± 8.74	34.56 ± 12.67	0.0692
Male age, CI 95%	38.3 ± 1.75	43.25 ± 2.75	41 ± 2.55	0.022

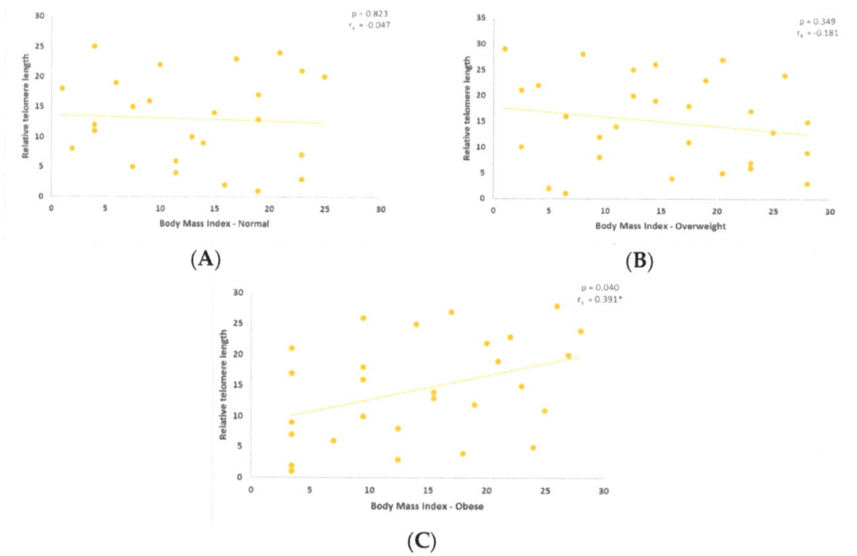

Figure 1. (**A**,**B**) Evaluation of the relative telomere length (TL) in the normal and overweight groups. The outcomes were not statistically significant with such p values, 0.823 and 0.349, respectively. (**C**) With a statistical significance level of 0.040, the measurement of the relative TL in the obese group revealed a positive association (correlation coefficient r_s = 0.391 *; is significant at the 0.05 level, two-tailed).

A negative association between BMI and relative TL was also observed in the overweight group, as indicated in the following graph (Figure 1B). Finally, relative TL demonstrated a positive correlation with BMI in the obese group (Figures 1C, A1a). The figures below depict the results of the Spearman's correlation coefficient conducted to examine the relationship between relative TL and BMI.

3.1. Correlation between Mitochondrial DNA Content and the Relative Telomere Length

Additionally, the normal and overweight groups' correlations between mitochondrial content and TL revealed a negative association. The results, which are shown in the figures below, are not statistically significant, as indicated by the p-values. The p-value for the normal group was 0.204 (Figure 2A), while it was 0.183 for the overweight group (Figure 2B).

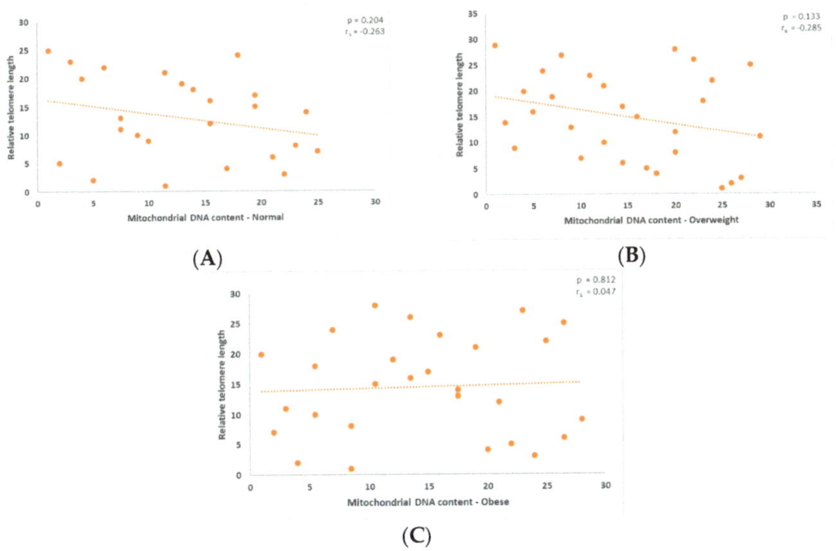

Figure 2. (**A**,**B**) For men in the normal and overweight groups, relative telomere length and mitochondrial DNA content did not show any statistically significant outcomes, $p = 0.204$ and $p = 0.133$, respectively. (**C**) In the obese group, relative TL and mitochondrial DNA load did not show any statistical significance, $p = 0.812$.

The comparison of mitochondrial content and relative telomere length for males who range into the obese category showed a positive connection. The graph below reflects this further (Figures 2C, A1b). The outcome in this instance was statistically significant, $p = 0.812$.

3.2. Correlation between mtDNA-to-nDNA Ratio and the Relative Telomere Length

Next, we assessed the correlation between relative telomere length and the ratio of nuclear to mitochondrial DNA. The diagram demonstrates the first finding, which is that there was a negative correlation between those with normal and overweight BMIs. The findings ($p = 0.189$ and $p = 0.36$, respectively) did not demonstrate any statistical significance (Figures 3A and 3B, respectively).

Nevertheless, the outcomes did not reach statistical significance for the group classified as obese. In particular, the ratio displayed a modest positive correlation with the relative length of telomeres in the obese group; however, the p-value is only $p = 0.763$ (Figures 3C, A1c). The results obtained were not statistically significant.

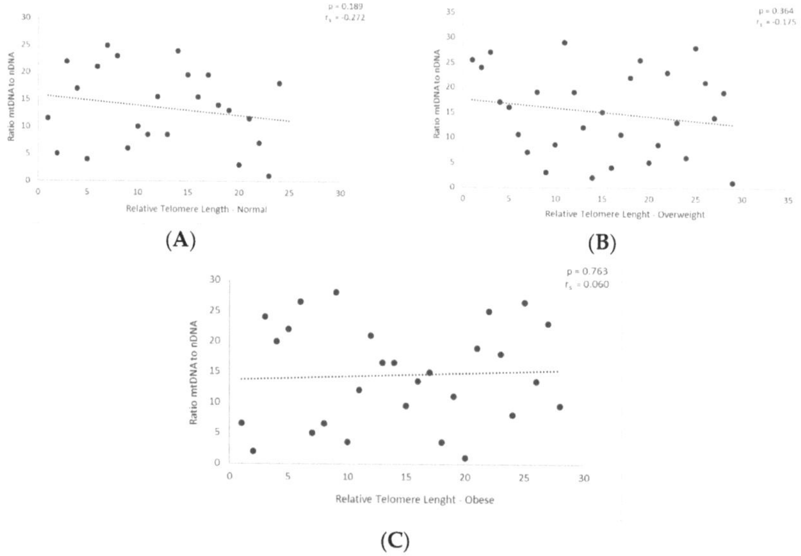

Figure 3. (**A**,**B**) Males with normal and overweight BMI showed no statistically significant differences in the ratio of mitochondrial to nuclear DNA with relative telomere length. (**C**) The ratio of mitochondrial to nuclear DNA and the relative telomere length of obese males indicates that the results are not statistically significant.

4. Discussion

Obesity has long been thought to have a deleterious impact on male fertility [30]. The precise processes and consequences of these instances on male fertility remain unclear despite significant advancements in the research. Consequently, this study offered a novel viewpoint on the connection between male fertility and mitochondria, telomere length, and body mass index. Initially, the relationship between relative telomere length and body mass index was investigated. It was found that the only group with a positive correlation and statistically significant results was the obese group, suggesting that weight affects telomere length and consequently sperm quality. Regarding the normal and overweight categories, no association was noticed.

Additionally, we noted that the obese group's average relative telomere length was lower than that of the normal group. The overweight population is covered by this as well. However, the average relative telomere length was higher in the obese group than in the overweight group. This result is consistent with a different study that used an adequate number of participants [31]. While we recruited patients with obesity (BMI $\geq$ 30 kg/m^2) from the general population and not just the infertile category, the previously mentioned study recruited patients from infertile couples undergoing their first fresh IVF cycle with male BMI of more than 28 (which includes both overweight and obese patients) [31]. Consideration should be given to a complex mechanism comprising confounding variables, as telomere shortening in obese individuals may not be a direct result of obesity. Weight-related OS and increased ROS levels, which cause telomere shortening, could be one of the main reasons for this [32].

Telomeres, telomerase subunits, and mitochondria have been intimately linked in recent years. Telomerase's primary function is to prevent telomere shortening and preserve telomere length. Furthermore, telomeres are involved in maintaining cell viability. It has been discovered that telomerase is the enzyme that catalyzes the removal of the oxidative stress-stimulated subunit TERT from the nuclei and deposits it in the mitochondria. By lowering mitochondrial ROS generation, this co-localization of TERT and mitochondria maintains mitochondrial function and mitigates nuclear DNA damage and apoptosis [33,34]. Interestingly, there is either no or very little DNA damage in cells that entirely eliminate telomerase. On the other hand, telomerase levels in cells rise in response to damage to cellular DNA that has not been entirely eliminated. Telomerase, according to the authors, may negatively impact cell nuclei's repair enzymes, potentially leading to increased DNA damage [35]. This also clarifies why, to some extent, telomerase is unable to resume its function following DNA damage.

Telomere damage results in the reprogramming of mitochondrial biosynthesis and mitochondrial dysfunction, which have significant consequences for aging and diseases. Nonetheless, mitochondrial dysfunction causes telomere attrition [18]. In our study, the findings obtained when comparing mitochondrial content and relative telomere length based on BMI were not statistically significant. However, it appears that there is a positive correlation for the obese group and a negative correlation for the normal and overweight groups. Lastly, we investigated the relationship between the ratio of mitochondrial DNA to nuclear DNA and the relative telomere length for each group of participants. The correlation was positive for the obese group and negative for the normal and overweight groups. However, for all the groups under investigation (normal, overweight, and obese), neither case showed statistically significant outcomes.

Telomere shortening and mitochondrial dysfunction are features of cellular senescence. They are tightly associated, with the former influencing mitochondrial function through p53-PGC-1α signaling pathways. While aging is unavoidable, growing older may shorten life expectancy due to elevated risk factors for chronic diseases. Different studies suggest that telomere attrition is modifiable, as substantial variability exists in the rate of telomere shortening that is independent of chronological age [36]. Telomere attrition has also been linked with other potentially modifiable lifestyle factors, such as poor nutrition and physical inactivity, indicating the plasticity of TL [37,38]. Findings from different studies show that a healthy diet, low stress, exercise, and a good sleep pattern are related to longer telomeres [39,40]. In the absence of direct evidence, the positive correlation between sperm telomere length (STL) and sperm DNA fragmentation in young individuals may be due to the activation of telomerase by a low-level adverse factor, such as mild OS, which causes genomic damage in addition to STL extension [41–43].

The normal process of fertilization may be affected by alterations in the mitochondrial DNA (mtDNA) [44–47]. Nonetheless, not much research has been conducted on potential correlations between telomeres and mitochondrial characteristics in human sperm. It is widely acknowledged that mtDNA is especially prone to cumulative mutation and deletion, either as a result of its proximity to the respiratory chains, which produce ROS, or because it lacks protective histones [48]. Oxidative insults are known to affect both nuclear and mitochondrial DNA [49]. A body of evidence has been gathered demonstrating that telomerase can also function in telomere-independent ways and that, under OS, the TERT transfers between the nucleus and mitochondria, and the TERC is processed, imported into mitochondria, and exported back to the cytosol [18].

Telomere length and structure are essential for maintaining the integrity of the nuclear genome, and spermatogenesis and conception are specifically linked to the maintenance of telomeres in germ cells [50]. An essential component of the dynamic maintenance of telomere length homeostasis is the existence of telomerase activity in spermatogenic cells. Previous research, however, has demonstrated that both endogenous and exogenous variables, including OS, inflammation, exposure to the environment, and lifestyle choices, may disrupt telomere homeostasis [51–54]. According to several studies, telomerase may even be triggered in some circumstances, leading to telomere elongation [51–53]. Low levels of arsenic exposure and oxidative stress have both been shown to boost telomerase activity and lengthen telomeres [54–56]. Given that early research is starting to reveal associations between sperm TL and reproductive outcomes, TL is a desirable topic for further research. Future research on these topics should be conducted in depth.

5. Conclusions

This investigation into the relationship between relative TL and mitochondrial DNA content has shed light on the complex interactions between these two vital aspects of cellular health and aging [49]. The findings highlight the significance of preserving mitochondrial health and telomere integrity as critical elements in promoting lifespan and general well-being, even though further study is required to clarify the specific nature of this link. This discovery could influence future medical therapies and methods meant to maintain cellular vitality and lengthen healthy lifespans as our understanding of these interrelated processes continues to advance.

6. Limitations of This Study

When evaluating this study's findings, one should take into account a number of its shortcomings. Firstly, a smaller sample size may have limited how broadly the results may be applied to the public. Furthermore, answer bias and recall errors may have been introduced by the data collection strategy, which mostly relied on self-report surveys. This study was also limited by the geographic area in which it was carried out; thus, contextual and cultural factors may have a different effect on the findings elsewhere. Relative measurements are often obtained by PCR-based methods, which are the most widely used approaches for measuring mtDNA-CN and telomere length. Furthermore, no research has been conducted that focuses on population-based studies and systematically examines the relationship between telomere length, mtDNA-CN, and sperm prevalence, incidence, and death. Finally, logistical and ethical limitations may have affected this study's methods and results, as they do with any research involving human beings. These restrictions highlight the need for additional investigation to strengthen and improve the understanding that this study has provided.

Author Contributions: Data curation, A.Z. (Athanasios Zikopoulos), C.S., S.S. and P.D.; Methodology, A.Z. (Athanasios Zikopoulos), C.S., S.S. and P.D.; Project administration, I.G. and A.Z. (Athanasios Zachariou); Resources, S.D., K.D., I.G. and A.Z. (Athanasios Zachariou); Supervision, I.G.; Writing—original draft, E.M.; Writing—review and editing, E.M., A.Z. (Athanasios Zikopoulos) and I.G. All authors have read and agreed to the published version of the manuscript.

Funding: This research received no external funding.

Institutional Review Board Statement: Academic research is monitored and licensed by the University Hospital, ethical approval number: 27657/10 November 2019.

Informed Consent Statement: Patient consent was waived due to in vitro fertilization (IVF).

Data Availability Statement: Data are unavailable due to privacy or ethical restrictions.

Conflicts of Interest: The authors declare no conflicts of interest.

Appendix A

We offer a thorough summary of all the variables examined in this research in this appendix. To improve transparency and reproducibility for readers and other researchers, we hope that this information will be presented in an orderly and systematic way, enabling a greater understanding of the variables and their impact on our study.

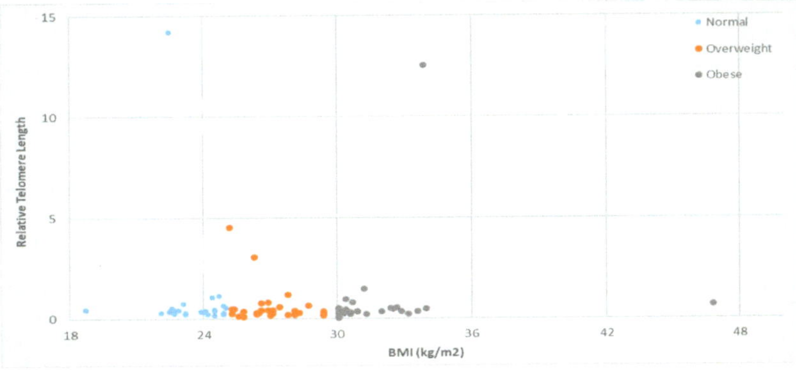

(**a**)

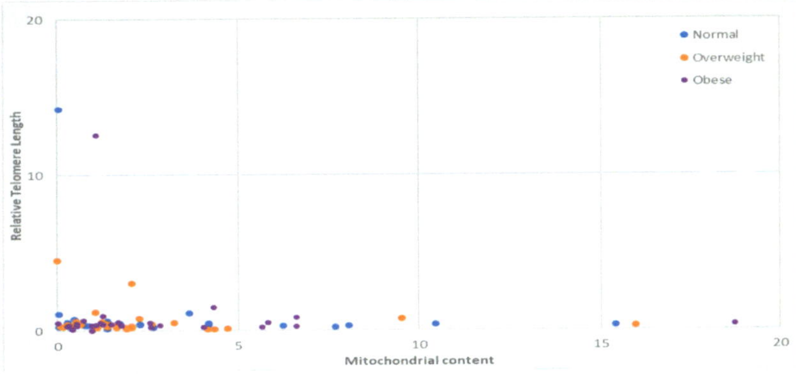

(**b**)

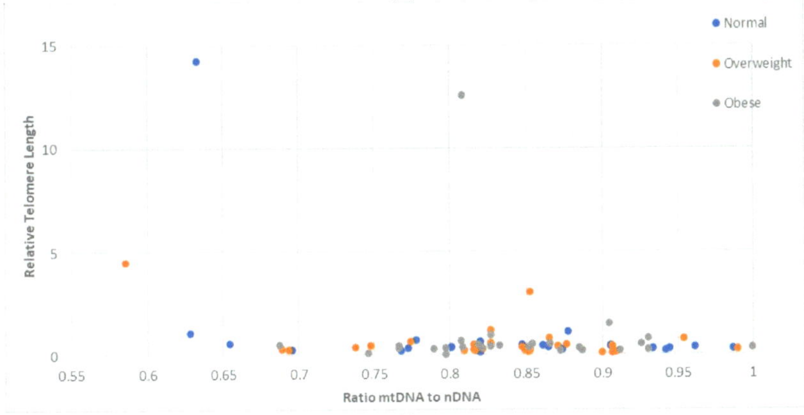

(**c**)

Figure A1. A comprehensive representation of the variables examined in this research. (**a**) Body mass index-based variation in relative telomere length. (**b**) Distribution of the mitochondrial content based on the relative telomere length. (**c**) Correlation between nuclear to mitochondrial DNA ratio and relative telomere length.

References

1. Cheng, L.; Wang, J.; Dai, H.; Duan, Y.; An, Y.; Shi, L.; Lv, Y.; Li, H.; Wang, C.; Ma, Q.; et al. Brown and beige adipose tissue: A novel therapeutic strategy for obesity and type 2 diabetes mellitus. *Adipocyte* **2021**, *10*, 48–65. [CrossRef] [PubMed]

2. Kawai, T.; Autieri, M.V.; Scalia, R. Adipose tissue inflammation and metabolic dysfunction in obesity. *Am. J. Physiol.-Cell Physiol.* **2021**, *320*, C375–C391. [CrossRef] [PubMed]
3. Roberto, C.A.; Swinburn, B.; Hawkes, C.; Huang, T.T.-K.; Costa, S.A.; Ashe, M.; Zwicker, L.; Cawley, J.H.; Brownell, K.D. Patchy progress on obesity prevention: Emerging examples, entrenched barriers, and new thinking. *Lancet* **2015**, *385*, 2400–2409. [CrossRef]
4. Santos, A.L.; Sinha, S. Obesity and aging: Molecular mechanisms and therapeutic approaches. *Ageing Res. Rev.* **2021**, *67*, 101268. [CrossRef] [PubMed]
5. Burton, D.G.A.; Faragher, R.G.A. Obesity and type-2 diabetes as inducers of premature cellular senescence and ageing. *Biogerontology* **2018**, *19*, 447–459. [CrossRef] [PubMed]
6. Welendorf, C.; Nicoletti, C.F.; Pinhel, M.A.D.S.; Noronha, N.Y.; De Paula, B.M.F.; Nonino, C.B. Obesity, weight loss, and influence on telomere length: New insights for personalized nutrition. *Nutrition* **2019**, *66*, 115–121. [CrossRef] [PubMed]
7. García-Calzón, S.; Moleres, A.; Marcos, A.; Campoy, C.; Moreno, L.A.; Azcona-Sanjulián, M.C.; Martínez-González, M.A.; Martínez, J.A.; Zalba, G.; Marti, A.; et al. Telomere length as a biomarker for adiposity changes after a multidisciplinary intervention in overweight/obese adolescents: The EVASYON study. *PLoS ONE* **2014**, *9*, e89828. [CrossRef] [PubMed]
8. Lee, M.; Martin, H.; Firpo, M.A.; Demerath, E.W. Inverse association between adiposity and telomere length: The Fels Longitudinal Study. *Am. J. Hum. Biol. Off. J. Hum. Biol. Counc.* **2011**, *23*, 100–106. [CrossRef]
9. Rode, L.; Nordestgaard, B.G.; Weischer, M.; Bojesen, S.E. Increased Body Mass Index, Elevated C-Reactive Protein, and Short Telomere Length. *J. Clin. Endocrinol. Metab.* **2014**, *99*, E1671–E1675. [CrossRef]
10. Narasimhan, A.; Flores, R.R.; Camell, C.D.; Bernlohr, D.A.; Robbins, P.D.; Niedernhofer, L.J. Cellular Senescence in Obesity and Associated Complications: A New Therapeutic Target. *Curr. Diab. Rep.* **2022**, *22*, 537–548. [CrossRef]
11. Hayflick, L.; Moorhead, P.S. The serial cultivation of human diploid cell strains. *Exp. Cell Res.* **1961**, *25*, 585–621. [CrossRef] [PubMed]
12. van Deursen, J.M. The role of senescent cells in ageing. *Nature* **2014**, *509*, 439–446. [CrossRef] [PubMed]
13. Bhari, V.K.; Kumar, D.; Kumar, S.; Mishra, R. Shelterin complex gene: Prognosis and therapeutic vulnerability in cancer. *Biochem. Biophys. Rep.* **2021**, *26*, 100937. [CrossRef] [PubMed]
14. Yuan, X.; Xu, D. Telomerase Reverse Transcriptase (TERT) in Action: Cross-Talking with Epigenetics. *Int. J. Mol. Sci.* **2019**, *20*, 3338. [CrossRef]
15. Yuan, X.; Larsson, C.; Xu, D. Mechanisms underlying the activation of TERT transcription and telomerase activity in human cancer: Old actors and new players. *Oncogene* **2019**, *38*, 6172–6183. [CrossRef] [PubMed]
16. Griffith, J.D.; Comeau, L.; Rosenfield, S.; Stansel, R.M.; Bianchi, A.; Moss, H.; De Lange, T. Mammalian Telomeres End in a Large Duplex Loop. *Cell* **1999**, *97*, 503–514. [CrossRef] [PubMed]
17. Vaiserman, A.; Krasnienkov, D. Telomere Length as a Marker of Biological Age: State-of-the-Art, Open Issues, and Future Perspectives. *Front. Genet.* **2021**, *11*, 630186. [CrossRef] [PubMed]
18. Zheng, Q.; Huang, J.; Wang, G. Mitochondria, Telomeres and Telomerase Subunits. *Front. Cell Dev. Biol.* **2019**, *7*, 274. [CrossRef]
19. Green, P.D.; Sharma, N.K.; Santos, J.H. Telomerase Impinges on the Cellular Response to Oxidative Stress Through Mitochondrial ROS-Mediated Regulation of Autophagy. *Int. J. Mol. Sci.* **2019**, *20*, 1509. [CrossRef]
20. Huang, J.; Liu, P.; Wang, G. Regulation of mitochondrion-associated cytosolic ribosomes by mammalian mitochondrial ribonuclease T2 (RNASET2). *J. Biol. Chem.* **2018**, *293*, 19633–19644. [CrossRef]
21. Cheng, Y.; Liu, P.; Zheng, Q.; Gao, G.; Yuan, J.; Wang, P.; Huang, J.; Xie, L.; Lu, X.; Tong, T.; et al. Mitochondrial Trafficking and Processing of Telomerase RNA TERC. *Cell Rep.* **2018**, *24*, 2589–2595. [CrossRef] [PubMed]
22. Liu, H.; Yang, Y.; Ge, Y.; Liu, J.; Zhao, Y. TERC promotes cellular inflammatory response independent of telomerase. *Nucleic Acids Res.* **2019**, *47*, 8084–8095. [CrossRef] [PubMed]
23. Chan, S.R.W.L.; Blackburn, E.H. Telomeres and telomerase. *Philos. Trans. R. Soc. Lond. B. Biol. Sci.* **2004**, *359*, 109–122. [CrossRef] [PubMed]
24. Kaltsas, A.; Moustakli, E.; Zikopoulos, A.; Georgiou, I.; Dimitriadis, F.; Symeonidis, E.N.; Markou, E.; Michaelidis, T.M.; Tien, D.M.B.; Giannakis, I.; et al. Impact of Advanced Paternal Age on Fertility and Risks of Genetic Disorders in Offspring. *Genes* **2023**, *14*, 486. [CrossRef] [PubMed]
25. Kimura, M.; Cherkas, L.F.; Kato, B.S.; Demissie, S.; Hjelmborg, J.B.; Brimacombe, M.; Cupples, A.; Hunkin, J.L.; Gardner, J.P.; Lu, X.; et al. Offspring's leukocyte telomere length, paternal age, and telomere elongation in sperm. *PLoS Genet.* **2008**, *4*, e37. [CrossRef] [PubMed]
26. Baird, D.M.; Britt-Compton, B.; Rowson, J.; Amso, N.N.; Gregory, L.; Kipling, D. Telomere instability in the male germline. *Hum. Mol. Genet.* **2006**, *15*, 45–51. [CrossRef] [PubMed]
27. Turner, K.J.; Watson, E.M.; Skinner, B.M.; Griffin, D.K. Telomere Distribution in Human Sperm Heads and Its Relation to Sperm Nuclear Morphology: A New Marker for Male Factor Infertility? *Int. J. Mol. Sci.* **2021**, *22*, 7599. [CrossRef] [PubMed]
28. Quiros, P.M.; Goyal, A.; Jha, P.; Auwerx, J. Analysis of mtDNA/nDNA Ratio in Mice. *Curr. Protoc. Mouse Biol.* **2017**, *7*, 47–54. [CrossRef] [PubMed]
29. Livak, K.J.; Schmittgen, T.D. Analysis of relative gene expression data using real-time quantitative PCR and the 2(-Delta Delta C(T)) Method. *Methods San Diego Calif* **2001**, *25*, 402–408. [CrossRef]
30. Zia, S. Obesity: Impact and Outcome on Infertility—A Literature Review. *Open J. Obstet. Gynecol.* **2023**, *13*, 214–240. [CrossRef]

31. Yang, Q.; Zhao, F.; Hu, L.; Bai, R.; Zhang, N.; Yao, G.; Sun, Y. Effect of paternal overweight or obesity on IVF treatment outcomes and the possible mechanisms involved. *Sci. Rep.* **2016**, *6*, 29787. [CrossRef] [PubMed]
32. Raee, P.; Shams Mofarahe, Z.; Nazarian, H.; Abdollahifar, M.-A.; Ghaffari Novin, M.; Aghamiri, S.; Ghaffari Novin, M. Male obesity is associated with sperm telomere shortening and aberrant mRNA expression of autophagy-related genes. *Basic Clin. Androl.* **2023**, *33*, 13. [CrossRef] [PubMed]
33. Qi, H.; Chen, Y.; Fu, X.; Lin, C.-P.; Zheng, X.F.S.; Liu, L.F. TOR Regulates Cell Death Induced by Telomere Dysfunction in Budding Yeast. *PLoS ONE* **2008**, *3*, e3520. [CrossRef]
34. Ahmed, S.; Passos, J.F.; Birket, M.J.; Beckmann, T.; Brings, S.; Peters, H.; Birch-Machin, M.A.; von Zglinicki, T.; Saretzki, G. Telomerase does not counteract telomere shortening but protects mitochondrial function under oxidative stress. *J. Cell Sci.* **2008**, *121*, 1046–1053. [CrossRef] [PubMed]
35. Singhapol, C.; Pal, D.; Czapiewski, R.; Porika, M.; Nelson, G.; Saretzki, G.C. Mitochondrial Telomerase Protects Cancer Cells from Nuclear DNA Damage and Apoptosis. *PLoS ONE* **2013**, *8*, e52989. [CrossRef] [PubMed]
36. Du, M.; Prescott, J.; Kraft, P.; Han, J.; Giovannucci, E.; Hankinson, S.E.; De Vivo, I. Physical Activity, Sedentary Behavior, and Leukocyte Telomere Length in Women. *Am. J. Epidemiol.* **2012**, *175*, 414–422. [CrossRef]
37. Cassidy, A.; De Vivo, I.; Liu, Y.; Han, J.; Prescott, J.; Hunter, D.J.; Rimm, E.B. Associations between diet, lifestyle factors, and telomere length in women. *Am. J. Clin. Nutr.* **2010**, *91*, 1273–1280. [CrossRef] [PubMed]
38. Puterman, E.; Lin, J.; Blackburn, E.; O'Donovan, A.; Adler, N.; Epel, E. The Power of Exercise: Buffering the Effect of Chronic Stress on Telomere Length. *PLoS ONE* **2010**, *5*, e10837. [CrossRef] [PubMed]
39. Farzaneh-Far, R. Association of Marine Omega-3 Fatty Acid Levels with Telomeric Aging in Patients with Coronary Heart Disease. *JAMA* **2010**, *303*, 250. [CrossRef]
40. Ornish, D.; Lin, J.; Daubenmier, J.; Weidner, G.; Epel, E.; Kemp, C.; Magbanua, M.J.M.; Marlin, R.; Yglecias, L.; Carroll, P.R.; et al. Increased telomerase activity and comprehensive lifestyle changes: A pilot study. *Lancet Oncol.* **2008**, *9*, 1048–1057. [CrossRef]
41. Wyrobek, A.J.; Eskenazi, B.; Young, S.; Arnheim, N.; Tiemann-Boege, I.; Jabs, E.W.; Glaser, R.L.; Pearson, F.S.; Evenson, D. Advancing age has differential effects on DNA damage, chromatin integrity, gene mutations, and aneuploidies in sperm. *Proc. Natl. Acad. Sci. USA* **2006**, *103*, 9601–9606. [CrossRef] [PubMed]
42. Vagnini, L.; Baruffi, R.L.R.; Mauri, A.L.; Petersen, C.G.; Massaro, F.C.; Pontes, A.; Oliveira, J.B.A.; Franco, J.G. The effects of male age on sperm DNA damage in an infertile population. *Reprod. Biomed. Online* **2007**, *15*, 514–519. [CrossRef]
43. Gunes, S.; Hekim, G.N.T.; Arslan, M.A.; Asci, R. Effects of aging on the male reproductive system. *J. Assist. Reprod. Genet.* **2016**, *33*, 441–454. [CrossRef] [PubMed]
44. Kim, J.-H.; Kim, H.K.; Ko, J.-H.; Bang, H.; Lee, D.-C. The relationship between leukocyte mitochondrial DNA copy number and telomere length in community-dwelling elderly women. *PLoS ONE* **2013**, *8*, e67227. [CrossRef] [PubMed]
45. Qiu, C.; Enquobahrie, D.A.; Gelaye, B.; Hevner, K.; Williams, M.A. The association between leukocyte telomere length and mitochondrial DNA copy number in pregnant women: A pilot study. *Clin. Lab.* **2015**, *61*, 363–369. [CrossRef] [PubMed]
46. Alegría-Torres, J.A.; Velázquez-Villafaña, M.; López-Gutiérrez, J.M.; Chagoyán-Martínez, M.M.; Rocha-Amador, D.O.; Costilla-Salazar, R.; García-Torres, L. Association of Leukocyte Telomere Length and Mitochondrial DNA Copy Number in Children from Salamanca, Mexico. *Genet. Test. Mol. Biomark.* **2016**, *20*, 654–659. [CrossRef] [PubMed]
47. Melicher, D.; Illés, A.; Littvay, L.; Tárnoki, Á.D.; Tárnoki, D.L.; Bikov, A.; Kunos, L.; Csabán, D.; Buzás, E.I.; Molnár, M.J.; et al. Positive association and future perspectives of mitochondrial DNA copy number and telomere length—A pilot twin study. *Arch. Med. Sci. AMS* **2021**, *17*, 1191–1199. [CrossRef] [PubMed]
48. Giorgi, C.; Marchi, S.; Simoes, I.C.M.; Ren, Z.; Morciano, G.; Perrone, M.; Patalas-Krawczyk, P.; Borchard, S.; Jędrak, P.; Pierzynowska, K.; et al. Mitochondria and Reactive Oxygen Species in Aging and Age-Related Diseases. *Int. Rev. Cell Mol. Biol.* **2018**, *340*, 209–344.
49. Moustakli, E.; Zikopoulos, A.; Sakaloglou, P.; Bouba, I.; Sofikitis, N.; Georgiou, I. Functional association between telomeres, oxidation and mitochondria. *Front. Reprod. Health* **2023**, *5*, 1107215. [CrossRef]
50. Fice, H.; Robaire, B. Telomere Dynamics throughout Spermatogenesis. *Genes* **2019**, *10*, 525. [CrossRef]
51. Yim, H.W.; Slebos, R.J.C.; Randell, S.H.; Umbach, D.M.; Parsons, A.M.; Rivera, M.P.; Detterbeck, F.C.; Taylor, J.A. Smoking is associated with increased telomerase activity in short-term cultures of human bronchial epithelial cells. *Cancer Lett.* **2007**, *246*, 24–33. [CrossRef] [PubMed]
52. Ferrario, D.; Collotta, A.; Carfi, M.; Bowe, G.; Vahter, M.; Hartung, T.; Gribaldo, L. Arsenic induces telomerase expression and maintains telomere length in human cord blood cells. *Toxicology* **2009**, *260*, 132–141. [CrossRef] [PubMed]
53. Mo, J.; Xia, Y.; Ning, Z.; Wade, T.J.; Mumford, J.L. Elevated human telomerase reverse transcriptase gene expression in blood cells associated with chronic arsenic exposure in Inner Mongolia, China. *Environ. Health Perspect.* **2009**, *117*, 354–360. [CrossRef] [PubMed]
54. López-Diazguerrero, N.E.; Pérez-Figueroa, G.E.; Martínez-Garduño, C.M.; Alarcón-Aguilar, A.; Luna-López, A.; Gutiérrez-Ruiz, M.C.; Königsberg, M. Telomerase activity in response to mild oxidative stress. *Cell Biol. Int.* **2012**, *36*, 409–413. [CrossRef] [PubMed]

55. Wang, Z.; Rhee, D.B.; Lu, J.; Bohr, C.T.; Zhou, F.; Vallabhaneni, H.; de Souza-Pinto, N.C.; Liu, Y. Characterization of oxidative guanine damage and repair in mammalian telomeres. *PLoS Genet.* **2010**, *6*, e1000951. [CrossRef]
56. Mishra, S.; Kumar, R.; Malhotra, N.; Singh, N.; Dada, R. Mild oxidative stress is beneficial for sperm telomere length maintenance. *World J. Methodol.* **2016**, *6*, 163. [CrossRef]

Journal of
Clinical Medicine

MDPI

Article

ANRIL rs4977574 Gene Polymorphism in Women with Recurrent Pregnancy Loss

Panagiotis Cherouveim [1], Despoina Mavrogianni [2], Eirini Drakaki [2], Anastasios Potiris [3,*], Athanasios Zikopoulos [4], Myrto Papamentzelopoulou [2], Konstantina Kouvoutsaki [2], Nikolaos Machairiotis [3], Theodoros Karampitsakos [3], Chara Skentou [5], Ekaterini Domali [2], Nikolaos Vrachnis [3], Peter Drakakis [2,3] and Sofoklis Stavros [3]

1 Division of Reproductive Endocrinology and Infertility, Obstetrics and Gynecology, Massachusetts General Hospital, Harvard Medical School, Boston, MA 02114, USA; pcherouveim@mgh.harvard.edu
2 First Department of Obstetrics and Gynecology, Alexandra Hospital, Medical School of the National and Kapodistrian University of Athens, 11528 Athens, Greece; dmavrogianni@med.uoa.gr (D.M.); eirinidrak@med.uoa.gr (E.D.); mpntua@yahoo.gr (M.P.); konskouv@med.uoa.gr (K.K.); kdomali@med.uoa.gr (E.D.); pdrakakis@med.uoa.gr (P.D.)
3 Third Department of Obstetrics and Gynecology, University General Hospital "ATTIKON", Medical School of the National and Kapodistrian University of Athens, 12462 Athens, Greece; nikolaosmachairiotis@gmail.com (N.M.); theokarampitsakos@hotmail.com (T.K.); nvrachnis@med.uoa.gr (N.V.); sfstavrou@med.uoa.gr (S.S.)
4 Department of Obstetrics and Gynecology, Royal Cornwall Hospital, Treliske, Truro TR1 3LQ, UK; thanzik92@gmail.com
5 Department of Obstetrics and Gynecology, Medical School of the University of Ioannina, 45110 Ioannina, Greece; haraskentou@gmail.com
* Correspondence: apotiris@med.uoa.gr; Tel.: +30-(210)-5832237

Abstract: Background: *ANRIL* rs4977574 gene polymorphism has been associated with arterial thrombosis and cardiovascular disease development. *ANRIL* rs4977574 gene polymorphism could also be associated with recurrent pregnancy loss (RPL) since there is increasing evidence in favor of a potential shared pathophysiological mechanism with cardiovascular disease, potentially through arterial thrombosis. This study's goal is to investigate the differences in *ANRIL* rs4977574 gene polymorphism between women with and without RPL, if any, as well as a potential association with the number of pregnancy losses. Methods: DNA was isolated from peripheral blood samples, and the sequence containing the polymorphism of interest was amplified with PCR. Results were visualized under UV light following electrophoresis in 3% agarose gel with ethidium bromide. *ANRIL* rs4977574 (A>G) prevalence was compared between 56 women with and 69 without RPL. Results were adjusted for women's age and BMI, while a stratified analysis was performed according to number of pregnancy losses. Results: Allele A was significantly more prevalent in the control group compared to RPL women [31 (44.9%) vs. 14 (25%), p = 0.021]. Although not reaching statistical significance, a gradually decreasing prevalence of allele A with an increasing number of pregnancy losses was observed [31 (44.9%) in control, eight (30.7%) with two, six (23.1%) with three, and 0 (0.0%) with four pregnancy losses, p = 0.078]. Results were also similar following adjustment. Conclusions: This is the first study that demonstrates an association between RPL presence and *ANRIL* rs4977574 gene polymorphism (lower prevalence of allele A), while a difference according to the number of pregnancy losses cannot be excluded.

Keywords: *ANRIL*; recurrent pregnancy loss; pregnancy loss; polymorphism; rs4977574

1. Introduction

Recurrent pregnancy loss (RPL) affects approximately 1–4% of women attempting pregnancy in Europe and the United States [1,2]. Despite its wide prevalence, shedding light on RPL pathophysiology and risk factors remains a challenge.

Many factors could interfere with the complex process of embryo–endometrium interaction and lead to pregnancy loss [3,4]. Amongst them, the role of vascular thrombosis in RPL pathophysiology has been recognized for more than 25 years [5]. Pregnancy, being a prothrombotic state, favors blood coagulation, which in turn could lead to pregnancy loss or other placenta-mediated complications [6]. Arterial thrombosis might have a more predominant role in RPL pathophysiology compared to venous thrombosis. Previous data suggest that even in diagnosed cases of venous thromboembolic disease, there is no clear benefit of a diagnostic workup and treatment [7]. On the other hand, many conditions leading to arterial thromboses have been linked to RPL. Lupus anticoagulant or anticardiolipin antibodies have been associated with arterial thromboses and may increase the risk of RPL [8]. The European Society of Human Reproduction and Embryology (ESHRE) and the American Society for Reproductive Medicine (ASRM) recommend investigating the presence of such antibodies in women with RPL, while they do not recommend investigating potential inherited thrombophilias [3,4]. Finally, a recent multicenter study found a correlation between pregnancy loss and cardiovascular risk [9], implying a shared underlying pathophysiological mechanism, at least partially, between the two disease processes.

A non-coding region in chromosome 9 (9p21) containing the Antisense Non-coding RNA in the INK4 Locus the CDKN2B antisense RNA 1 gene (*CDKN2B-AS1* or *ANRIL*) was discovered following Genome-Wide Association Studies (GWAS) that investigated the genetic basis of atheromatosis [10]. The *ANRIL* gene can form at least 20 circular or linear transcripts through alternative splicing [11–13], and its discovery remains very promising with many disease associations and implications [14–21]. One of its most prominent correlations seems to be with cardiovascular disease [10,14]. Ever since it was first described, there has been a body of steadily increasing evidence suggesting the critical role of *ANRIL* in the formation and progression of atheromatous plaques through vascular endothelial, smooth muscular, and mononuclear cells [22–25]. More specifically, rs4977574 polymorphism has been associated with atheromatosis in various arterial locations [26–28], leading to blood flow impediment to the heart [29,30] or the brain [31] and resulting in acute myocardial infarction [29,30] or ischemic stroke [31], respectively. Likewise, a similar event might lead to blood flow impediment in the uterine vessels, leading to the clinical manifestations of RPL. Congrains et al. reported an abnormal expression of *CDKN2A/B* and a decrease in cell growth when *ANRIL* was knocked down in cells of vascular smooth muscle [32]. According to Jarinova et al. and Congrains et al., the genetic variants of *ANRIL* influence atherosclerosis mechanisms such as thrombogenesis, vascular repair, and plaque stability by altering *ANRIL* expression and cell proliferation [32,33]. Xu Bing proposes that *ANRIL* changes the expression of the corresponding coding-related genes via mechanisms such as RNAi, gene silencing, or DNA methylation [30]. These data suggest that *ANRIL* rs4977574 gene polymorphism involvement in vascular disease and arterial thrombosis pathophysiology could provide a link to RPL development, further supporting the hypothesis of a shared underlying mechanism with cardiovascular disease.

One hypothesis would be *ANRIL* rs4977574 gene polymorphism being associated with arterial thrombosis, uterine blood flow restriction, and RPL manifestation. Consequently, the aim of our study is to investigate whether *ANRIL* rs4977574 gene polymorphism prevalence differs between women with or without RPL, as well as according to the number of pregnancy losses.

2. Materials and Methods

2.1. Study Design

This study included 125 women from the Alexandra University Hospital, First Department of Obstetrics and Gynecology, Medical School of the National and Kapodistrian University of Athens. The study protocol was approved by the scientific and ethics committee of the institution (Protocol Number 91970). Fifty-six women who had at least 2 prior pregnancy losses and who were aged less than 40 years old were included in the recurrent pregnancy loss (RPL) group. Sixty-nine women who had already had at least one livebirth without any prior pregnancy loss were included in the control group. Patient characteristics, such as age and BMI, were registered for the RPL group. The age and the BMI of the control group were matched to those in the RPL group. *ANRIL* rs4977574 gene polymorphism (A>G) prevalence was compared between the two groups. Data were not available for all partners and, consequently, were not included.

2.2. DNA Isolation and Detection of ANRIL rs4977574 Gene Polymorphism

Peripheral blood samples (2–3 mL) were collected, and DNA extraction was performed using the PureLink® Genomic DNA Mini Kit (Invitrogen by Life Technologies, Waltham, MA, USA). Primers used for *ANRIL* polymorphism detection (rs4977574) were forward 5′-TTGAGGGTACATCAAAAGCATTCTATATCG-3′ and reverse 5′-TTTATTAGAGTGACTTGA ACATCCCGT-3′. The conditions of the PCR were as follows: 95 °C for 1 min, 65 °C for 1 min, and 72 °C for 1 min. PCR products were visualized using agarose gel electrophoresis, and different fragments at 226 for allele G and 166 for allele A were detected.

2.3. Statistical Analysis

T-test, Mann–Whitney U-test, ANOVA, and Kruskal–Wallis H-test were used for numerical variables depending on each variable's distribution and the number of groups compared. Chi-square test and Fisher exact test were used to compare categorical variables as appropriate. *ANRIL* rs4977574 gene polymorphism results were compared between controls and RPL, as well as after stratification of the RPL group according to the number of pregnancy losses. Odds ratios (ORs) and their respective 95% confidence intervals (CIs) were calculated using logistic regression to compare the odds of allele A prevalence between women with 2 and 3 pregnancy losses. The group of women with 4 pregnancy losses was not separately included in the regression models since it was comprised of only 4 women. OR results were adjusted for maternal age and BMI. Statistical significance was determined as a p-value < 0.05. Statistical analysis was performed using R (v4.1.0; R foundation for statistical programming).

3. Results

3.1. Baseline Characteristics

Table 1 summarizes baseline characteristics for the RPL group. In total, there were 56 women with RPL included in our analysis. The mean age was 35 for the women and 37.9 for their partners, while the mean women's BMI was 23. Following stratification according to number of pregnancy losses, mean ages were 33.1, 36.7, and 35.8 years, their partner's ages were 34.5, 40.7, and 36.5 years, and women's BMI was 23.1, 22.8, and 24.7, among women with 2, 3, and 4 pregnancy losses, respectively. Both women (33.1 vs. 36.7 years, p = 0.019) and their partners (34.5 vs. 40.7 years, p = 0.027) with 2 pregnancy losses were younger compared to those with 3.

Table 1. RPL group baseline characteristics.

Variable	All RPL (N = 56)	2 Losses (N = 26)	3 Losses (N = 26)	4 Losses (N = 4)	p-Value *
Women's age *(years)*					
Mean (SD)	35.0 (5.7)	33.1 (5.6)	36.7 (5.2)	35.8 (7.3)	
Median (IQR)	35.0 (31.0, 40.0)	33.0 (30.0, 38.0)	38.0 (32.0, 41.0)	34.0 (30.0, 43.3)	0.019
BMI *(kg/m²)*					
Mean (SD)	23.0 (3.1)	23.1 (3.2)	22.8 (3.1)	24.7 (0.4)	
Median (IQR)	22.5 (20.3, 25.1)	22.7 (20.7, 24.2)	22.1 (20.2, 25.7)	24.7 (24.7, -)	0.914

Table 1. *Cont.*

Variable	All RPL (N = 56)	2 Losses (N = 26)	3 Losses (N = 26)	4 Losses (N = 4)	*p*-Value *
Partner's age *(years)*					
Mean (SD)	37.9 (5.8)	34.5 (3.7)	40.7 (6.7)	36.5 (0.7)	
Median (IQR)	37.0 (34.0, 40.0)	34.5 (31.8, 38.5)	37 (36, 46)	36.5 (36.0, -)	0.027

* 2 vs. 3 pregnancy losses; (-): not able to calculate. RPL: recurrent pregnancy loss; BMI: body mass index.

3.2. *ANRIL rs4977574 Gene Polymorphism in RPL and Control Groups*

The results presented were classified according to specific zones following electrophoresis (Figure 1). The *ANRIL* rs4977574 gene polymorphism results between the control and RPL groups are shown in Table 2. Women in the control group had allele A in a significantly higher frequency compared to RPL [31 (44.9%) control vs. 14 (25%) RPL, $p = 0.021$]. Of them, nine women (13.0%) in the control group and three (5.4%) in the RPL were homozygous for allele A (genotype A/A). When analysis was based on specific genotypes, the results did not reach statistical significance ($p = 0.062$) (Figure 2).

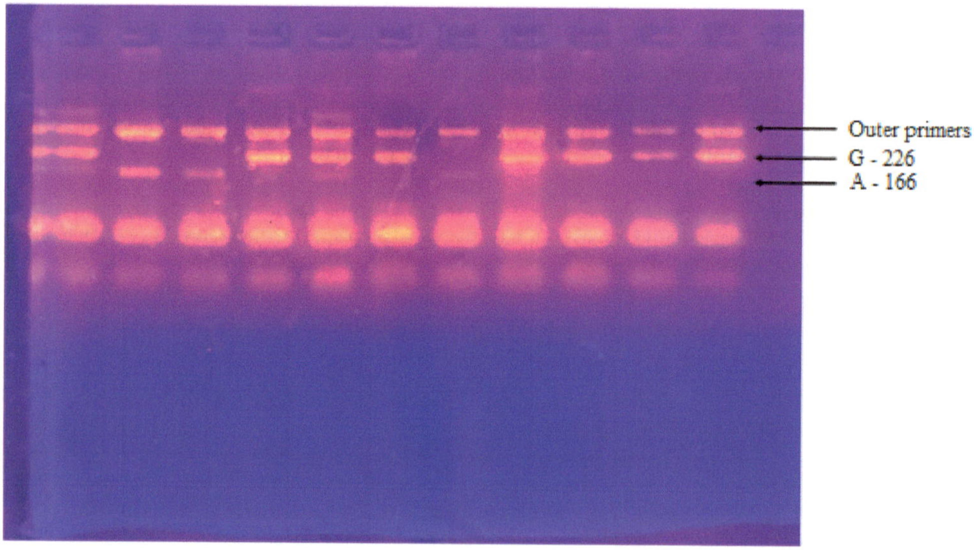

Figure 1. Agarose electrophoresis after PCR reaction. Lanes 1–11 show amplification of PCR products. A 226bp PCR product corresponds to a G allele. A 166bp PCR product corresponds to A allele. A 330bp PCR product is visualized after amplification with an outer primer pair.

Table 2. *ANRIL* rs4977574 polymorphism results between control and RPL.

ANRIL rs4977574 Polymorphism	Controls (n = 69)	RPL (n = 56)	*p*-Value
G/G	38 (55.1%)	42 (75.0%)	
G/A	22 (31.9%)	11 (19.6%)	0.062, for genotype
A/A	9 (13.0%)	3 (5.4%)	0.021, for allele A

ANRIL: Antisense non-coding RNA in the INK4 Locus; RPL: recurrent pregnancy loss.

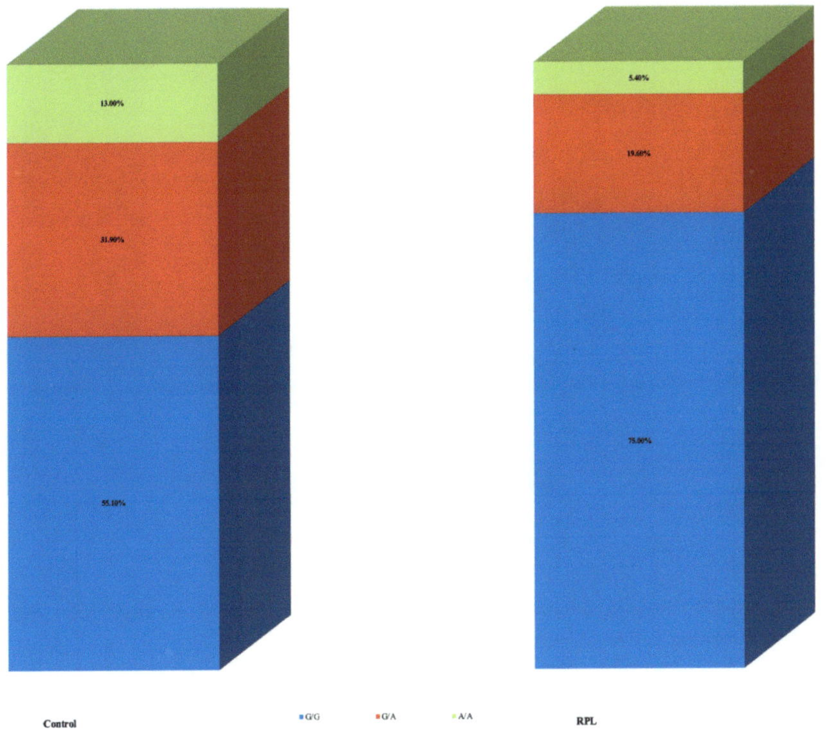

Figure 2. *ANRIL* (Antisense non-coding RNA in the INK4 Locus) rs4977574 polymorphism results between control and RPL (recurrent pregnancy loss).

3.3. *ANRIL rs4977574 Gene Polymorphism Depending on Number of Pregnancy Losses*

Table 3 summarizes the results following stratification according to the number of pregnancy losses. The first group (None) represents the control group, which included women with no pregnancy losses. Even though results did not reach statistical significance (p = 0.078), there was a pattern of gradually decreased prevalence of allele A with an increasing number of pregnancy losses. Thirty-one (44.9%) of women in the control group had at least one allele A, eight (30.7%) with two pregnancy losses, six (23.1%) with three, and none with four pregnancy losses. Of them, nine women (13.0%) in the control group, three (11.5%) with two pregnancy losses, and none with three were homozygous for allele A (genotype A/A) (Figure 3).

Table 3. *ANRIL* rs4977574 polymorphism results according to number of pregnancy losses.

ANRIL rs4977574 Polymorphism	None (n = 69)	Two (n = 26)	Three (n = 26)	Four (n = 4)	p-Value
G/G	38 (55.1%)	18 (69.3%)	20 (76.9%)	4 (100%)	
G/A	22 (31.9%)	5 (19.2%)	6 (23.1%)	0 (0.0%)	0.188, for genotype
A/A	9 (13.0%)	3 (11.5%)	0 (0.0%)	0 (0.0%)	0.078, for allele A

ANRIL: Antisense non-coding RNA in the INK4 Locus.

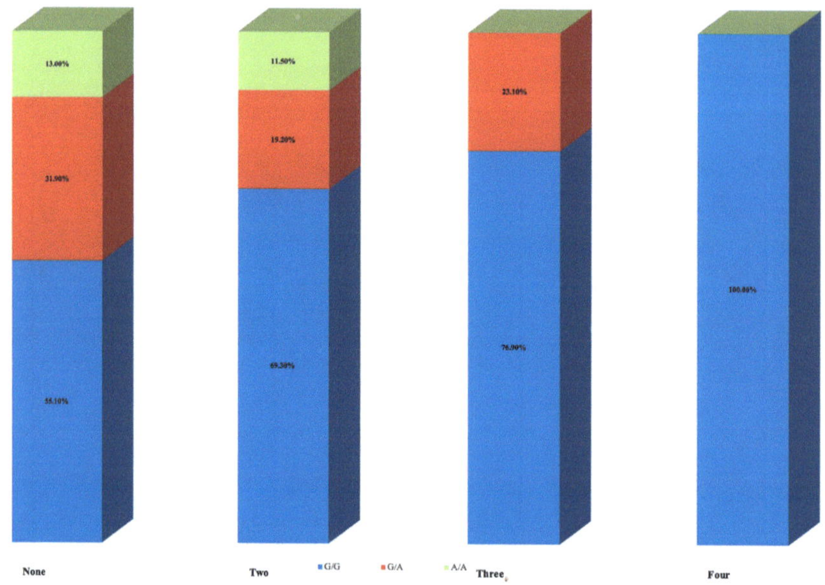

Figure 3. *ANRIL* (Antisense Non-coding RNA in the INK4 Locus) rs4977574 polymorphism results according to number of pregnancy losses.

3.4. ANRIL rs4977574 Gene Polymorphism in Women with 2 and 3 Pregnancy Losses

Finally, OR for allele A presence between women with 2 and 3 pregnancy losses was not significant neither before [OR (95%CI): 0.68(0.20–2.32), $p = 0.533$], nor after adjustment [adjOR(95%CI): 0.54(0.14–2.13), $p = 0.375$].

4. Discussion

Our study investigated whether *ANRIL* rs4977574 gene polymorphism prevalence differs between women with or without RPL, as well as according to the number of pregnancy losses. The results suggest that allele A was more prevalent among women with RPL compared to those without, with a high percentage of heterozygosity (G/A) in both groups. After stratification according to the number of pregnancy losses, even though the results did not reach statistical significance, allele A prevalence decreased with an increasing number of pregnancy losses both before and after accounting for women's age and BMI. Thus, our results suggest that there might be an association of *ANRIL* rs4977574 gene polymorphism with RPL diagnosis, while an association with the number of pregnancy losses could not be excluded.

Since there are no studies investigating polymorphism rs4977574 in the setting of RPL, we will focus on the literature related to cardiovascular disease and potential molecular mechanisms implicated in the formation, rupture, and thrombosis of the atheromatous plaque. These processes are partially mediated by *ANRIL* gene expression in vascular endothelial, smooth muscle, and mononuclear cells [22–25]. *ANRIL* mediates inflammatory response and enhances vascular endothelial damage through TNF-α-NF-κB-*ANRIL*/YY1-IL6/8 pathway [34], caspase recruitment domain-containing protein 8 [35], and vascular endothelial growth factor [36] expression increase. Moreover, *ANRIL* has been associated with abnormal proliferation, migration, aging, and apoptosis of vascular smooth muscle cells [32,37–39]. *ANRIL* has also been found to regulate cyclin-dependent kinase inhibitor 2A and 2B expression, which have a major role in the regulation of the cell cycle, apoptosis, and cell aging [37,40]. Finally, Alu elements, a family of short interspersed repeat elements, are associated with atheromatosis by facilitating mononuclear cell adhesion and proliferation [41] and have been found to be functionally related to *ANRIL* in knock-out studies [42,43]. Taken together, this evidence highlights the role of *ANRIL* in many aspects of atheromatosis and cardiovascular disease pathophysiology, which might also be associated with RPL.

To the best of our knowledge, there are no published data about *ANRIL* gene polymorphism prevalence in women with RPL. Therefore, we provide the first preliminary data on *ANRIL* rs4977574 gene polymorphism among women with RPL as part of a novel investigation of the common pathophysiology shared between RPL and cardiovascular disease. We found a significant association between *ANRIL* rs4977574 gene polymorphism and RPL diagnosis. Two recent metanalyses have found an association between *ANRIL* rs4977574 gene polymorphism and a higher risk for coronary artery disease [30,44]. Both studies concluded that allele G was associated with increased risk [30,44]. Similarly, our results suggest a higher prevalence of allele G in women with RPL. Taking into consideration the higher probability of cardiovascular disease development later in life among women with pregnancy loss [9], these results further support the hypothesis of a shared underlying pathophysiological mechanism that contributes to both conditions.

Formation and progression of the atheromatous plaque might explain, at least partially, the basis of the shared underlying mechanism. *ANRIL* rs4977574 gene polymorphism has been associated with atheromatosis in coronary [27] and carotid arteries [26,28], which is probably independent of hypertension [45]. Additionally, consumption of vegetables, wine [46], and smoking [47] seem to further modify the risk for cardiovascular disease associated with the polymorphism. The ultimate result is atheromatous plaque rupture and vessel thrombosis [27]. Depending on the location of the affected vessel, there is the respective clinical manifestation of acute myocardial infarction [29,30] or ischemic stroke [31]. Therefore, one potential explanation would be that the presence of allele G in rs4977574 increases the risk for atheromatosis [26–28] and, thus, arterial thrombosis, leading to RPL.

Our study is the first to investigate *ANRIL* gene polymorphisms in women with RPL. The number of pregnancy losses, age, and BMI have been found to be correlated to RPL [2,48] and adjusting for them enhances the validity of our results. Nevertheless, there were no available demographic data for women or their partners in the control group, restricting relevant analyses. Additionally, we do not have consistent data available on other factors that might also contribute to RPL development, such as the presence of thrombophilia, chromosomal abnormalities, or autoimmune diseases.

Future studies could aim at investigating the underlying molecular mechanisms that might explain a potential *ANRIL* and RPL correlation. In addition to utilizing next-generation sequencing, including more baseline demographic characteristics of the couples could help establish useful RPL biomarkers.

5. Conclusions

In summary, this study provides the first possible association between *ANRIL* gene polymorphism and recurrent abortions. Our results suggest that rs4977574 is associated with RPL prevalence, while an association with the number of pregnancy losses cannot be excluded. Although the mechanisms underlying the aforementioned association are not clarified, the present study proposes that a shared pathophysiological mechanism is possible for both RPL and cardiovascular disease, potentially through atheromatosis and arterial thrombosis as genetic variants of *ANRIL* influence atherosclerosis mechanisms such as thrombogenesis, vascular repair, and plaque stability by altering *ANRIL* expression and cell proliferation. Consequently, the studied polymorphism could be proposed as a possible biomarker of recurrent abortions, and additionally, future studies may focus on the genes interfering with *ANRIL* and also on genes in linkage disequilibrium with the studied polymorphism.

Author Contributions: Conceptualization, P.C., E.D. (Ekaterini Domali) and S.S.; methodology, D.M. and C.S.; validation, D.M. and A.Z.; formal analysis, M.P.; data curation, K.K.; writing—original draft preparation, P.C. and E.D. (Eirini Drakaki); writing—review and editing, A.P., N.M. and T.K.; visualization, A.P.; supervision, N.V., E.D. (Ekaterini Domali) and P.D.; project administration, S.S. All authors have read and agreed to the published version of the manuscript.

Funding: This research received no external funding.

Institutional Review Board Statement: The present study was conducted according to the Declaration of Helsinki for Medical Research involving Human Subjects and approved by the Ethics and Scientific Committee of Alexandra University Hospital, Medical School of the National and Kapodistrian University of Athens with protocol identification number 91970.

Informed Consent Statement: Informed consent was obtained from all subjects involved in the study.

Data Availability Statement: Not applicable.

Acknowledgments: We would like to thank all the members of the First Department of Obstetrics and Gynecology in Alexandra University Hospital for their help, as well as all the women and their partners who took part in our study.

Conflicts of Interest: The authors declare no conflict of interest.

References

1. Rasmark Roepke, E.; Matthiesen, L.; Rylance, R.; Christiansen, O.B. Is the incidence of recurrent pregnancy loss increasing? A retrospective register-based study in Sweden. *Acta Obstet. Gynecol. Scand.* **2017**, *96*, 1365–1372. [CrossRef] [PubMed]
2. Magnus, M.C.; Wilcox, A.J.; Morken, N.H.; Weinberg, C.R.; Haberg, S.E. Role of maternal age and pregnancy history in risk of miscarriage: Prospective register based study. *BMJ* **2019**, *364*, l869. [CrossRef]
3. The ESHRE Guideline Group on RPL; Bender Atik, R.; Christiansen, O.B.; Elson, J.; Kolte, A.M.; Lewis, S.; Middeldorp, S.; Nelen, W.; Peramo, B.; Quenby, S.; et al. ESHRE guideline: Recurrent pregnancy loss. *Hum. Reprod. Open* **2018**, *2018*, hoy004. [CrossRef] [PubMed]
4. Practice Committee of the American Society for Reproductive Medicine. Evidence-based treatments for couples with unexplained infertility: A guideline. *Fertil. Steril.* **2020**, *113*, 305–322. [CrossRef]
5. Preston, F.E.; Rosendaal, F.R.; Walker, I.D.; Briet, E.; Berntorp, E.; Conard, J.; Fontcuberta, J.; Makris, M.; Mariani, G.; Noteboom, W.; et al. Increased fetal loss in women with heritable thrombophilia. *Lancet* **1996**, *348*, 913–916. [CrossRef]
6. Kutteh, W.H.; Triplett, D.A. Thrombophilias and recurrent pregnancy loss. *Semin. Reprod. Med.* **2006**, *24*, 54–66. [CrossRef] [PubMed]
7. Bates, S.M.; Middeldorp, S.; Rodger, M.; James, A.H.; Greer, I. Guidance for the treatment and prevention of obstetric-associated venous thromboembolism. *J. Thromb. Thrombolysis* **2016**, *41*, 92–128. [CrossRef]
8. Jauniaux, E.; Farquharson, R.G.; Christiansen, O.B.; Exalto, N. Evidence-based guidelines for the investigation and medical treatment of recurrent miscarriage. *Hum. Reprod.* **2006**, *21*, 2216–2222. [CrossRef]
9. Murugappan, G.; Leonard, S.A.; Farland, L.V.; Lau, E.S.; Shadyab, A.H.; Wild, R.A.; Schnatz, P.; Carmichael, S.L.; Stefanick, M.L.; Parikh, N.I. Association of infertility with atherosclerotic cardiovascular disease among postmenopausal participants in the Women's Health Initiative. *Fertil. Steril.* **2022**, *117*, 1038–1046. [CrossRef] [PubMed]
10. Samani, N.J.; Erdmann, J.; Hall, A.S.; Hengstenberg, C.; Mangino, M.; Mayer, B.; Dixon, R.J.; Meitinger, T.; Braund, P.; Wichmann, H.E.; et al. Genomewide association analysis of coronary artery disease. *N. Engl. J. Med.* **2007**, *357*, 443–453. [CrossRef]
11. Burd, C.E.; Jeck, W.R.; Liu, Y.; Sanoff, H.K.; Wang, Z.; Sharpless, N.E. Expression of linear and novel circular forms of an INK4/ARF-associated non-coding RNA correlates with atherosclerosis risk. *PLoS Genet.* **2010**, *6*, e1001233. [CrossRef]
12. Hubberten, M.; Bochenek, G.; Chen, H.; Hasler, R.; Wiehe, R.; Rosenstiel, P.; Jepsen, S.; Dommisch, H.; Schaefer, A.S. Linear isoforms of the long noncoding RNA CDKN2B-AS1 regulate the c-myc-enhancer binding factor RBMS1. *Eur. J. Hum. Genet.* **2019**, *27*, 80–89. [CrossRef]
13. Rivera, N.V.; Carreras-Torres, R.; Roncarati, R.; Viviani-Anselmi, C.; De Micco, F.; Mezzelani, A.; Koch, W.; Hoppmann, P.; Kastrati, A.; Stewart, A.F.; et al. Assessment of the 9p21.3 locus in severity of coronary artery disease in the presence and absence of type 2 diabetes. *BMC Med. Genet.* **2013**, *14*, 11. [CrossRef]
14. Broadbent, H.M.; Peden, J.F.; Lorkowski, S.; Goel, A.; Ongen, H.; Green, F.; Clarke, R.; Collins, R.; Franzosi, M.G.; Tognoni, G.; et al. Susceptibility to coronary artery disease and diabetes is encoded by distinct, tightly linked SNPs in the ANRIL locus on chromosome 9p. *Hum. Mol. Genet.* **2008**, *17*, 806–814. [CrossRef]
15. Burdon, K.P.; Macgregor, S.; Hewitt, A.W.; Sharma, S.; Chidlow, G.; Mills, R.A.; Danoy, P.; Casson, R.; Viswanathan, A.C.; Liu, J.Z.; et al. Genome-wide association study identifies susceptibility loci for open angle glaucoma at TMCO1 and CDKN2B-AS1. *Nat. Genet.* **2011**, *43*, 574–578. [CrossRef]

16. Cugino, D.; Gianfagna, F.; Santimone, I.; de Gaetano, G.; Donati, M.B.; Iacoviello, L.; Di Castelnuovo, A. Type 2 diabetes and polymorphisms on chromosome 9p21: A meta-analysis. *Nutr. Metab. Cardiovasc. Dis.* **2012**, *22*, 619–625. [CrossRef] [PubMed]
17. Emanuele, E.; Lista, S.; Ghidoni, R.; Binetti, G.; Cereda, C.; Benussi, L.; Maletta, R.; Bruni, A.C.; Politi, P. Chromosome 9p21.3 genotype is associated with vascular dementia and Alzheimer's disease. *Neurobiol. Aging* **2011**, *32*, 1231–1235. [CrossRef] [PubMed]
18. Kong, Y.; Hsieh, C.H.; Alonso, L.C. ANRIL: A lncRNA at the CDKN2A/B Locus With Roles in Cancer and Metabolic Disease. *Front. Endocrinol.* **2018**, *9*, 405. [CrossRef] [PubMed]
19. Ramdas, W.D.; van Koolwijk, L.M.; Lemij, H.G.; Pasutto, F.; Cree, A.J.; Thorleifsson, G.; Janssen, S.F.; Jacoline, T.B.; Amin, N.; Rivadeneira, F.; et al. Common genetic variants associated with open-angle glaucoma. *Hum. Mol. Genet.* **2011**, *20*, 2464–2471. [CrossRef]
20. Schaefer, A.S.; Richter, G.M.; Groessner-Schreiber, B.; Noack, B.; Nothnagel, M.; El Mokhtari, N.E.; Loos, B.G.; Jepsen, S.; Schreiber, S. Identification of a shared genetic susceptibility locus for coronary heart disease and periodontitis. *PLoS Genet.* **2009**, *5*, e1000378. [CrossRef]
21. Uno, S.; Zembutsu, H.; Hirasawa, A.; Takahashi, A.; Kubo, M.; Akahane, T.; Aoki, D.; Kamatani, N.; Hirata, K.; Nakamura, Y. A genome-wide association study identifies genetic variants in the CDKN2BAS locus associated with endometriosis in Japanese. *Nat. Genet.* **2010**, *42*, 707–710. [CrossRef]
22. Consortium, E.P. An integrated encyclopedia of DNA elements in the human genome. *Nature* **2012**, *489*, 57–74. [CrossRef] [PubMed]
23. Nanda, V.; Downing, K.P.; Ye, J.; Xiao, S.; Kojima, Y.; Spin, J.M.; DiRenzo, D.; Nead, K.T.; Connolly, A.J.; Dandona, S.; et al. CDKN2B Regulates TGFbeta Signaling and Smooth Muscle Cell Investment of Hypoxic Neovessels. *Circ. Res.* **2016**, *118*, 230–240. [CrossRef] [PubMed]
24. Papait, R.; Kunderfranco, P.; Stirparo, G.G.; Latronico, M.V.; Condorelli, G. Long noncoding RNA: A new player of heart failure? *J. Cardiovasc. Transl. Res.* **2013**, *6*, 876–883. [CrossRef] [PubMed]
25. Zollbrecht, C.; Grassl, M.; Fenk, S.; Hocherl, R.; Hubauer, U.; Reinhard, W.; Esslinger, U.B.; Ebert, S.; Langmann, T.; Stark, K.; et al. Expression pattern in human macrophages dependent on 9p21.3 coronary artery disease risk locus. *Atherosclerosis* **2013**, *227*, 244–249. [CrossRef]
26. Jin, W.; Wu, W.; Yang, K.; Shen, F.; Fu, N.; Feng, Y.; Fu, Y. The Single Nucleotide Polymorphisms of Chromosome 9p21 and CD147 Were Relevant with the Carotid Plaque Risk in Acute Cerebral Infarction Patients Among Chinese Han Population. *J. Mol. Neurosci.* **2020**, *70*, 1282–1292. [CrossRef] [PubMed]
27. Liu, R.; Song, L.; Jiang, L.; Tang, X.; Xu, L.; Gao, Z.; Zhao, X.; Xu, J.; Gao, R.; Yuan, J. Susceptible gene polymorphism in patients with three-vessel coronary artery disease. *BMC Cardiovasc. Disord.* **2020**, *20*, 172. [CrossRef]
28. Lu, Z.; Zhang, Y.; Maimaiti, Y.; Feng, Y.; Sun, J.; Zhuang, J.; Zeng, L.; Fu, Y. Variants on Chromosome 9p21 Confer Risks of Noncardioembolic Cerebral Infarction and Carotid Plaque in the Chinese Han Population. *J. Atheroscler. Thromb.* **2015**, *22*, 1061–1070. [CrossRef]
29. Sakalar, C.; Gurbuz, E.; Kalay, N.; Kaya, M.G. Higher frequency of rs4977574 (the G Allele) on chromosome 9p21.3 in patients with myocardial infarction as revealed by PCR-RFLP analysis. *Tohoku J. Exp. Med.* **2013**, *230*, 171–176. [CrossRef]
30. Xu, B.; Fang, Z.; He, S.; Wang, J.; Yang, X. ANRIL polymorphism rs4977574 is associated with increased risk of coronary artery disease in Asian populations: A meta-analysis of 12,005 subjects. *Medicine* **2018**, *97*, e12641. [CrossRef]
31. Lasek-Bal, A.; Kula, D.; Urbanek, T.; Puz, P.; Szymszal, J.; Jarzab, M.; Halczok, M.; Cyplinska, R.; Bal, W.; Labuz-Roszak, B.; et al. The Association of SNPs Located in the CDKN2B-AS1 and LPA Genes With Carotid Artery Stenosis and Atherogenic Stroke. *Front. Neurol.* **2019**, *10*, 1170. [CrossRef]
32. Congrains, A.; Kamide, K.; Oguro, R.; Yasuda, O.; Miyata, K.; Yamamoto, E.; Kawai, T.; Kusunoki, H.; Yamamoto, H.; Takeya, Y.; et al. Genetic variants at the 9p21 locus contribute to atherosclerosis through modulation of ANRIL and CDKN2A/B. *Atherosclerosis* **2012**, *220*, 449–455. [CrossRef]
33. Jarinova, O.; Stewart, A.F.; Roberts, R.; Wells, G.; Lau, P.; Naing, T.; Buerki, C.; McLean, B.W.; Cook, R.C.; Parker, J.S.; et al. Functional analysis of the chromosome 9p21.3 coronary artery disease risk locus. *Arterioscler. Thromb. Vasc. Biol.* **2009**, *29*, 1671–1677. [CrossRef]
34. Zhou, X.; Han, X.; Wittfeldt, A.; Sun, J.; Liu, C.; Wang, X.; Gan, L.M.; Cao, H.; Liang, Z. Long non-coding RNA ANRIL regulates inflammatory responses as a novel component of NF-kappaB pathway. *RNA Biol.* **2016**, *13*, 98–108. [CrossRef]
35. Bai, Y.; Nie, S.; Jiang, G.; Zhou, Y.; Zhou, M.; Zhao, Y.; Li, S.; Wang, F.; Lv, Q.; Huang, Y.; et al. Regulation of CARD8 expression by ANRIL and association of CARD8 single nucleotide polymorphism rs2043211 (p.C10X) with ischemic stroke. *Stroke* **2014**, *45*, 383–388. [CrossRef]
36. Thomas, A.A.; Feng, B.; Chakrabarti, S. ANRIL: A Regulator of VEGF in Diabetic Retinopathy. *Investig. Ophthalmol. Vis. Sci.* **2017**, *58*, 470–480. [CrossRef] [PubMed]
37. Aguilo, F.; Di Cecilia, S.; Walsh, M.J. Long Non-coding RNA ANRIL and Polycomb in Human Cancers and Cardiovascular Disease. *Curr. Top. Microbiol. Immunol.* **2016**, *394*, 29–39. [CrossRef] [PubMed]
38. Katsiki, N.; Tziomalos, K.; Chatzizisis, Y.; Elisaf, M.; Hatzitolios, A.I. Effect of HMG-CoA reductase inhibitors on vascular cell apoptosis: Beneficial or detrimental? *Atherosclerosis* **2010**, *211*, 9–14. [CrossRef] [PubMed]

39. Wang, P.; Xu, T.Y.; Guan, Y.F.; Zhao, Y.; Li, Z.Y.; Lan, X.H.; Wang, X.; Yang, P.Y.; Kang, Z.M.; Vanhoutte, P.M.; et al. Vascular smooth muscle cell apoptosis is an early trigger for hypothyroid atherosclerosis. *Cardiovasc. Res.* **2014**, *102*, 448–459. [CrossRef] [PubMed]
40. Gil, J.; Peters, G. Regulation of the INK4b-ARF-INK4a tumour suppressor locus: All for one or one for all. *Nat. Rev. Mol. Cell Biol.* **2006**, *7*, 667–677. [CrossRef]
41. Rudiger, N.S.; Gregersen, N.; Kielland-Brandt, M.C. One short well conserved region of Alu-sequences is involved in human gene rearrangements and has homology with prokaryotic chi. *Nucleic Acids Res.* **1995**, *23*, 256–260. [CrossRef] [PubMed]
42. Chi, J.S.; Li, J.Z.; Jia, J.J.; Zhang, T.; Liu, X.M.; Yi, L. Long non-coding RNA ANRIL in gene regulation and its duality in atherosclerosis. *J. Huazhong Univ. Sci. Technol. Med. Sci.* **2017**, *37*, 816–822. [CrossRef] [PubMed]
43. Hueso, M.; Cruzado, J.M.; Torras, J.; Navarro, E. ALUminating the Path of Atherosclerosis Progression: Chaos Theory Suggests a Role for Alu Repeats in the Development of Atherosclerotic Vascular Disease. *Int. J. Mol. Sci.* **2018**, *19*, 1734. [CrossRef]
44. Li, Y.Y.; Wang, H.; Zhang, Y.Y. CDKN2B-AS1 gene rs4977574 A/G polymorphism and coronary heart disease: A meta-analysis of 40,979 subjects. *J. Cell Mol. Med.* **2021**, *25*, 8877–8889. [CrossRef] [PubMed]
45. Kunnas, T.; Piesanen, J.; Nikkari, S.T. Association of a Chromosome Locus 9p21.3 CDKN2B-AS1 Variant rs4977574 with Hypertension: The TAMRISK Study. *Genet. Test. Mol. Biomark.* **2018**, *22*, 327–330. [CrossRef]
46. Hindy, G.; Ericson, U.; Hamrefors, V.; Drake, I.; Wirfalt, E.; Melander, O.; Orho-Melander, M. The chromosome 9p21 variant interacts with vegetable and wine intake to influence the risk of cardiovascular disease: A population based cohort study. *BMC Med. Genet.* **2014**, *15*, 1220. [CrossRef]
47. Hamrefors, V.; Hedblad, B.; Hindy, G.; Smith, J.G.; Almgren, P.; Engstrom, G.; Sjogren, M.; Gransbo, K.; Orho-Melander, M.; Melander, O. Smoking modifies the associated increased risk of future cardiovascular disease by genetic variation on chromosome 9p21. *PLoS ONE* **2014**, *9*, e85893. [CrossRef]
48. Boots, C.; Stephenson, M.D. Does obesity increase the risk of miscarriage in spontaneous conception: A systematic review. *Semin. Reprod. Med.* **2011**, *29*, 507–513. [CrossRef]

Journal of
Clinical Medicine

MDPI

Article

Detection of zeb1 Gene in Granulosa Cells in Women Undergoing IVF Treatment

Ioannis Chrysanthopoulos [1], Despoina Mavrogianni [1], Eirini Drakaki [1], Anastasios Potiris [2,*], Athanasios Zikopoulos [3], Athanasios Zachariou [4], Ekaterini Domali [1], Peter Drakakis [1,2] and Sofoklis Stavros [2]

1 First Department of Obstetrics and Gynecology, Alexandra Hospital, Medical School, National and Kapodistrian University of Athens, 115 28 Athens, Greece; johnchrysan@med.uoa.gr (I.C.); dmavrogianni@med.uoa.gr (D.M.); eirinidrak@med.uoa.gr (E.D.); kdomali@med.uoa.gr (E.D.); pdrakakis@med.uoa.gr (P.D.)

2 Third Department of Obstetrics and Gynecology, University General Hospital "ATTIKON", Medical School, National and Kapodistrian University of Athens, 12462 Athens, Greece; sfstavrou@med.uoa.gr

3 Department of Obstetrics and Gynecology, Royal Cornwall Hospital, Treliske, Truro TR1 3LQ, UK; thanzik92@gmail.com

4 Laboratory of Spermatology, Department of Urology, School of Health Sciences, University of Ioannina, 451 10 Ioannina, Greece; zahariou@otenet.gr

* Correspondence: apotiris@med.uoa.gr; Tel.: +30-(210)5832237

Abstract: Background: ZEB1 plays a role in epithelial-to-mesenchymal transition and acts as a repressor of E-cadherin, TGF-β, and Wnt/β-catenin. Since ZEB1 protein is expressed in estrogen-responsive tissues, and expression of the gene in the normal ovary and endometrium is positively correlated with high estrogen levels, we performed a direct analysis of granulosa cell samples to determine whether there are any significant changes in zeb1 expression during folliculogenesis. Methods: ZEB1 expression levels were measured in the granulosa cells of 56 infertile women undergoing IVF treatment. RNA extraction from granulosa cells was performed along with reverse transcription quantitative polymerase chain reaction (RT-qPCR) with SYBR Green I to determine zeb1 gene expression levels. Statistical analysis was performed by using *t*-test, while possible correlations of the expression of ZEB1 protein with body mass index (BMI), age, number of oocytes, and oocyte maturation were investigated. Results: Zeb1 gene expression levels correlate significantly with body mass index (BMI) and age, but not with oocyte number and oocyte maturation stage. Obese women demonstrate a higher expression level of zeb1 gene compared to normal and overweight women. Moreover, zeb1 gene is overexpressed in women aged 35–40 years old and is under-expressed in women >40 years old. Conclusions: ZEB1 expression should be further investigated as it may unveil new potential findings of the zeb1 gene's role in female fertility and its use as a biomarker in fertility workups.

Keywords: infertility; in vitro fertilization (IVF); ZEB1 gene; granulosa cells; body mass index (BMI); age; oocyte number; oocyte maturation

1. Introduction

The current clinical definition of infertility is the inability to conceive after 12 months of systematic and unprotected coitus. Infertility prevalence is approximately 13% among women and 10% among men. It is estimated through demographic data that 9% of couples worldwide lack the ability to conceive naturally, and approximately 180 million couples are characterized by infertility problems [1,2]. There are several causal and contributory factors that include hormonal inadequacies or imbalances, pathophysiological deviation in the reproductive anatomy and function, genetics, and lifestyle factors among others, while a significant percentage of infertility is attributed to unknown or idiopathic factors [3].

ZEB1 is a protein encoded by the zeb1 gene which is located on chromosome 10p11.2. In humans, ZEB1 protein is expressed in estrogen-responsive tissues such as the breast, bone, uterus, endometrium, ovary, and cardiovascular system. The overexpression of the gene in normal ovary and endometrium is correlated with high estrogen levels [4].

The zinc-finger E homeobox (ZEB) protein family of transcription factors consists of two members: ZEB1 and ZEB2 [5]. The ZEB family, as a transcription factor, regulates its transcription by binding to the E-promoter DNA sequence (5′-CANNTG-3′), In humans, ZEB1 contains more than a thousand amino acids and consists of two zinc-finger clusters at the N- and C-terminal ends of the protein. The middle region consists of a homeodomain, a Smad interaction domain, and a C-terminal binding protein (CtBP) interaction domain. CtBP cannot directly bind to DNA and participates in the regulation of ZEB1 function by interacting with other regulatory factors [6,7].

Epithelial-to-mesenchymal transition (EMT) defines a process during which cells lose their epithelial characteristics and acquire typical properties of mesenchymal cells. This transition requires complex changes in cell shape that happen concomitantly to gene expression reprogramming [8]. While EMT is an essential process during embryogenesis for delamination of neural crest from the neural tube, it is a major pathological event in cancer progression, causing invasion and metastasis, which are the primary causes of morbidity and mortality in human cancer [4].

The main hallmark of EMT is the downregulation of the adherens junction protein E-cadherin due to transcriptional repression [8]. Downregulation of E-cadherin, and the resulting release of cell–cell adhesion in tumors, is thought to contribute to a motile phenotype that facilitates metastasis. Conversely, mesenchymal genes including vimentin and smooth muscle actin, as well as various matrix and matrix-degrading enzymes, are induced during EMT [9]. In addition, it has been reported that the ZEB1 protein appears to inhibit the expression of cell polarity factors, suppresses basement membrane synthesis, and activates the expression of basement membrane metalloproteases (matrix metalloproteases (MMPs), such as MMP-1, MMP-9, and MMP-14. It also promotes basement membrane remodeling and invasion into adjacent tissues. The functions of ZEB1 protein are not limited in regulating the EMT, they are also considered a central switch that controls many cellular functions such as differentiation, proliferation, response to DNA damage, and cell survival with a strong impact on tumor growth in the early stages of tumorigenesis [10].

EMT-inducing pathways, such as transforming growth factor-β (TGFβ) and Wnt signaling trigger epithelial dedifferentiation by impairing the expression/ function of the epithelial adhesion protein E-cadherin [6,9,11,12]. Repression of E-cadherin is mediated by distinct transcription factors, including Snail1 (Snail), Snail2 (Slug), and SIP1(ZEB2). ZEB1 is also tightly controlled by micro-RNAs such as miR-200 (along with miR-200 family members miR-200a, miR-200c, and miR-141), which are involved in a negative feedback loop to control EMT during normal development and tumorigenesis [13].

Both transcription and post-transcriptional mechanisms are used to regulate Zeb1. Snail1 and TGF-β lower the levels of miR-200, which stabilizes ZEB1 RNA and Zeb1 protein. A second effect of EMT is the stimulation of ZEB1 gene transcription, which is dependent on the actions of Twist and Ets1. Snail1 boosts the function of these two factors in a unique way. More specifically, it increases Twist protein levels and facilitates Ets1 translocation to the nucleus. As a result, there is an increase in the binding of these two proteins to the ZEB1 promoter. Numerous effects of this multiple upregulation of zeb1 gene expression are possible. Consequently, it is proposed that Zeb1 upregulation might be cell-dependent. Thus, whereas the effect might be mainly transcriptional in some cells, the downregulation of miRNA might be predominant in other cells [8]. EMT is one of the main mechanisms involved in both cancer and endometriosis [9].

Endometriosis is one of the main causes of female infertility and increases the risk of ovarian cancer in nearly 10% of women in reproductive age [14]. One of the main mechanisms involved in both cancer and endometriosis is the epithelial-mesenchymal transition (EMT) [9]. The main fact of the epithelial-to-mesenchymal transition (EMT) is the down regulation of E-cadherin, a protein that plays a major role in cell-to-cell adhesion. ZEB1 protein is the main regulator of EMT, through direct or indirect inhibitory action on various downstream targets such as E-cadherin [7,10]. ZEB1 protein is expressed at high levels in the epithelial cells of endometriotic tissue, while it is not expressed in normal endometrium, which makes the epithelial expression of ZEB1 a hallmark of endometriosis [15,16].

Considering the relationship between the transcription factor ZEB1 in EMT and its expression levels in women with endometriosis, we decided to study its expression in granulosa cells derived from infertile women undergoing IVF treatment. Moreover, regarding the relationship between age and infertility, it has been shown that fertility decreases with increasing age in both men and women. However, the risk of infertility has a strong correlation with maternal age. Reproductive aging is a normal process of declining fertility as a woman goes through the stages of puberty, reproductive age, transition to menopause, and menopause [17].

The aim of the present study is to focus on the interaction between zeb1 gene expression and oocyte characteristics. More specifically, we try to determine whether there is any significance in zeb1 expression during folliculogenesis and, overall, the female fertility dynamics, since ZEB1 protein is expressed in estrogen-responsive tissues such as the breast, uterus, endometrium, and ovary, while expression of the gene in the normal ovary and endometrium is positively correlated with high estrogen levels.

2. Materials and Methods

2.1. Study Design, Population, and Participant Characteristics

The study was conducted in accordance with the Declaration of Helsinki and approved by the Institutional Review Board of the Medical School of the National and Kapodistrian University of Athens with protocol identifier 56353/26.11.2020. The study was conducted in the Assisted Reproduction Unit of the First Department of Obstetrics and Gynecology through a 7-month period. The data were retrospectively collected from 56 women diagnosed with infertility, aged 20–47 years old, who underwent IVF treatment. Informed consent was obtained from all patients involved in the study during their second visit in the Unit. For each patient, data were collected regarding body mass index (BMI), age, oocyte number, and oocyte maturation. The women were separated in three groups according to their BMI: normal weight, BMI = 18.5–24.99 kg/m^2 (n = 38); overweight, BMI = 25.00–29.99 kg/m^2 (n = 11); obese, BMI $\geq$30.00 kg/m^2 (n = 7). Underweight women (BMI < 18.5 kg/m^2) were not detected in our study. The division of these BMI groups was carried out in accordance with World Health Organization (WHO) criteria.

For the comparison of zeb1 gene expression according to age, the women were separated into three groups: Group A, 20–34 years old (n = 23); Group B, 35–40 years old (n = 17); Group C, over 40 years old (n = 16). Female participants had an average age of 34.85 years (min = 20 years; max = 47 years) and median age of 37 years. We also performed a secondary analysis to investigate the effect of zeb1 expressed according to ovarian stimulation response; thus, we divided the cohort into normal responders and poor responders. According to the number of oocytes resulting from the ovarian response, women were separated in two groups: normal responders (n = 46) including women with more than 4 oocytes, and poor responders (n = 10) including women with less than 3 oocytes. Regarding oocyte maturation, the 56 women were separated in two groups: Group 1 with oocyte maturation 30–75% (n = 19), and Group 2 with oocyte maturation over 75% (n = 37). Cases with oocyte maturation less than 30% were not detected in this study. All groups (age, responders, and oocyte maturation) were divided according to Bologna and Poseidon criteria [18,19].

Exclusion criteria included female participants with any endometrial or endocrinological pathology and/or any medical history of endometriosis, hydrosalpinx, or autoimmune disorders.

2.2. Oocyte Retrieval, Denudation, and Maturity Evaluation

Pituitary suppression was achieved by daily injection of 0.25 mg gonadotrophin-releasing hormone (GnRH) antagonist (Orgalutran; Organon, Oss, Netherlands, Cetrotide; Merck, Merk KGaA, Darmstadt, Germany). Gonadotropin stimulation consisted of recombinant FSH (Gonal F, Merk KGaA, Darmstadt, Germany; or Puregon (MSD, Kenilworth, NJ, USA), alone or in combination with urinary gonadotropins (hMG) (Menopur, Ferring, Saint-Prex Switzerland). Ovarian response was monitored by transvaginal ultrasound measurements of follicular growth and of serum estradiol and progesterone levels every 1–3 days. FSH and hMG dosages were adjusted accordingly. The trigger for final oocyte maturation with 250 µg of human chorionic gonadotrophin (Ovitrelle, Merck Serono Europe Limited, London, UK) was administrated when the two leading follicles reached a diameter of ≥17 mm. The dosage of the HCG trigger was determined on a sliding scale based on the estradiol levels of the patient. Transvaginal oocyte retrieval was performed under conscious sedation 35–37 h after HCG administration. Following oocyte aspiration procedure, oocytes were incubated in pre-equilibrated culture medium dishes (Universal IVF Medium, Origio a/s, Malov, Denmark). For the determination of ZEB1 expression, cumulus cells were collected on the day of oocyte retrieval. More specifically, the cells were segregated from cumulus oocyte complexes (COCs) by applying the process of stripping using 40 IU/mL hyaluronidase (Cumulase) [20]. To enhance the enzymatic removal of the cumulus and corona cells, the oocytes were aspirated in and out of a calibrated pipette stripper with an approximate inner dimeter of 200 µm.

The oocyte maturation/nuclear maturity is morphologically computable, and it is validated by the extrusion of the first polar body [21]. After the removal of the cumulus/corona cells around the oocytes, these cells were kept in a deep freezer at −80 °C.

2.3. RNA Isolation and Reverse Transcription

Total RNA was extracted from granulosa cells using Monarch Total RNA Miniprep Kit (New England Biolabs Inc., Ipswich, MA, USA). Single-stranded complementary DNA (cDNA) was synthetized from 100 ng of total RNA as a template using LunaScript RT SuperMix Kit (New England Biolabs Inc.) and according to the manufacturer's protocol.

2.4. Quantitative Real-Time PCR (qRT-PCR) Analysis

The real-time quantitative PCR reaction was performed using a SYBR Luna Universal qPCR Master Mix kit (New England Biolabs Inc.) and the Light Cycler 480II (Roche Molecular Biochemicals, Mannheim Germany), according to the manufacturers protocol. The sequences of the qRT-PCR primer were as follows: zeb1 forward (5′-CAGCCCTGCAGTCCAAGAAC-3′), zeb1 reverse (5′-TTGTCTTTCATCCTGATTTCCATTT-3′), G6PD forward (5′-TGGACCTGACCTACGGCAACAGATA-3′), and G6PD reverse (5′-GCCCTCATACTGGAAACCC-3′). The qRT-PCR reaction was 30 s at 95 °C, 1 cycle, 5 s at 95 °C, and 30 s at 60 °C, 40 cycles. The $2^{-\Delta\Delta CT}$ method was used to calculate the relative transcript abundance. All qRT-PCR reactions were repeated twice.

2.5. Statistical Analysis

Data are presented as the mean ± standard error (SE). Comparisons of dCt between groups were performed using Student's F-test to ascertain if the variances were equal or unequal and then using a two-sample *t*-test assuming equal variances or unequal variances. Results were considered statistically significant when reaching $p < 0.05$ (5%) or tended to be statistically significant when reaching $p < 0.1$ (10%).

3. Results

3.1. Correlation of Zeb1 Expression Levels with BMI

Obese women with BMI ≥ 30.00 kg/m^2 seemed to have a higher dCt compared to the other two groups. Obese women demonstrated a higher expression level of zeb1 gene compared women with normal weight, BMI = 18.5–24.99 kg/m^2 ($p = 0.036$) and overweight women with statistically significant differences ($p = 0.055$). Women with normal weight and overweight women had no statistically significant difference in zeb1 expression levels ($p = 0.385$) (Table 1).

Table 1. Mean dCt of each BMI group and its correlation with zeb1 gene expression levels.

BMI Group	Mean dCt
Normal	1.147631579
Overweight	1.405454545
Obese	3.18
Compared Groups	***p*-Value (5%)**
Normal vs. obese	0.0364868
Overweight vs. obese women	0.0558143
Normal vs. overweight	0.3874018

3.2. Correlation of Zeb1 Expression Levels with Age

Women aged 35–40 years old had higher zeb1 expression levels in the granulosa cell samples following oocyte retrieval, compared to other age groups. Moreover, women over 40 years old had reduced expression levels of zeb1 gene compared to the other age groups (Table 2). Comparing two age groups, 35–40 years and >40 years, zeb1 gene was overexpressed in women aged 35–40 years old and under-expressed in women >40 years old, and this result was statistically significant ($p = 0.014 < 0.05$) (Table 2).

Table 2. Mean dCt of each age group and its correlation with zeb1 gene expression levels.

Age Group	Mean dCt
Group A (20–34 years)	1.44913043
Group B (35–40 years)	2.41411765
Group C (>40 years)	0.41625
Compared Groups	***p*-Value (5%)**
Group A—Group B	0.14036174
Group A—Group C	0.09724657
Group B—Group C	0.01430555

The difference in expression levels of zeb1 gene between women aged 20–34 years old and >40 years old tended to be statistically significant ($p = 0.097 < 0.1$). However, between women aged 20–34 years old and 35–40 years old, the difference in zeb1 gene expression levels was not statistically significant ($p = 0.14 > 0.05$) (Table 2).

3.3. Zeb1 Expression Levels in Granulosa Cells

The correlation of Zeb1 expression with the ovarian response was also studied. Women were divided into two groups: normal responders and poor responders. After the comparison of mean dCt of these two groups, we found no statistically significant difference in zeb1 expression levels between normal responders and poor responders ($p = 0.34$) (Table 3). We also investigated if there was a correlation between zeb1 gene expression levels in granulosa cells and oocyte maturation. As shown in Table 4, there was no significant difference in mean dCt when comparing Group 1 with Group 2 ($p = 0.263$); thus, zeb1 gene expression levels seemed not to affect oocyte maturation rate.

Table 3. Correlation of Zeb1 expression with oocyte number.

Groups Based on Oocyte Number	Mean dCt
Normal responders	1.515869565
Poor responders	1.15
Compared Groups	***p*-Value (5%)**
Normal responders vs. poor responders	0.3467274

Table 4. Correlation of Zeb1 expression with oocyte maturation.

Groups Based on Oocyte Maturation (%)	Mean dCt
Group 1 (30–75%)	1.13947368
Group 2 (>75%)	1.61297297
Compared Groups	***p*-Value (5%)**
Group 1 vs. Group 2	0.26379416

4. Discussion

Infertility is the state of a diminished capacity to conceive and bear offspring. It is estimated to affect 8–12% of couples of reproductive age [22]. Endometriosis is one of the main causes of female infertility and increases the risk of ovarian cancer in nearly 10% of women of reproductive age [14]. ZEB1 protein is expressed at high levels in the epithelial cells of endometriotic tissue, while it is not expressed in the normal endometrium, which makes the epithelial expression of ZEB1 a hallmark of endometriosis [15,16].

One of the main mechanisms involved in both cancer and endometriosis is the epithelial-to-mesenchymal transition (EMT) [9]. The main aspect of epithelial-to-mesenchymal transition (EMT) is the downregulation of E-cadherin, a protein that plays a major role in cell-to-cell adhesion. ZEB1 protein is the main regulator of the progress of EMT, from its initiation and tumorigenesis up to metastasis through direct or indirect inhibitory action on various downstream targets such as E-cadherin [4,9,11].

On the basis of the above conclusions, regarding the role of the transcription factor ZEB1 in EMT and the relation of its expression levels in women with endometriosis, which makes them infertile, we decided to study the expression levels of this specific protein in granulosa cells derived from infertile women undergoing IVF.

Regarding the relationship between age and infertility, it has been shown that fertility decreases with increasing age in both men and women. However, the risk of infertility has a strong correlation with maternal age. Accordingly, reproductive aging is a normal process of declining fertility [17]. Interestingly, we found that, in women aged 35–40 years, zeb1 gene had increased expression, while, in women over 40 years old, its expression levels decreased.

Furthermore, it has been proven that BMI and obesity have a strong association with infertility. Studies have also shown that, in obese women, the fertility rate decreases with a simultaneous increase in BMI, while obese women have a three times greater risk of infertility compared to non-obese women [23,24]. We demonstrated that zeb1 gene had increased expression levels in granulosa cells of obese women compared to overweight and normal-weight women.

Obesity also appears to affect oocyte quality by altering oocyte maturation and developmental capacity [23]. Our study also demonstrated that the expression of zeb1 gene could not directly affect the oocyte number and, therefore, the response of each woman to ovarian stimulation, nor did the maturation rate of the retrieved oocytes seem to correlate with zeb1 gene expression.

Zinc finger E-box binding homeobox 1 (ZEB1) promotes epithelial-to-mesenchymal transition (EMT) in carcinogenesis, but its role in embryo implantation has not yet been identified. The initial stage allowing the blastocyst to adhere to the endometrium during implantation is the migration of endometrial epithelial cells (EECs). During the mid-secretory phase of the menstrual cycle, ZEB1 was significantly expressed in the human endometrium at both mRNA and protein levels. ZEB1 knockdown prevented in vitro embryo implantation while altering EMT markers. ZEB1 may modify endometrial receptivity by promoting EMT, which may be essential for the embryo implantation process [25].

After parturition, menstruation, and, in certain cases, injury, the human uterine endometrium experiences considerable remodeling and regeneration on a regular basis. Successful human reproduction depends on the adult endometrium's capacity for cyclic regeneration, differentiation, and decidualization. The endometrium must undergo processes known as mesenchymal-to-epithelial transition (MET) and epithelial-to-mesenchymal transition (EMT) in order for its cells to switch between mesenchymal and epithelial phenotypes. MET/EMT processes have been extensively studied in the context of cancer and embryonic development, but growing evidence shows how crucial they are for giving the endometrium the phenotypic and functional flexibility required for successful decidualization, regeneration/re-epithelialization, and embryo implantation [26,27].

Endometrial stromal fibroblasts develop epithelioid phenotypes in response to estrogen, progesterone, and numerous other stimuli. The maternal luminal epithelium and the decidualized stromal cells acquire mesenchymal characteristics of increased migration/motility during embryo implantation in response to both maternal and embryonic-derived signals undergoing EMT in order to accommodate the invading trophoblast [27]. Regulation of the EMT/MET processes required in the maternal endometrium during implantation depends on communication between the maternal and embryonic compartments. Molecular signals from the mother's endometrium that have been linked to unsuccessful embryo implantation have also been demonstrated to control the EMT procedure. Most notably, microRNAs (miRNAs) have been found to play a role. Many aspects of embryo implantation have also been linked to miRNAs [28].

Additionally, compared to the peri-implantation interval, miR-30a-3p is considerably downregulated throughout the implantation period. Its expression depends on the status and presence of blastocysts in addition to endometrial decidualization. Furthermore, Snail2 expression appears to be reverse-regulated by miR-30a-3p. While downregulation accelerates embryo implantation by inducing EMT, upregulation of miR-30a-3p significantly decreases implantation sites both in vivo and in vitro. Thus, dysregulation of miR-30a-3p alters the ability of cells to migrate and invade by affecting EMT-related indicators, such as Zeb1 protein [29]. Therefore, miR-429, another miRNA, has an impact on embryo implantation. A gain of function for MiR-429 significantly decreases the number of implantation sites while having little effect on fertilization. MiR-429 suppresses migratory and invasive ability, as well as mesenchymal markers, which are indicators of miR-429's ability to decrease the EMT in vivo and in vitro. Therefore, miR-429 downregulation may help in embryo implantation by promoting EMT [30].

In conclusion, our study demonstrated that the expression levels of the transcription factor ZEB1 in granulosa cells are influenced by two factors. Firstly, BMI, mainly in obese women, plays an important role, as the zeb1 gene demonstrates a statistically significant higher expression level compared to women with normal weight and overweight women. In addition, the age of women affects zeb1 gene expression levels, with the main changes being found in women over 35 years old. It is proposed to further explore ZEB1 protein expression levels, as its expression in estrogen-responsive tissues and its correlation with BMI and age may unveil new potential findings of the zeb1 gene's role in female fertility and its use as a surrogate biomarker in fertility workups.

Author Contributions: Conceptualization, E.D. (Ekaterini Domali), P.D., and S.S.; methodology, I.C. and D.M.; validation, E.D. (Eirini Drakaki), A.P., and A.Z. (Athanasios Zachariou); formal analysis, I.C. and D.M.; writing—original draft preparation, I.C. and D.M.; writing—review and editing, A.P., E.D. (Eirini Drakaki), and A.Z. (Athanasios Zikopoulos); supervision, E.D. (Ekaterini Domali) and P.D.; project administration, S.S. All authors have read and agreed to the published version of the manuscript.

Funding: This research received no external funding.

Institutional Review Board Statement: The study was conducted in accordance with the Declaration of Helsinki and approved by the Institutional Review Board of the Medical School of the National and Kapodistrian University of Athens with protocol identifier 56353 and approval date 26 November 2020.

Informed Consent Statement: Informed consent was obtained from all subjects involved in the study.

Data Availability Statement: Not applicable.

Acknowledgments: The authors would like to acknowledge the contribution of all recruited patients in the present study.

Conflicts of Interest: The authors declare no conflict of interest.

References

1. Agarwal, A.; Farkouh, A.; Saleh, R.; Abdel-Meguid Hamoda, T.A.; Harraz, A.M.; Kavoussi, P.; Arafa, M.; Salvio, G.; Rambhatla, A.; Toprak, T.; et al. Controversy and Consensus on Indications for Sperm DNA Fragmentation Testing in Male Infertility: A Global Survey, Current Guidelines, and Expert Recommendations. *World J. Mens Health* **2023**, *41*, 575–602. [CrossRef] [PubMed]
2. Henkel, R.; Morris, A.; Vogiatzi, P.; Saleh, R.; Sallam, H.; Boitrelle, F.; Garrido, N.; Arafa, M.; Gul, M.; Rambhatla, A.; et al. Predictive value of seminal oxidation-reduction potential analysis for reproductive outcomes of ICSI. *Reprod. Biomed. Online* **2022**, *45*, 1007–1020. [CrossRef]
3. Carson, S.A.; Kallen, A.N. Diagnosis and Management of Infertility: A Review. *JAMA* **2021**, *326*, 65–76. [CrossRef] [PubMed]
4. Aigner, K.; Dampier, B.; Descovich, L.; Mikula, M.; Sultan, A.; Schreiber, M.; Mikulits, W.; Brabletz, T.; Strand, D.; Obrist, P.; et al. The transcription factor ZEB1 (deltaEF1) promotes tumour cell dedifferentiation by repressing master regulators of epithelial polarity. *Oncogene* **2007**, *26*, 6979–6988. [CrossRef] [PubMed]
5. Scott, C.L.; Omilusik, K.D. ZEBs: Novel Players in Immune Cell Development and Function. *Trends Immunol.* **2019**, *40*, 431–446. [CrossRef]
6. Llorens, M.C.; Lorenzatti, G.; Cavallo, N.L.; Vaglienti, M.V.; Perrone, A.P.; Carenbauer, A.L.; Darling, D.S.; Cabanillas, A.M. Phosphorylation Regulates Functions of ZEB1 Transcription Factor. *J. Cell. Physiol.* **2016**, *231*, 2205–2217. [CrossRef]
7. Zhang, Y.; Xu, L.; Li, A.; Han, X. The roles of ZEB1 in tumorigenic progression and epigenetic modifications. *Biomed. Pharmacother.* **2019**, *110*, 400–408. [CrossRef]
8. Dave, N.; Guaita-Esteruelas, S.; Gutarra, S.; Frias, A.; Beltran, M.; Peiro, S.; de Herreros, A.G. Functional cooperation between Snail1 and twist in the regulation of ZEB1 expression during epithelial to mesenchymal transition. *J. Biol. Chem.* **2011**, *286*, 12024–12032. [CrossRef]
9. Liu, Y.; El-Naggar, S.; Darling, D.S.; Higashi, Y.; Dean, D.C. Zeb1 links epithelial-mesenchymal transition and cellular senescence. *Development* **2008**, *135*, 579–588. [CrossRef]
10. Caramel, J.; Ligier, M.; Puisieux, A. Pleiotropic Roles for ZEB1 in Cancer. *Cancer Res.* **2018**, *78*, 30–35. [CrossRef]
11. Zhang, H.; Li, G.; Sheng, X.; Zhang, S. Upregulation of miR-33b promotes endometriosis via inhibition of Wnt/beta-catenin signaling and ZEB1 expression. *Mol. Med. Rep.* **2019**, *19*, 2144–2152. [CrossRef] [PubMed]
12. Zhang, P.; Sun, Y.; Ma, L. ZEB1: At the crossroads of epithelial-mesenchymal transition, metastasis and therapy resistance. *Cell Cycle* **2015**, *14*, 481–487. [CrossRef] [PubMed]
13. Madany, M.; Thomas, T.; Edwards, L.A. The Curious Case of ZEB1. *Discoveries* **2018**, *6*, e86. [CrossRef] [PubMed]
14. Xiao, Y.Y.; Lin, L.; Li, Y.H.; Jiang, H.P.; Zhu, L.T.; Deng, Y.R.; Lin, D.; Chen, W.; Zeng, C.Y.; Wang, L.J.; et al. ZEB1 promotes invasion and metastasis of endometrial cancer by interacting with HDGF and inducing its transcription. *Am. J. Cancer Res.* **2019**, *9*, 2314–2330.
15. Eggers, J.C.; Martino, V.; Reinbold, R.; Schafer, S.D.; Kiesel, L.; Starzinski-Powitz, A.; Schuring, A.N.; Kemper, B.; Greve, B.; Gotte, M. microRNA miR-200b affects proliferation, invasiveness and stemness of endometriotic cells by targeting ZEB1, ZEB2 and KLF4. *Reprod. Biomed. Online* **2016**, *32*, 434–445. [CrossRef] [PubMed]
16. Furuya, M.; Masuda, H.; Hara, K.; Uchida, H.; Sato, K.; Sato, S.; Asada, H.; Maruyama, T.; Yoshimura, Y.; Katabuchi, H.; et al. ZEB1 expression is a potential indicator of invasive endometriosis. *Acta Obs. Gynecol. Scand.* **2017**, *96*, 1128–1135. [CrossRef]
17. Crawford, N.M.; Steiner, A.Z. Age-related infertility. *Obs. Gynecol. Clin. N. Am.* **2015**, *42*, 15–25. [CrossRef]
18. Younis, J.S.; Ben-Ami, M.; Ben-Shlomo, I. The Bologna criteria for poor ovarian response: A contemporary critical appraisal. *J. Ovarian Res.* **2015**, *8*, 76. [CrossRef]

19. Roque, M.; Haahr, T.; Esteves, S.C.; Humaidan, P. The POSEIDON stratification—Moving from poor ovarian response to low prognosis. *JBRA Assist. Reprod.* **2021**, *25*, 282–292. [CrossRef]
20. Neri, Q.V.; Lee, B.; Rosenwaks, Z.; Machaca, K.; Palermo, G.D. Understanding fertilization through intracytoplasmic sperm injection (ICSI). *Cell Calcium* **2014**, *55*, 24–37. [CrossRef]
21. Grondahl, C. Oocyte maturation. Basic and clinical aspects of in vitro maturation (IVM) with special emphasis of the role of FF-MAS. *Dan. Med. Bull.* **2008**, *55*, 1–16.
22. Vander Borght, M.; Wyns, C. Fertility and infertility: Definition and epidemiology. *Clin. Biochem.* **2018**, *62*, 2–10. [CrossRef] [PubMed]
23. Bala, R.; Singh, V.; Rajender, S.; Singh, K. Environment, Lifestyle, and Female Infertility. *Reprod. Sci.* **2021**, *28*, 617–638. [CrossRef] [PubMed]
24. Imterat, M.; Agarwal, A.; Esteves, S.C.; Meyer, J.; Harlev, A. Impact of Body Mass Index on female fertility and ART outcomes. *Panminerva Med.* **2019**, *61*, 58–67. [CrossRef] [PubMed]
25. Ran, J.; Yang, H.H.; Huang, H.P.; Huang, H.L.; Xu, Z.; Zhang, W.; Wang, Z.X. ZEB1 modulates endometrial receptivity through epithelial-mesenchymal transition in endometrial epithelial cells in vitro. *Biochem. Biophys. Res. Commun.* **2020**, *525*, 699–705. [CrossRef]
26. Jena, S.K.; Das, S.; Chakraborty, S.; Ain, R. Molecular determinants of epithelial mesenchymal transition in mouse placenta and trophoblast stem cell. *Sci. Rep.* **2023**, *13*, 10978. [CrossRef]
27. Owusu-Akyaw, A.; Krishnamoorthy, K.; Goldsmith, L.T.; Morelli, S.S. The role of mesenchymal-epithelial transition in endometrial function. *Hum. Reprod. Update* **2019**, *25*, 114–133. [CrossRef]
28. Jimenez, P.T.; Mainigi, M.A.; Word, R.A.; Kraus, W.L.; Mendelson, C.R. miR-200 Regulates Endometrial Development During Early Pregnancy. *Mol. Endocrinol.* **2016**, *30*, 977–987. [CrossRef]
29. Li, L.; Gou, J.; Yi, T.; Li, Z. MicroRNA-30a-3p regulates epithelial-mesenchymal transition to affect embryo implantation by targeting Snai2dagger. *Biol. Reprod.* **2019**, *100*, 1171–1179. [CrossRef]
30. Li, Z.; Gou, J.; Jia, J.; Zhao, X. MicroRNA-429 functions as a regulator of epithelial-mesenchymal transition by targeting Pcdh8 during murine embryo implantation. *Hum. Reprod.* **2015**, *30*, 507–518. [CrossRef]

Journal of
Clinical Medicine

MDPI

Review

The Effect of Bisphenol and Its Cytotoxicity on Female Infertility and Pregnancy Outcomes: A Narrative Review

Eirini Drakaki [1], Sofoklis Stavros [2,†], Dimitra Dedousi [1,†], Anastasios Potiris [2,*], Despoina Mavrogianni [1], Athanasios Zikopoulos [2], Efthalia Moustakli [3], Charikleia Skentou [4], Nikolaos Thomakos [1], Alexandros Rodolakis [1], Peter Drakakis [2] and Ekaterini Domali [1]

1 First Department of Obstetrics and Gynecology, Alexandra Hospital, Medical School, National and Kapodistrian University of Athens, 115 28 Athens, Greece; eirinidrak@med.uoa.gr (E.D.); dimitradedousi@hotmail.com (D.D.); dmavrogianni@med.uoa.gr (D.M.); nthomakos@med.uoa.gr (N.T.); arodolak@med.uoa.gr (A.R.); kdomali@yahoo.fr (E.D.)

2 Third Department of Obstetrics and Gynecology, University General Hospital "ATTIKON", Medical School, National and Kapodistrian University of Athens, 124 62 Athens, Greece; sfstavrou@med.uoa.gr (S.S.); thanzik92@gmail.com (A.Z.); pdrakakis@med.uoa.gr (P.D.)

3 Laboratory of Medical Genetics, Faculty of Medicine, School of Health Sciences, University of Ioannina, 451 10 Ioannina, Greece; thaleia.moustakli@gmail.com

4 Department of Obstetrics and Gynecology, Medical School, University of Ioannina, 451 10 Ioannina, Greece; haraskentou@uoi.gr

* Correspondence: apotiris@med.uoa.gr; Tel.: +30-(210)-5832237

† These authors contributed equally to this work.

Abstract: Bisphenols, particularly bisphenol A (BPA), are among the most thoroughly investigated endocrine disrupting chemicals (EDCs). BPA was the first synthetic estrogen to be identified, exerting its estrogenic effects through interaction with human estrogen receptors (ERs). The aim of the present narrative review is to summarize the most recent literature regarding the adverse effects of bisphenols on female fertility and pregnancy outcomes. A review of the literature in the PubMed/Medline and Scopus databases was conducted in November 2024 and 15 studies were included in the present review. BPA levels were higher in women with diminished ovarian reserve, polycystic ovary syndrome, and recurrent miscarriages. Furthermore, one study showed a significant association between BPA levels and the onset of gestational diabetes mellitus. Higher levels of BPA are associated with disruptions to the female reproductive system, such as ovarian function, reduced number of antral follicles, and lower anti-Müllerian hormone (AMH) levels. Bisphenols A and S were associated with an increased risk of developing gestational diabetes mellitus. Bisphenols A and F were correlated with an increased risk of lower birth weight and bisphenol F seemed to be associated with an increased risk of preterm delivery. Ultimately, further research is necessary to fully understand the extent of the harmful effects that bisphenols have separately and as mixtures on the female reproductive system.

Keywords: bisphenols; bisphenol A (BPA); endocrine disrupting compounds (EDCs); female infertility; perinatal outcomes

1. Introduction

Infertility constitutes a major medical condition with profound personal and societal implications [1]. According to the latest definition by the American Society of Reproductive Medicine, infertility is a disease, condition, or status of the reproductive system characterized by the failure to achieve a pregnancy after regular and unprotected sexual intercourse or the need for medical intervention [2]. Globally, infertility is estimated to affect approximately 8 to 12% of couples of reproductive age [3]. The rate of fertility reduction has accelerated significantly over the past few decades [1]. Unfortunately, fertility is expected to continue to decrease in the near future.

Infertility is classified into primary and secondary infertility. Primary infertility refers to couples who have never succeeded in conceiving, whereas secondary infertility describes difficulties in conceiving after having previously achieved pregnancy, whether resulting in a live birth or miscarriage [4]. Secondary infertility is the most frequent type of female infertility and it is more prevalent in areas with high rates of unsafe abortions and inadequate maternal healthcare [3]. In developed countries, approximately one in seven women of reproductive age experience infertility, while, in developing countries, the rate is about one in four couples. Roughly half of all cases of infertility are attributed to female reproductive issues [5]. Female infertility could result from the advanced age of women at the time of conception, as well as from various medical conditions including premature ovarian failure, polycystic ovary syndrome (PCOS), endometriosis, uterine fibroids, or endometrial polyps [6,7]. Additional conditions that have the potential to impact female fertility include reproductive tract infections, lifestyle related factors, and various exposures to environmental chemicals [3]. Over the past few decades, there has been increasing interest in the impact of endocrine disruptors on the female reproductive system and pregnancy [8].

Endocrine disrupting chemicals (EDCs) are exogenous chemical substances that can interfere with normal endocrine functions. EDCs can disrupt hormonal balance by mimicking natural hormones such as estrogens and/or androgens, blocking their actions, or altering the concentrations of endogenous hormones within the body. In particular, EDCs can trigger tissue-specific estrogenic effects by acting as either agonists or antagonists of estrogen receptors (ERs), disrupting ERα-dependent transcriptional signaling pathways [9]. They may also interfere with ERα-mediated transcription by influencing interactions between ERs and other nuclear receptors, as well as through modulation of growth factors [9]. This disruption can lead to a variety of health issues such as reproductive and developmental disorders [8,10]. Thorough research has shown that EDCs can negatively impact distinct characteristics of female fertility, including the number of follicles, ovulation, meiosis, and uterine implantation of the embryo [3]. High levels of endocrine disruptors could be found in various sources including industrial chemicals, pesticides, plastic bottles, food packages, cosmetics, and even in some natural products [11]. Exposure to these chemicals can occur through ingestion of contaminated food, inhalation, or skin contact. Among the major endocrine disruptors are bisphenols, which have the potential to affect the progression of pregnancy and the development of the fetus [8,12].

Bisphenols (BPs), and especially bisphenol A (BPA), are widely used in the production of polycarbonate plastics and epoxy resins. Therefore, BPs are present as ingredients in various everyday products including food packaging, baby plastic bottles, dental materials, and the inner lining of food cans [13]. Consequently, the main route of exposure to BPs is through dietary intake [14]. BPA (2,2-bis (4-hydroxyphenyl) propane) is synthesized through a condensation reaction between phenol and acetone in the presence of an ion-exchange catalyst. BPA was the first synthetic estrogen to be identified, exerting its estrogenic effects through interaction with human estrogen receptors (ERs), particularly estrogen receptor alpha (ERα) [14]. BPA activates signaling pathways associated with estrogen receptors ER-α (alpha) and ER-β (beta), mimicking the activity of natural estrogen [9]. These estrogenic effects could cause cellular changes in estrogen-sensitive tissues, potentially leading to disruptions in normal hormonal functions and health issues, especially within the reproductive and endocrine systems. BPA can also cross the placenta and amniotic fluid, leading to its accumulation in fetal tissues. Exposure to this endocrine disruptor can potentially affect the development and health of the fetus [15,16]. It is worth noting that several studies have demonstrated that exposure to high levels of BPA, which can be detected in both serum and urine, is associated with disruptions to the female reproductive system, such as disruption of ovarian function, irregular menstrual cycles, reduced number of antral follicles, and lower anti-Müllerian hormone (AMH) levels. These factors could potentially contribute to infertility [13].

Due to its cytotoxicity and reproductive toxicity, BPA has been removed from many products and substituted by alternatives such as BPS (4,40-sulfonyldiphenol) and BPF

(4,40-dihydroxydiphenylmethane), which are considered to be less detrimental to the human body. BPS is produced by combining phenol with sulfur trioxide, while in the synthesis of BPF, formaldehyde acts as the solvent and a Brønsted acidic ionic liquid serves as the catalyst [17,18]. However, because of their structural resemblance to BPA, these analogues have a negative impact on the reproductive system by exerting estrogenic and antiandrogenic effects [13]. The present review aims to summarize the most recent literature regarding the negative effects of BPs on female fertility and pregnancy outcomes. The studies included in this review provide additional information regarding the most recent data that associate exposure to BPs with the occurrence of female infertility and adverse pregnancy outcomes.

2. Literature Research

A thorough literature investigation was performed in the Medline/Pubmed and Scopus databases in November 2024 with the aim of identifying relevant studies and articles regarding the negative impact of bisphenols on female fertility and pregnancy outcomes. The search query used included keywords like "Bisphenol*", "Bisphenol A", "BPA", "Bisphenol S", "Bisphenol F", "Endocrine Disrupting Chemicals", "EDCs", "Female infertility", "ovarian reserve", "polycystic ovary syndrome", "PCOS", "Pregnancy outcomes", "preterm birth", "birth weight", and "gestational diabetes mellitus". These search terms were either used as presented, separately, or in combination with the help of the Boolean administrators (OR, AND). Neither time limit nor other filters were applied in either database. The search was further refined by including studies that directly investigated the impact of bisphenol exposure. Additionally, the "snowball literature searching method" was applied to identify further relevant sources from the reference lists of selected articles. A formal risk of bias and quality assessment was not performed due to narrative nature of this review.

The inclusion criteria for the present review included studies that met the following criteria: (1) examined the cytotoxicity of bisphenols and their effects on female fertility and pregnancy outcomes; (2) were patient-control studies, cohort studies, and cross-sectional studies with adequate primary data (number of subjects per population and statistical for comparison p-value or q-value and/or foldchange). Similarly, the exclusion criteria included studies that (1) did not relate to bisphenols or their effects on female reproductive system, (2) did not provide adequate data (number of subjects per population and statistical for comparison p-value or q-value and/or foldchange) for extraction, and (3) were written in a language other than English.

3. Results

The present review includes fifteen studies. Regarding the effect of bisphenols in female infertility, two cross-sectional and two cohort studies assess the impact of BPA exposure on ovarian reserve, two case-control studies demonstrate the association between bisphenols and the occurrence of PCOS, and there is one cross-sectional study regarding the possible correlation between exposure to BPA and BPS and the occurrence of oxidative stress along with homeostatic imbalance. Regarding the impact of bisphenols on pregnancy outcomes, there are two case-control studies and one cohort study that examine the association between exposure to BPA and BPS during pregnancy and the occurrence of GDM; four cohort studies exploring the impact of bisphenols A, S, and F on birth weight; and one cohort study demonstrating the impact of BPF exposure on the risk of preterm delivery. These studies were published between 2020 and 2024. Table 1 summarizes the key clinical outcomes of each study included in this review.

Table 1. Studies included in this review.

Authors, Year	Study Design	Study Location	Sample	Sample Size	Mean Age	Ethnicity	Main Outcome
Studies investigating the effect of bisphenols on female fertility							
Park et al., 2021 [19]	Cross-sectional study	Ewha Womans University Mokdong Hospital in Seoul of Korea	Urine samples	307 women	36.8 ± 4.4 years	Korean women	BPA concentration was significantly elevated in the DOR group.
Czubacka et al., 2021 [20]	Cross-sectional study	Fertility clinic	Urine samples	511 women	33.30 ± 3.69 years	Polish women	Significant association between BPA levels and diminished ovarian reserve.
Zhang et al., 2023 [21]	Cohort study	Shenyang, China	Urine samples	111 women	32.0 (interquartile range 4.1)	Chinese population	- BPA and BPS were significantly associated with an increased risk of diminished ovarian reserve. - BPS concentrations were negatively associated with AMH (β = 0.287, 95% CI: 0.505–0.070, p = 0.010).
Zhang et al., 2024 [22]	Cohort study	Shenyang, China	Urine samples	111 women	32.0 (interquartile range 4.1)	Chinese population	Higher urinary concentrations of BPA, BPF, and BPS were associated with lower AFC (β = 0.016; 95% CI: 0.025, 0.006 in BPA; β = 0.017; 95% CI: 0.029, 0.004 in BPF; β = 0.128; 95% CI: 0.197, 0.060 in BPS).
Zhan et al., 2023 [23]	Case-control study	Shandong, Shanghai, and Zhejiang Provinces, China	Urine samples	733 women	29 years	Chinese women	Exposure to BPA and its analog is correlated with a significantly higher risk of developing PCOS.
Patel et al., 2024 [24]	Case-control study	Ahmedabad, India	Blood samples in early follicular phase	130 women (80 women in the PCOS group and 50 controls)	29.16 ± 4.15 in the PCOS group and 24.34 ± 5.11 in Control group	Indian population	BPA levels of the PCOS group were significantly higher compared to the controls (102.15 ± 0.1 ng/mL vs. 61.35 ± 50.13 ng/mL, p < 0.0001).
Liang et al., 2020 [25]	Cross-sectional study	Center for Reproductive Medicine of Shandong University	Urine samples	111 women	28 years	Chinese women	Association between exposure to bisphenol A and S and oxidative stress as well as immune system imbalance in women with unexplained recurrent spontaneous abortion (URSA).
Studies investigating the effect of bisphenols on pregnancy outcomes							
Soomro et al., 2024 [26]	Cohort study	Calgary or Edmonton, Alberta, Canada	Urine samples	420 women	50.71% were in the 30 to 34 age range and 113 26.90% were over the age of 35	Canadian women	Significant association between BPA and the onset of gestational diabetes mellitus (GDM).
Tang et al., 2023 [27]	Case-control Study	Guangxi, China	Serum samples collected during the first trimester	500 women (100 women with GDM and 400 matched controls)	30.62 ± 6.46 for the cases and 30.6 ± 6.41 for controls	Chinese population	Bisphenol S exposure in first trimester is statistically significantly associated with an increased risk of developing gestational diabetes mellitus.
Zhu et al., 2022 [28]	Case-control Study	United States, Pregnancy Environment and Lifestyle Study (PETALS) cohort	Urine samples collected during the first and second trimester	333 women (111 women with GDM and 222 matched controls)	31.2 ± 4.6	Asian/Pacific Islander 39.6%, Black 9%, Hispanic 33.3%, White 14.1% and Other 3.9%	- GDM case subjects had a higher detection frequency of BPA in the second trimester (79.6 vs. 66.7%) and higher cumulative levels of BPS across the two trimesters (145.7 vs. 103.9 ng/mL × day). - First trimester urinary BPS was associated with higher risk of developing GDM (aOR: 2.12, 95% CI 1.00–4.50).

Table 1. *Cont.*

Authors, Year	Study Design	Study Location	Sample	Sample Size	Mean Age	Ethnicity	Main Outcome
Trasande et al., 2024 [29]	Cohort study	United States, The NIH Environmental influences on Child Health Outcomes (ECHO) Program	Urine samples	3619 women	22.9% were less than 25 years old, 58.8% were between 25 and 34 years old, and 18.3% were more than 35 years old.	Non-Hispanic White (41.3%), Non-Hispanic Black (13.4%), Hispanic (34.5%) and Other (10.8%)	- Bisphenol S in third trimester was associated with Small for Gestational Age (OR 1.52, 95% CI 1.08, 2.13). - Bisphenol F in first and third trimester was significantly associated with Low Birth Weight.
Li et al., 2024 [30]	Cohort Study	Shenyang, China	Urine samples in the third trimester	113 women	56.6% were less than 30 years old and 43.4% were older than 30 years old	Han 84.1% and Other 15.9%	BPA and BPF exposure during pregnancy was significantly associated with lower birth weight (standardized regression coefficients (β = −0.081 kg, 95% CI: −0.134 to −0.027; β = −0.049 kg, 95% CI: −0.097 to −0.001)).
Hong et al., 2024 [31]	Cohort Study	Seoul, Republic of Korea	Maternal urine samples and cord blood samples	146 women	50.0% were less than 35 years old and 50.0% were older than 35 years old	Korean population	The asymmetric FGR group showed significantly higher maternal and fetal BPA levels compared to normal growth ($p < 0.05$ in both maternal urine and cord blood BPA).
Sol et al., 2021 [32]	Cohort Study	Rotterdam, The Netherlands	Maternal urine samples in all three trimesters	1379 women	30.5 (SD: 4.8)	European population	- First trimester bisphenol S was associated with larger fetal head circumference and fetal weight. - Bisphenol S and F in first trimester were also associated with a lower risk of being born at a small size for gestational age (OR = 0.56, 95% CI: 0.38–0.74 and OR = 0.55, 95% CI: 0.36–0.85, respectively).
Liang et al., 2021 [33]	Cohort Study	Guangxi, China	Maternal blood samples in first trimester	2023 women (113 in the preterm group and 1910 in term group)	28.2 ± 5.5 for the term group and 29.1 ± 5.9 for the preterm group	Chinese population	Bisphenol F (BPF) concentrations were positively associated with the risk of PTB (OR = 1.73, 95% CI: 1.18, 2.55).

BPA: Bisphenol A, BPF: Bisphenol F, BPS: Bisphenol S, DOR: diminished ovarian reserve, PCOS: polycystic ovarian syndrome, AMH: Anti-Müllerian Hormone, AFC: Antral Follicle Count, GDM: Gestational Diabetes Mellitus, PTB: Preterm Birth, FGR: Fetal Growth Restriction, SD: Standard Deviation, OR: Odds Ratio, aOR: adjusted Odds Ratio, CI: Confidence Interval.

The study conducted by Park et al., published in 2021 [19], aimed to assess the potential correlation between exposure to bisphenol A (BPA) among women and diminished ovarian reserve (DOR). In this cross-sectional study, 307 Korean women of reproductive age were included. Participants were classified into two groups, determined by anti-Müllerian hormone (AMH) percentiles corresponding to age-specific serum AMH concentrations. The DOR group consisted of 93 women with AMH levels lower than 25%, while the non-DOR group included 214 women who had serum AMH levels greater than 25%. Individuals had an average age of 36.8 ± 4.4 years, and their mean BMI was 22.4 ± 3.1 kg/m^2. The researchers further evaluated the mean BPA levels in both groups. In the DOR group, the mean concentration of urinary BPA ranged from 1.89 ± 2.17 μg/g, while, in the non-DOR group, the average BPA concentration was 1.58 ± 1.08 μg/g. Therefore, the average BPA concentration was observed to be significantly elevated in the group that included women with diminished ovarian reserve. Furthermore, the researchers detected that BPA levels were elevated while serum AMH concentrations adjusted for BMI decreased mainly in women aged 40 to 44 years. The results of the logistic regression analysis suggested a higher incidence of infertility among women with BPA levels at or above the 90th percentile, with the odds ratio (4.248) being statistically significant after accounting for factors such as age, first menstruation age, oral contraceptives, number of pregnancies, and waist measurement. Finally, no association was observed between participants' exposure to BPA and the occurrence of fibroids, endometriomas in the ovaries, or adenomyosis [19].

Another cross-sectional study, published in 2021 by Czubacka et al. [20], aimed to determine the effects of environmental exposure to BPA on ovarian reserve. A total of 511 women who visited a fertility clinic due to difficulties in conceiving were included in the study. Women with long-term conditions that could affect ovarian function such Fragile X syndrome or chromosomal abnormalities were excluded from the research. The main cause of infertility was attributed to male factors, with idiopathic infertility and female factors following. The mean age of the participants was 33.30 ± 3.69 years, while their average BMI was 23.18 ± 3.80 kg/m^2. Blood and urine samples were collected from all subjects. The researchers evaluated the ovarian reserve by determining the antral follicle count (AFC) as well as the levels of estradiol (E2), follicle-stimulating hormone (FSH), and anti-Müllerian hormone (AMH) between the second and fourth day of the menstrual cycle. BPA levels in urine were determined using gas chromatography ion-trap mass spectrometry. The study results revealed that BPA was present in 97% of the participants' urine samples with BPA levels recorded at 1.38 ± 2.34 ng/mL and SG-adjusted BPA levels at 1.60 ± 2.15 ng/mL. The levels of bisphenol A in urine showed a negative correlation with the levels of AMH ($p = 0.02$) and AFC ($p = 0.03$). However, the BPA urinary concentration did not correlate with other evaluated ovarian reserve factors such as FSH and E2 [20].

Similar results regarding the effect of bisphenols A, F, and S on ovarian reserve were presented in a cohort study from Shenyang, China. The authors showed that higher BPA (OR = 7.112, 95% CI: 1.247–40.588, $p = 0.027$) and BPS (OR = 6.851, 95% CI: 1.241, 37.818, $p = 0.027$) concentrations were significantly associated with a seven-fold higher risk of diminished ovarian reserve. Furthermore, the authors showed that there was a significant negative association between BPS levels and AMH ($p = 0.010$) [21]. The same results also applied also to the antral follicle count. The authors in another publication from the same study sample demonstrated that higher urinary concentrations of BPA, BPF, and BPS were significantly associated with lower AFC (β = 0.016; 95% CI: 0.025, 0.006 in BPA; β = 0.017; 95% CI: 0.029, 0.004 in BPF; β = 0.128; 95% CI: 0.197, 0.060 in BPS). Furthermore, a quantile increase in the bisphenols mixture was negatively associated with AFC [22].

In a 2023 study, the scientific team of Zhan et al. [23], aimed to determine the effects of BPs on female fertility focusing on their association with the occurrence of polycystic ovary syndrome (PCOS). A multi-center hospital-based case-control study was performed, including a total of 733 Chinese women. The participants were classified into two groups. The first group was defined as cases, consisting of 321 women who had been diagnosed with infertility due to PCOS according to the Rotterdam diagnostic criteria. The age of the cases ranged from 20 to 40 years (mean age 29 years). The control group included 412 women without reproductive disorders who had visited the same fertility clinics because of male infertility and underwent donor artificial insemination (AID). The mean body mass index (BMI) of the participants was 23.06 kg/m^2, while approximately 33% of these women were overweight or obese. The BMI of the cases was significantly higher compared to the control group ($p < 0.01$). Using liquid–liquid extraction paired with high-performance liquid chromatography–tandem mass spectrometry (HPLC-MS/MS), the concentrations of seven bisphenol variants were measured in urine samples. The examined bisphenol analogs were BPA, BPAF, BPAP, BPB, BPP, BPS, and BPZ. Additionally, the researchers analyzed the levels of FSH, LH, prolactin, estradiol, and testosterone in the serum from venous blood samples taken during the first three days of the menstrual cycle. The age of the women, their body mass index (BMI), alcohol intake, smoking, educational and occupational status, and the location of the study were identified as potential confounding factors in the relationship between the occurrence of polycystic ovary syndrome and exposure to bisphenols. The research team used odds ratios with a 95% confidence interval to demonstrate the association between bisphenol levels and the increased risk of developing PCOS. The analysis revealed that the urine samples of the cases exhibited statistically significant higher levels of the seven bisphenol analogs compared to those of the control group. Bisphenol A (BPA) presented the highest concentration with a measurement of 1.14 μg/g Cr. The researchers observed that there was a statistically significant relationship between the presence of the bisphenols BPA (aOR 1.09; 1.05–1.14), BPAF (aOR = 1.07; 1.02–1.13), BPS (aOR = 1.18; 1.10–1.25), and BPZ (aOR = 1.15; 1.08–1.22) in urine samples and the risk of developing polycystic ovary syndrome (PCOS). Quantile-based g computation (QGC) analysis was performed, revealing that exposure to a combination of seven bisphenol analogs was significantly linked to an increased risk of PCOS (aOR = 1.26; 1.12–1.45), largely attributed to BPS, BPZ, and BPAF. Hormonal analysis revealed that women with PCOS had significantly increased levels of LH and testosterone, but significantly decreased FSH and estradiol levels compared to the control group ($p < 0.01$). Furthermore, a significant positive correlation between BPA, BPF, BPS, and testosterone levels was demonstrated. Finally, women classified as overweight or obese exhibited a stronger link between bisphenol variants and PCOS compared to those who maintained a normal body weight. There was no significant relationship between the concentrations of bisphenol variants and the use of plastic household items [23].

A similar negative association between BPA and PCOS was presented in the case-control study by Patel et al. The authors demonstrated that the BPA levels in the peripheral blood sampling of the PCOS group were significantly higher than the controls (102.15 ± 0.1 ng/mL vs. 61.35 ± 50.13 ng/mL, $p < 0.0001$). Furthermore, a significant positive correlation between bisphenol A and luteinizing hormone (LH) levels (r = 0.23, $p = 0.03$) was observed [24].

The study by Liang et al., published in 2020 [25], sought to investigate the possible correlation between exposure to BPA and BPS and the occurrence of oxidative stress along with homeostatic imbalance, which represent factors linked to the occurrence of recurrent spontaneous miscarriage. A total of 111 women with a history of recurrent spontaneous abortion participated in this cross-sectional study. Women who experienced recurrent miscarriages due to other causes, such as active infections, chromosomal or anatomical anomalies, endocrine disorders, and autoimmune diseases, were excluded from the study. The mean age of the women who were included in the study was 28 years (range 26 to 31 years) with a BMI of 22.0 kg/m^2 (range 20.0 to 24.7 kg/m^2). Among them, 88.3% (98/111) had a regular menstrual cycle, while 25.2% (28/111) had previously given birth. The concentrations of BPA and BPS were determined in urine samples using ultra-performance liquid chromatography with tandem mass spectrometry (UPLC-MS/MS). The detection limits (LOD) were 0.1 ng/mL for BPA and 0.01 ng/mL for BPS, respectively. Furthermore, the concentrations of two major biomarkers of oxidative stress, 8-hydroxy-deoxyguanosine (8-OHdG) and 8-isoprostane, were identified in the specific urine samples. The serum levels of a range of cytokines which serve as biomarkers of immune homeostasis were also evaluated through ECL-ELISA. BPA was present in 99.1% of the urinary samples collected from the 111 women. On average, the concentrations of urinary BPA and creatinine-adjusted BPA were 0.95 ng/mL and 1.41 mg/g creatinine, respectively. 8-hydroxy-deoxyguanosine (8-OHdG) was detected in 100% of the urinary samples, while 8-isoprostane was present in 98.2%, with median concentrations of 0.02 mg/g creatinine for 8-OHdG and 1.49 mg/g creatine for 8-isoprostane. Levels of cytokines, both inflammatory and anti-inflammatory, were detectable in between 9.0% and 100% of the serum samples from all studied women. To evaluate the association between bisphenol exposure levels and biomarkers of oxidative stress and immune balance, multivariable linear regression models were utilized. BPA demonstrated a significant correlation with elevated concentrations of both 8-isoprostane and IFN-γ, while no statistical relationship was noted between BPA and 8-OHdG. Additionally, no significant association was observed between BPS concentrations and oxidative stress or immunology [25].

The cohort study by Soomro et al., published in 2024 [26], examined the association between exposure to bisphenol A and other endocrine disrupting chemicals (EDCs) in pregnant women during the second trimester and the occurrence of gestational diabetes mellitus (GDM). Among the 420 women involved in the research, 15 (3.57%) were diagnosed with diabetes during pregnancy. Regarding the participants' ages, 213 women (50.71%) were in the 30 to 34 age range and 113 (26.90%) were over the age of 35. A total of 223 women reported that they were experiencing their first pregnancy. Almost all women refrained from smoking during their pregnancy, while only 4.52% reported alcohol consumption. Urine samples were collected to determine the concentrations of bisphenol A and S. The participants' blood sugar levels were evaluated between the 24th and 28th weeks using the recommended screening for GDM. Childbearing history, maternal age, BMI, and the educational background of the pregnant women were considered as potential adjustment variables. The results of the study showed that bisphenol A (BPA) had a detection ratio of 92.3%, whereas bisphenol S (BPS) had a detection ratio of 58.6%. Moreover, the minimum detectable concentrations of BPA and BPS were found to be 0.32 μg/L and 0.10 μg/L, respectively. In models examining single exposures, multiple logistic regression analysis indicated a significant link between bisphenol A (BPA) and a greater risk of developing gestational diabetes mellitus (GDM) in both unadjusted (OR: 1.69, 95% CI: 1.03–2.78) and adjusted analyses (AOR: 1.70, 95% CI: 1.00–2.91). On the other hand, no association was found between bisphenol S and the occurrence of diabetes during the second trimester of pregnancy [26].

On the contrary, a cohort study from China examined the effect of bisphenol exposure during pregnancy and the development of GDM. In this study, 500 women were included (100 women with GDM and 400 matched controls) and bisphenol exposure was measured via blood sampling in the first trimester. The study results showed a statistically significant positive correlation between BPS exposure and the development of GDM, especially in medium- and high-exposure cases (for medium exposure: OR: 1.71, 95% CI: 0.99–2.96 and aOR: 1.77, 95% CI: 1.01–3.13; for high exposure: OR: 1.68, 95% CI: 0.96–2.94 and aOR: 1.68, 95% CI: 0.95–2.99). It should be noted that, in this study, BPA exposure was negatively correlated with GDM [27].

The negative effects of BPS exposure regarding the development of GDM were reported by another case-control study with a population from the United States. In this study, urine samples taken in the first and second trimester from 333 pregnant women (111 with GDM and 222 matched controls) were assessed. Study results showed that GDM cases had higher detection frequency of BPA in the second trimester (79.6 vs. 66.7%) and higher cumulative levels of BPS across the two trimesters (145.7 vs. 103.9 ng/mL × day) compared to the control group. Regarding the odds of developing GDM, the authors showed that first-trimester urinary BPS was associated with higher risk (aOR: 2.12, 95% CI 1.00–4.50) [28].

Regarding the effect of bisphenols on birth weight, a recent cohort study from the NIH Environmental influences on Child Health Outcomes (ECHO) Program included 3619 singleton pregnancies with at least one bisphenol measurement during pregnancy. The authors showed that bisphenol S exposure in the third trimester was associated with an increased risk of delivering a small for gestational age newborn (OR 1.52, 95% CI 1.08, 2.13). Furthermore, the study results revealed a significant association between bisphenol F exposure in first and third trimester and Low Birth Weight (less than 2500 g). Interestingly, this study showed no positive association between BPA exposure and birth weight, mainly due to the increased usage of replacement bisphenols F and S [29]. In a cohort study from China, both BPA and BPF exposure, measured in the third trimester, were significantly correlated with lower birth weight. BPS exposure showed no significant correlation [30].

Hong et al. [31], in their cohort study, showed that BPA levels in the fetal cord blood had a significant linear association with the head circumference to abdominal circumference ratio. Furthermore, in the same study the authors showed that maternal and fetal BPA levels were significantly higher in the fetal growth restricted group than in the normal birthweight group [31]. Lastly, Sol et al. [32], in a population-based cohort which was embedded in the Generation R Study, demonstrated that bisphenol S was associated with larger fetal head circumference and fetal weight. Furthermore, bisphenol S and F exposure in the first trimester were also associated with a lower risk of being born small for gestational age [32].

Finally, regarding the effect of BPF on preterm birth, Liang et al., in their study, showed that bisphenol F (BPF) was positively correlated with an increased risk of preterm birth (OR = 1.73, 95% CI: 1.18–2.55). Moreover, the authors showed that BPA concentrations were also associated with preterm birth, especially in the subgroup of female infants (OR = 1.30, 95% CI: 1.02–1.64) [33].

4. Discussion

In modern societies, the rapid development of industry has led to the daily exposure of individuals to several toxic chemical compounds that may adversely affect the endocrine system. Among these substances, bisphenols, and especially bisphenol A, are frequently used in plastic production and can be found in high concentrations in numerous consumer products, making them some of the most well-studied endocrine disrupting chemicals (EDCs). Lately, there has been increasing concern regarding the negative impact of bisphenols on female fertility. In the present review, we aim to summarize the most recent data regarding the effects of bisphenols on the female reproductive system and pregnancy outcomes.

The study conducted by Park et al. [19], revealed that the exposure of reproductive-age Korean women to BPA could have detrimental effects on ovarian reserve, leading to infertility. The scientific team demonstrated that the mean urinary BPA concentration was significantly elevated in the group that included women with diminished ovarian reserve (DOR group). These findings are in agreement with those of Zhou et al., which demonstrated that higher BPA levels in urine correlated with a decrease in antral follicle count (AFC) [34]. However, their findings were not statistically significant. It is important to note that bisphenols, particularly bisphenol A, exert a toxic effect on the ovaries by interfering with various pathways, such as those of oxidative stress, apoptosis, and folliculogenesis [35]. Furthermore, BPA has been associated with alterations in the structure of the fallopian tubes and uterus, along with disruptions in the expression of GnRH and kisspeptin which play a crucial role in the reproductive hormonal system [35,36]. The results of this research could be limited by the small sample size and the fact that bisphenol A has a brief half-life, while exposure to different endocrine disruptors occurs over a long period. However, it is worth mentioning that the study by Park et al. consisted of women who participated voluntarily and did not comprise patients from infertility clinics. Therefore, they could be seen as more representative of the general population.

The findings of the above study are also supported by Czubacka et al. [20], who presented the adverse effects of bisphenol A on ovarian reserve. The researchers evaluated the relationship between BPA exposure and four indicators of ovarian reserve, including AMH, AFC, E2, and FSH. A negative correlation was observed between AMH, AFC, and BPA levels, while no association was found between E2 and FSH with BPA concentrations. It is worth mentioning that anti-Müllerian hormone (AMH) and antral follicle count (AFC) are considered the most specific and reliable indicators of ovarian sufficiency [37]. The findings of Czubacka et al. [20] are consistent with the results of previous studies that attempted to determine the effects of BPA exposure on the ovarian reserve of reproductive-age women. Specifically, Souter et al., through a prospective cohort study that included women undergoing infertility treatment, observed a significant correlation between high BPA levels and a reduction in AFC [38]. Moreover, Cao et al. reached a similar deduction in their study demonstrating that, in the follicular fluid of women with diminished ovarian reserve, BPA concentrations were significantly increased, while the levels of AMH and E2 were decreased compared to healthy women [39]. Although the study by Czubacka et al. [20] involves a considerable number of participants, its findings might be limited and not generalizable in the broad population since it focuses on women experiencing infertility problems from a particular clinic. Finally, the study does not describe the mechanisms by which bisphenol A exerts its harmful effects on the ovarian reserve parameters.

The research conducted by Zhan et al. [23] indicates that exposure to bisphenol A (BPA) and its analogs, such as BPAF, BPAP, BPP, BPS, and BPZ, is correlated with a significantly higher risk of developing polycystic ovary syndrome (PCOS), especially among women who are overweight or obese. However, it should be mentioned that the BMI in the case group was significantly higher than the controls. These results are supported by the studies of Konieczna et al. and Jurewicz et al., which concluded that bisphenol A and bisphenol S levels are associated with increased odds of developing polycystic ovary syndrome, respectively [40,41]. Given its estrogenic activity, BPA may interact with various endocrine systems and metabolic pathways, while bisphenol analogs may exert similar effects on metabolic pathways, promoting insulin resistance and hyperinsulinemia through chronic inflammation, which in turn leads to increased secretion of GnRH and LH, as seen in PCOS [42]. Polycystic ovary syndrome (PCOS) is the most common endocrine disorder of women of reproductive age and its prevalence ranges between 5% and 21% globally [23]. According to the Rotterdam criteria, polycystic ovary syndrome (PCOS) could be diagnosed when at least two of the following three criteria are present: (1) clinical or biochemical hyperandrogenism, (2) irregular or absent ovulation, (3) presence of polycystic ovarian morphology observed via ultrasound imaging [43]. The researchers also noted a significant positive correlation between BPA, BPF, BPS, and testosterone levels. These findings are consistent with the results of the study conducted by Kandaraki et al., which demonstrated that women with PCOS exhibited significantly elevated BPA serum levels, which were also positively correlated with serum levels of testosterone and androstenedione [44]. The findings of Jurewicz et al. further support the association between higher bisphenol A concentrations and increased serum testosterone levels [40]. In vitro studies have shown that BPA and its analogs induce the production of androgens by the ovaries through disruptions to the activity of 17α-hydroxylase, leading to hyperandrogenism, which is a typical trait of PCOS [45,46].

According to Liang et al., exposure to bisphenols A and S may be associated with oxidative stress and immune system imbalance in women with unexplained recurrent spontaneous abortion (URSA). Based on the latest definition provided by the American Society for Reproductive Medicine and the European Society of Human Reproduction and Embryology, recurrent pregnancy loss is defined as the loss of two or more consecutive pregnancies before the 24th week of pregnancy [47,48]. Among the factors that have been implicated in the incidence of recurrent miscarriage, recent studies have focused on the potential impact of various chemical substances on the occurrence of this major reproductive health issue. The researchers observed that BPA levels were associated with increased levels of a biomarker of oxidative stress, 8-isoprostane. In the case of 8OHdG, no similar positive correlation was found. At the same time, the research team concluded that the increased concentrations of BPA were also related to the elevated levels of the pro-inflammatory cytokine IFN-γ. The study showed that BPA concentration in the urine samples of women experiencing unexplained recurrent abortion was 1.41 mg/g creatinine, which was higher than those in the control group. These results are consistent with the studies by Shen et al. and Peng et al., which support the higher levels of bisphenol A in women with URSA [49,50]. Although the mechanism by which exposure to bisphenols may lead to miscarriages has not been clarified yet, scientific evidence suggests that oxidative stress and immune imbalance are factors that could lead to various disorders in the female reproductive system. Specifically, BPA can activate estrogen receptors, leading to the production of reactive oxygen species (ROS) and several inflammatory cytokines, including IFN-γ [51]. The subsequent inflammatory responses mediated by these cytokines interfere with the normal development of the embryo and ultimately result in miscarriage [52]. According to the study, BPS levels in women with URSA were measured at 0.07 mg/g creatinine. Despite the lack of adequate evidence linking BPS exposure to an increased risk of miscarriage, further research is necessary to explore the potential role of BPS in miscarriage occurrence. The study showed that BPS, which is the main substitute for BPA, demonstrates a positive correlation with IL-10. IL-10 plays an important role in maintaining a normal pregnancy by suppressing the production of pro-inflammatory cytokines. However, elevated levels of IL-10 are associated with placental development disorders and consequently adverse pregnancy outcomes [53,54].

Another potential effect of bisphenols during pregnancy concerns their impact on the increased possibility of developing gestational diabetes mellitus (GDM). GDM, which is characterized by impaired glucose tolerance that occurs or is recognized for the first time during pregnancy, is one of the most frequent complications during pregnancy, with a growing prevalence observed worldwide. Gestational diabetes is linked to gynecological and neonatal complications resulting from elevated birth weight, as well as potential long-term health issues for both the mother and child, including type 2 diabetes and cardiovascular diseases [55]. Soomro et al. aimed to investigate the potential impact of bisphenols and other endocrine disrupting chemicals (EDCs) on the development of GDM. Their results revealed a significant correlation between BPA and the onset of diabetes during pregnancy [26]. These findings are consistent with the prospective study by Zhu et al., who observed a positive association between BPA levels and the development of GDM in early and mid-pregnancy [56]. In this study, a positive association was also found between BPS concentrations in the first trimester of pregnancy and the onset of diabetes [56]. In contrast to this finding, Soomro et al. [26] did not identify any association between bisphenol S and the occurrence of GDM. These differences may be attributed to variations in sample size or in the different levels of exposure to BPS. In addition, it should be noted that the limited number of women diagnosed with gestational diabetes (n = 15) in the present study could represent a limitation, as the researchers were unable to stratify the results by fetal gender. Finally, another limitation of the study by Soomro et al. could be the restriction of using a single urine or blood sample from each woman in the second trimester of pregnancy, which resulted in the inability to assess variability in bisphenol levels throughout the entire pregnancy, as well as to identify time points when the possibility of exposure of pregnant women to these endocrine disruptors could be greater and related to the onset of gestational diabetes. The same negative correlation between BPA exposure and GDM was reported by a case-control study with 301 pregnant women from the United States. In this case-control study, BPA was negatively associated with GDM (aOR: 0.61, 95% CI: 0.37–0.99). However, in this study the study sample was relatively small, and the two comparing groups were not matched [57].

The study conducted by Cantonwine et al., published in 2010 [58], suggested that women who delivered prematurely (<37 weeks) had higher concentrations of BPA in their urine samples compared to those who delivered after 37 weeks. However, the study has several limitations, including a small sample size, single urine collection, and the use of the participants' last menstrual period for determining gestational age [58]. A study by Ye et al., demonstrated that women who developed preeclampsia had significantly higher BPA levels in their serum samples between the 16th and 20th weeks of pregnancy. Preeclampsia is characterized by high blood pressure during pregnancy (systolic $\geq$ 140 mmHg and/or diastolic $\geq$ 90 mmHg) along with proteinuria (>300 mg/24 h) occurring after 20 weeks of gestation. However, additional research is necessary to further explore the link between BPA exposure and the development of preeclampsia [59].

Similar negative effects of bisphenol exposure have been also shown in analysis of the placenta of fetal growth restricted fetuses. Cao et al. showed that BPA levels and estrogen levels were significantly higher ($p < 0.001$) in the placenta of FGR fetuses compared to normal weight fetuses, pointing to the cytotoxic events induced by bisphenols [60].

Studies show conflicting results about the influence of BPA on steroidogenesis-related genes; Liu et al. [61], show that, in KGN cells, low concentrations of BPA induce increased expression of *FOXL2*, a transcription factor related to ovarian function. BPA is also associated with elevated aromatase expression and E2 production, according to Kwintkiewicz et al., [62] while Watanabe et al. [63] showed that higher concentrations of BPA (50 μM) downregulated *CYP19* gene transcription. Shi et al. [64] showed that exposure to BPA may induce a decrease in ferredoxin and ferredoxin reductase expression and consequently regulate progesterone synthesis. They also showed that exposure to BPA may also lead to the inhibition of the testosterone-related genes *HSD17B2* and *HSD17B3* and the E2 production-related gene *HSD17B* while simultaneously upregulating p450 oxidoreductase expression.

Additionally to hormone receptor binding, BPA may induce molecular changes in endocrine mechanisms by altering the epigenome [65]. Dolinoy et al. suggested that maternal exposure to BPA may influence offspring by altering their epigenome [66]. It is also known that, during embryonic development, the genome undergoes extensive epigenetic reprogramming. Zhang showed that DNA methylation of the imprinted genes *Igf2r*, *Peg3*, and *H19* showed a decrease of 12–30% in fetal mouse germ cells when they were treated with high doses of BPA [67], while Iqbal et al. found no changes in DNA methylation of germ cells following BPA in utero exposure [68]. Chao et al. tested the potential effects of BPA on DNA methylation during mouse oocyte growth and reported decreased DNA methylation at *Peg3* and *Igf2r* when oocytes were exposed to BPA [69].

Another organ related to disease risk in offspring is the placenta, as it acts as a barrier to maternal xenobiotics, hormones, and pathogens. Concentrations of 1–104.4 ng/gr were measured in the placenta tissue and male fetuses accumulated significantly higher levels of BPA compared to female fetuses [70]. BPA can directly influence the placenta, resulting in abnormal development of trophoblast cells. This disruption could impact hCG secretion from early trimester trophoblasts and increase cell apoptosis [71]. Consequently, if the placental function is impaired by EDCs, fetal development may be compromised. Kang et al. showed that in utero BPA exposure reduced the expression of *Rtl1* in the placenta [72], while Susiarjo et al. demonstrated that BPA exposure significantly reduced DNA methylation [73].

Although the results of the studies included in this review are consistent with findings from previous research, they could be limited by specific factors, including variations in the methods used to detect bisphenol levels, small sample sizes, and differences in the ethnic backgrounds of the participants. Additionally, the available literature on the effects of bisphenol analogues, such as BPS and BPF, on female fertility is limited, which could raise concerns about the reliability of the findings. Consequently, the effects of bisphenols on female fertility and pregnancy outcomes requires further study.

In the future, further research is required to investigate the effects of the substitutes of bisphenol A, such as bisphenols S and F, on female reproductive health, as they share structural similarities with BPA, which has been thoroughly studied for its toxic impact on the reproductive system. Additionally, greater emphasis should be placed on the molecular mechanisms through which BPA and bisphenol analogs exert their negative effects on the female reproductive system, affecting hormone functions, ovaries, or other procedures such as embryo implantation. Finally, future studies should also focus on the changes in lifestyle and nutrition that women of reproductive age or pregnant women could make in order to reduce their exposure to endocrine disrupting chemicals such as bisphenols.

5. Conclusions

Overall, the current research evidence presents a variety of effects of bisphenols, particularly bisphenol A, on female fertility and pregnancy outcomes. While the impact of BPA on both female infertility and pregnancy outcomes has been more extensively studied, the negative effects of other bisphenol analogues are debatable due to the limited number of studies. In the present review, we sought to provide the most recent evidence on the effects of analogues S and F on gestational diabetes, birth weight, and preterm birth. Nevertheless, further research is necessary to fully understand the extent of the harmful effects that bisphenols have separately and as mixtures on the female reproductive system.

Author Contributions: Conceptualization, E.D. (Eirini Drakaki) and S.S.; methodology, D.D. and A.P.; validation, D.M., A.Z. and E.M.; investigation, C.S.; data curation, N.T.; writing—original draft preparation, E.D. (Eirini Drakaki) and D.D.; writing—review and editing, S.S., A.P., D.M., A.Z., E.M., C.S., N.T., A.R., P.D. and E.D. (Ekaterini Domali); visualization, A.P.; supervision, N.T., A.R. and P.D.; project administration, E.D. (Ekaterini Domali). All authors have read and agreed to the published version of the manuscript.

Funding: This research received no external funding.

Institutional Review Board Statement: Not applicable.

Informed Consent Statement: Not applicable.

Data Availability Statement: No new data were created or analyzed in this study.

Conflicts of Interest: The authors declare no conflicts of interest.

References

1. Fertility, G.B.D.; Forecasting, C. Global fertility in 204 countries and territories, 1950–2021, with forecasts to 2100: A comprehensive demographic analysis for the Global Burden of Disease Study 2021. *Lancet* **2024**, *403*, 2057–2099. [CrossRef]
2. Chin, A.H.B.; Nguma, J.B.; Ahmad, M.F. The American Society for Reproductive Medicine's new and more inclusive definition of infertility may conflict with traditional and conservative religious-cultural values. *Fertil. Steril.* **2024**, *121*, 892. [CrossRef] [PubMed]
3. Vander Borght, M.; Wyns, C. Fertility and infertility: Definition and epidemiology. *Clin. Biochem.* **2018**, *62*, 2–10. [CrossRef] [PubMed]
4. Zegers-Hochschild, F.; Adamson, G.D.; Dyer, S.; Racowsky, C.; de Mouzon, J.; Sokol, R.; Rienzi, L.; Sunde, A.; Schmidt, L.; Cooke, I.D.; et al. The International Glossary on Infertility and Fertility Care, 2017. *Hum. Reprod.* **2017**, *32*, 1786–1801. [CrossRef] [PubMed]
5. Guerri, G.; Maniscalchi, T.; Barati, S.; Gerli, S.; Di Renzo, G.C.; Della Morte, C.; Marceddu, G.; Casadei, A.; Lagana, A.S.; Sturla, D.; et al. Non-syndromic monogenic female infertility. *Acta Biomed.* **2019**, *90*, 68–74. [CrossRef] [PubMed]
6. Potiris, A.; Perros, P.; Drakaki, E.; Mavrogianni, D.; Machairiotis, N.; Sfakianakis, A.; Karampitsakos, T.; Vrachnis, D.; Antonakopoulos, N.; Panagopoulos, P.; et al. Investigating the Association of Assisted Reproduction Techniques and Adverse Perinatal Outcomes. *J. Clin. Med.* **2024**, *13*, 328. [CrossRef]
7. Kyriakopoulos, K.; Domali, E.; Stavrou, S.; Rodolakis, A.; Loutradis, D.; Drakakis, P. Recurrent benign leiomyomas after total abdominal hysterectomy. Rich or poor estrogenic environment may lead to their recurrence? *Int. J. Surg. Case Rep.* **2018**, *44*, 191–193. [CrossRef]
8. Panagopoulos, P.; Mavrogianni, D.; Christodoulaki, C.; Drakaki, E.; Chrelias, G.; Panagiotopoulos, D.; Potiris, A.; Drakakis, P.; Stavros, S. Effects of endocrine disrupting compounds on female fertility. *Best Pract. Res. Clin. Obstet. Gynaecol.* **2023**, *88*, 102347. [CrossRef]
9. Lee, H.R.; Jeung, E.B.; Cho, M.H.; Kim, T.H.; Leung, P.C.; Choi, K.C. Molecular mechanism(s) of endocrine-disrupting chemicals and their potent oestrogenicity in diverse cells and tissues that express oestrogen receptors. *J. Cell. Mol. Med.* **2013**, *17*, 1–11. [CrossRef]
10. Land, K.L.; Miller, F.G.; Fugate, A.C.; Hannon, P.R. The effects of endocrine-disrupting chemicals on ovarian- and ovulation-related fertility outcomes. *Mol. Reprod. Dev.* **2022**, *89*, 608–631. [CrossRef]
11. Rolfo, A.; Nuzzo, A.M.; De Amicis, R.; Moretti, L.; Bertoli, S.; Leone, A. Fetal-Maternal Exposure to Endocrine Disruptors: Correlation with Diet Intake and Pregnancy Outcomes. *Nutrients* **2020**, *12*, 1744. [CrossRef] [PubMed]
12. Filardi, T.; Panimolle, F.; Lenzi, A.; Morano, S. Bisphenol A and Phthalates in Diet: An Emerging Link with Pregnancy Complications. *Nutrients* **2020**, *12*, 525. [CrossRef]
13. Srnovrsnik, T.; Virant-Klun, I.; Pinter, B. Polycystic Ovary Syndrome and Endocrine Disruptors (Bisphenols, Parabens, and Triclosan)—A Systematic Review. *Life* **2023**, *13*, 138. [CrossRef]
14. Mehlsen, A.; Hollund, L.; Boye, H.; Frederiksen, H.; Andersson, A.M.; Bruun, S.; Husby, S.; Jensen, T.K.; Timmermann, C.A.G. Pregnancy exposure to bisphenol A and duration of breastfeeding. *Environ. Res.* **2022**, *206*, 112471. [CrossRef]
15. Gorini, F.; Bustaffa, E.; Coi, A.; Iervasi, G.; Bianchi, F. Bisphenols as Environmental Triggers of Thyroid Dysfunction: Clues and Evidence. *Int. J. Environ. Res. Public Health* **2020**, *17*, 2654. [CrossRef]
16. Loukas, N.; Vrachnis, D.; Antonakopoulos, N.; Pergialiotis, V.; Mina, A.; Papoutsis, I.; Iavazzo, C.; Fotiou, A.; Stavros, S.; Valsamakis, G.; et al. Prenatal Exposure to Bisphenol A: Is There an Association between Bisphenol A in Second Trimester Amniotic Fluid and Fetal Growth? *Medicina* **2023**, *59*, 882. [CrossRef]
17. Wang, Q.; Wu, Z.M.; Li, Y.; Tan, Y.; Liu, N.; Liu, Y. The efficient hydroxyalkylation of phenol with formaldehyde to bisphenol F over a thermoregulated phase-separable reaction system containing a water-soluble Brønsted acidic ionic liquid. *RSC Adv.* **2014**, *4*, 33466–33473. [CrossRef]
18. Thoene, M.; Rytel, L.; Nowicka, N.; Wojtkiewicz, J. The state of bisphenol research in the lesser developed countries of the EU: A mini-review. *Toxicol. Res. Camb.* **2018**, *7*, 371–380. [CrossRef]
19. Park, S.Y.; Jeon, J.H.; Jeong, K.; Chung, H.W.; Lee, H.; Sung, Y.A.; Ye, S.; Ha, E.H. The Association of Ovarian Reserve with Exposure to Bisphenol A and Phthalate in Reproductive-aged Women. *J. Korean Med. Sci.* **2021**, *36*, e1. [CrossRef]
20. Czubacka, E.; Wielgomas, B.; Klimowska, A.; Radwan, M.; Radwan, P.; Karwacka, A.; Kaluzny, P.; Jurewicz, J. Urinary Bisphenol A Concentrations and Parameters of Ovarian Reserve among Women from a Fertility Clinic. *Int. J. Environ. Res. Public Health* **2021**, *18*, 8041. [CrossRef]

21. Zhang, N.; Zhao, Y.; Zhai, L.; Bai, Y.; Jia, L. Urinary bisphenol A and S are associated with diminished ovarian reserve in women from an infertility clinic in Northern China. *Ecotoxicol. Environ. Saf.* **2023**, *256*, 114867. [CrossRef]
22. Zhang, N.; Zhao, Y.; Zhai, L.; Bai, Y.; Wei, W.; Sun, Q.; Jia, L. Urinary concentrations of bisphenol A and its alternatives: Potential predictors of and associations with antral follicle count among women from an infertility clinic in Northern China. *Environ. Res.* **2024**, *249*, 118433. [CrossRef]
23. Zhan, W.; Tang, W.; Shen, X.; Xu, H.; Zhang, J. Exposure to bisphenol A and its analogs and polycystic ovarian syndrome in women of childbearing age: A multicenter case-control study. *Chemosphere* **2023**, *313*, 137463. [CrossRef]
24. Patel, J.; Chaudhary, H.; Panchal, S.; Parekh, B.; Joshi, R. Connecting Bisphenol A Exposure to PCOS: Findings from a Case-Control Investigation. *Reprod. Sci.* **2024**, *31*, 2273–2281. [CrossRef]
25. Liang, F.; Huo, X.; Wang, W.; Li, Y.; Zhang, J.; Feng, Y.; Wang, Y. Association of bisphenol A or bisphenol S exposure with oxidative stress and immune disturbance among unexplained recurrent spontaneous abortion women. *Chemosphere* **2020**, *257*, 127035. [CrossRef]
26. Soomro, M.H.; England-Mason, G.; Reardon, A.J.F.; Liu, J.; MacDonald, A.M.; Kinniburgh, D.W.; Martin, J.W.; Dewey, D.; APrON Study Team. Maternal exposure to bisphenols, phthalates, perfluoroalkyl acids, and trace elements and their associations with gestational diabetes mellitus in the APrON cohort. *Reprod. Toxicol.* **2024**, *127*, 108612. [CrossRef]
27. Tang, P.; Liang, J.; Liao, Q.; Huang, H.; Guo, X.; Lin, M.; Liu, B.; Wei, B.; Zeng, X.; Liu, S.; et al. Associations of bisphenol exposure with the risk of gestational diabetes mellitus: A nested case-control study in Guangxi, China. *Environ. Sci. Pollut. Res. Int.* **2023**, *30*, 25170–25180. [CrossRef]
28. Zhu, Y.; Hedderson, M.M.; Calafat, A.M.; Alexeeff, S.E.; Feng, J.; Quesenberry, C.P.; Ferrara, A. Urinary Phenols in Early to Midpregnancy and Risk of Gestational Diabetes Mellitus: A Longitudinal Study in a Multiracial Cohort. *Diabetes* **2022**, *71*, 2539–2551. [CrossRef]
29. Trasande, L.; Nelson, M.E.; Alshawabkeh, A.; Barrett, E.S.; Buckley, J.P.; Dabelea, D.; Dunlop, A.L.; Herbstman, J.B.; Meeker, J.D.; Naidu, M.; et al. Prenatal Phenol and Paraben Exposures and Adverse Birth Outcomes: A Prospective Analysis of U.S. Births. *Environ. Int.* **2024**, *183*, 108378. [CrossRef] [PubMed]
30. Li, X.; Chen, Q.; Wu, D.; Xiao, Z.; Shi, C.; Dong, Y.; Jia, L. High Levels of BPA and BPF Exposure during Pregnancy Are Associated with Lower Birth Weight in Shenyang in Northeast China. *Chem. Res. Toxicol.* **2024**, *37*, 1199–1209. [CrossRef] [PubMed]
31. Hong, S.; Kang, B.S.; Kim, O.; Won, S.; Kim, H.S.; Wie, J.H.; Shin, J.E.; Choi, S.K.; Jo, Y.S.; Kim, Y.H.; et al. The associations between maternal and fetal exposure to endocrine-disrupting chemicals and asymmetric fetal growth restriction: A prospective cohort study. *Front. Public Health* **2024**, *12*, 1351786. [CrossRef] [PubMed]
32. Sol, C.M.; van Zwol-Janssens, C.; Philips, E.M.; Asimakopoulos, A.G.; Martinez-Moral, M.P.; Kannan, K.; Jaddoe, V.W.V.; Trasande, L.; Santos, S. Maternal bisphenol urine concentrations, fetal growth and adverse birth outcomes: A population-based prospective cohort. *Environ. Health* **2021**, *20*, 60. [CrossRef]
33. Liang, J.; Yang, C.; Liu, T.; Tan, H.J.J.; Sheng, Y.; Wei, L.; Tang, P.; Huang, H.; Zeng, X.; Liu, S.; et al. Prenatal exposure to bisphenols and risk of preterm birth: Findings from Guangxi Zhuang birth cohort in China. *Ecotoxicol. Environ. Saf.* **2021**, *228*, 112960. [CrossRef]
34. Zhou, W.; Fang, F.; Zhu, W.; Chen, Z.J.; Du, Y.; Zhang, J. Bisphenol A and Ovarian Reserve among Infertile Women with Polycystic Ovarian Syndrome. *Int. J. Environ. Res. Public Health* **2016**, *14*, 18. [CrossRef]
35. Ziv-Gal, A.; Flaws, J.A. Evidence for bisphenol A—Induced female infertility: A review (2007–2016). *Fertil. Steril.* **2016**, *106*, 827–856. [CrossRef]
36. Hung, P.H.; Van Winkle, L.S.; Williams, C.J.; Hunt, P.A.; VandeVoort, C.A. Prenatal Bisphenol A Exposure Alters Epithelial Cell Composition in the Rhesus Macaque Fetal Oviduct. *Toxicol. Sci.* **2019**, *167*, 450–457. [CrossRef]
37. Practice Committee of the American Society for Reproductive Medicine. Testing and interpreting measures of ovarian reserve: A committee opinion. *Fertil. Steril.* **2020**, *114*, 1151–1157. [CrossRef]
38. Souter, I.; Smith, K.W.; Dimitriadis, I.; Ehrlich, S.; Williams, P.L.; Calafat, A.M.; Hauser, R. The association of bisphenol-A urinary concentrations with antral follicle counts and other measures of ovarian reserve in women undergoing infertility treatments. *Reprod. Toxicol.* **2013**, *42*, 224–231. [CrossRef]
39. Cao, Y.; Qu, X.; Ming, Z.; Yao, Y.; Zhang, Y. The correlation between exposure to BPA and the decrease of the ovarian reserve. *Int. J. Clin. Exp. Pathol.* **2018**, *11*, 3375–3382. [PubMed]
40. Jurewicz, J.; Majewska, J.; Berg, A.; Owczarek, K.; Zajdel, R.; Kaleta, D.; Wasik, A.; Rachon, D. Serum bisphenol A analogues in women diagnosed with the polycystic ovary syndrome—Is there an association? *Environ. Pollut.* **2021**, *272*, 115962. [CrossRef] [PubMed]
41. Konieczna, A.; Rachon, D.; Owczarek, K.; Kubica, P.; Kowalewska, A.; Kudlak, B.; Wasik, A.; Namiesnik, J. Serum bisphenol A concentrations correlate with serum testosterone levels in women with polycystic ovary syndrome. *Reprod. Toxicol.* **2018**, *82*, 32–37. [CrossRef] [PubMed]
42. Lewandowski, K.C.; Cajdler-Luba, A.; Salata, I.; Bienkiewicz, M.; Lewinski, A. The utility of the gonadotrophin releasing hormone (GnRH) test in the diagnosis of polycystic ovary syndrome (PCOS). *Endokrynol. Pol.* **2011**, *62*, 120–128. [PubMed]
43. Christ, J.P.; Cedars, M.I. Current Guidelines for Diagnosing PCOS. *Diagnostics* **2023**, *13*, 1113. [CrossRef] [PubMed]
44. Kandaraki, E.; Christakou, C.; Diamanti-Kandarakis, E. Metabolic syndrome and polycystic ovary syndrome... and vice versa. *Arq. Bras. Endocrinol. Metabol.* **2009**, *53*, 227–237. [CrossRef] [PubMed]

45. Ashraf, S.; Rasool, S.U.A.; Nabi, M.; Ganie, M.A.; Jabeen, F.; Rashid, F.; Amin, S. CYP17 gene polymorphic sequence variation is associated with hyperandrogenism in Kashmiri women with polycystic ovarian syndrome. *Gynecol. Endocrinol.* **2021**, *37*, 230–234. [CrossRef]
46. Ye, L.; Zhao, B.; Hu, G.; Chu, Y.; Ge, R.S. Inhibition of human and rat testicular steroidogenic enzyme activities by bisphenol A. *Toxicol. Lett.* **2011**, *207*, 137–142. [CrossRef]
47. ESHRE Guideline Group on RPL; Bender Atik, R.; Christiansen, O.B.; Elson, J.; Kolte, A.M.; Lewis, S.; Middeldorp, S.; McHeik, S.; Peramo, B.; Quenby, S.; et al. ESHRE guideline: Recurrent pregnancy loss: An update in 2022. *Hum. Reprod. Open* **2023**, *2023*, hoad002. [CrossRef]
48. Practice Committee of the American Society for Reproductive Medicine. Definitions of infertility and recurrent pregnancy loss: A committee opinion. *Fertil. Steril.* **2020**, *113*, 533–535. [CrossRef]
49. Peng, F.; Ji, W.; Zhu, F.; Peng, D.; Yang, M.; Liu, R.; Pu, Y.; Yin, L. A study on phthalate metabolites, bisphenol A and nonylphenol in the urine of Chinese women with unexplained recurrent spontaneous abortion. *Environ. Res.* **2016**, *150*, 622–628. [CrossRef]
50. Shen, Y.; Zheng, Y.; Jiang, J.; Liu, Y.; Luo, X.; Shen, Z.; Chen, X.; Wang, Y.; Dai, Y.; Zhao, J.; et al. Higher urinary bisphenol A concentration is associated with unexplained recurrent miscarriage risk: Evidence from a case-control study in eastern China. *PLoS ONE* **2015**, *10*, e0127886. [CrossRef]
51. Panchanathan, R.; Liu, H.; Leung, Y.K.; Ho, S.M.; Choubey, D. Bisphenol A (BPA) stimulates the interferon signaling and activates the inflammasome activity in myeloid cells. *Mol. Cell. Endocrinol.* **2015**, *415*, 45–55. [CrossRef]
52. Ren, H.; Li, Y.; Jiang, H.; Du, M. Porphyromonas gingivalis induces IL-8 and IFN-gamma secretion and apoptosis in human extravillous trophoblast derived HTR8/SVneo cells via activation of ERK1/2 and p38 signaling pathways. *Placenta* **2016**, *45*, 8–15. [CrossRef]
53. White, C.A.; Johansson, M.; Roberts, C.T.; Ramsay, A.J.; Robertson, S.A. Effect of interleukin-10 null mutation on maternal immune response and reproductive outcome in mice. *Biol. Reprod.* **2004**, *70*, 123–131. [CrossRef]
54. Stavros, S.; Panagopoulos, P.; Machairiotis, N.; Potiris, A.; Mavrogianni, D.; Sfakianakis, A.; Drakaki, E.; Christodoulaki, C.; Panagiotopoulos, D.; Sioutis, D.; et al. Association between cytokine polymorphisms and recurrent pregnancy loss: A review of current evidence. *Int. J. Gynaecol. Obstet.* **2024**, *167*, 45–57. [CrossRef]
55. Sweeting, A.; Wong, J.; Murphy, H.R.; Ross, G.P. A Clinical Update on Gestational Diabetes Mellitus. *Endocr. Rev.* **2022**, *43*, 763–793. [CrossRef]
56. Zhu, Y.; Zhang, C. Prevalence of Gestational Diabetes and Risk of Progression to Type 2 Diabetes: A Global Perspective. *Curr. Diabetes Rep.* **2016**, *16*, 7. [CrossRef]
57. Chen, W.J.; Robledo, C.; Davis, E.M.; Goodman, J.R.; Xu, C.; Hwang, J.; Janitz, A.E.; Garwe, T.; Calafat, A.M.; Peck, J.D. Assessing urinary phenol and paraben mixtures in pregnant women with and without gestational diabetes mellitus: A case-control study. *Environ. Res.* **2022**, *214*, 113897. [CrossRef]
58. Cantonwine, D.; Meeker, J.D.; Hu, H.; Sanchez, B.N.; Lamadrid-Figueroa, H.; Mercado-Garcia, A.; Fortenberry, G.Z.; Calafat, A.M.; Tellez-Rojo, M.M. Bisphenol a exposure in Mexico City and risk of prematurity: A pilot nested case control study. *Environ. Health* **2010**, *9*, 62. [CrossRef] [PubMed]
59. Ye, Y.; Zhou, Q.; Feng, L.; Wu, J.; Xiong, Y.; Li, X. Maternal serum bisphenol A levels and risk of pre-eclampsia: A nested case-control study. *Eur. J. Public Health* **2017**, *27*, 1102–1107. [CrossRef] [PubMed]
60. Cao, Y.; Chen, Z.; Zhang, M.; Shi, L.; Qin, S.; Lv, D.; Li, D.; Ma, L.; Zhang, Y. Maternal exposure to bisphenol A induces fetal growth restriction via upregulating the expression of estrogen receptors. *Chemosphere* **2022**, *287*, 132244. [CrossRef] [PubMed]
61. Liu, H.; Jin, H.; Kim, G.; Bae, J. A low dose of bisphenol A stimulates estradiol production by regulating beta-catenin-FOXL2-CYP19A1 pathway in human ovarian granulosa cells. *Biochem. Biophys. Res. Commun.* **2021**, *583*, 192–198. [CrossRef]
62. Kwintkiewicz, J.; Nishi, Y.; Yanase, T.; Giudice, L.C. Peroxisome proliferator-activated receptor-gamma mediates bisphenol A inhibition of FSH-stimulated IGF-1, aromatase, and estradiol in human granulosa cells. *Environ. Health Perspect.* **2010**, *118*, 400–406. [CrossRef]
63. Watanabe, M.; Ohno, S.; Nakajin, S. Effects of bisphenol A on the expression of cytochrome P450 aromatase (CYP19) in human fetal osteoblastic and granulosa cell-like cell lines. *Toxicol. Lett.* **2012**, *210*, 95–99. [CrossRef]
64. Shi, J.; Liu, C.; Chen, M.; Yan, J.; Wang, C.; Zuo, Z.; He, C. The interference effects of bisphenol A on the synthesis of steroid hormones in human ovarian granulosa cells. *Environ. Toxicol.* **2021**, *36*, 665–674. [CrossRef]
65. Bernal, A.J.; Jirtle, R.L. Epigenomic disruption: The effects of early developmental exposures. *Birth Defects Res. A Clin. Mol. Teratol.* **2010**, *88*, 938–944. [CrossRef]
66. Dolinoy, D.C. The agouti mouse model: An epigenetic biosensor for nutritional and environmental alterations on the fetal epigenome. *Nutr. Rev.* **2008**, *66* (Suppl. S1), S7–S11. [CrossRef]
67. Zhang, X.F.; Zhang, L.J.; Feng, Y.N.; Chen, B.; Feng, Y.M.; Liang, G.J.; Li, L.; Shen, W. Bisphenol A exposure modifies DNA methylation of imprint genes in mouse fetal germ cells. *Mol. Biol. Rep.* **2012**, *39*, 8621–8628. [CrossRef]
68. Iqbal, K.; Tran, D.A.; Li, A.X.; Warden, C.; Bai, A.Y.; Singh, P.; Wu, X.; Pfeifer, G.P.; Szabo, P.E. Deleterious effects of endocrine disruptors are corrected in the mammalian germline by epigenome reprogramming. *Genome Biol.* **2015**, *16*, 59. [CrossRef]
69. Chao, H.H.; Zhang, X.F.; Chen, B.; Pan, B.; Zhang, L.J.; Li, L.; Sun, X.F.; Shi, Q.H.; Shen, W. Bisphenol A exposure modifies methylation of imprinted genes in mouse oocytes via the estrogen receptor signaling pathway. *Histochem. Cell Biol.* **2012**, *137*, 249–259. [CrossRef]

70. Jalal, N.; Surendranath, A.R.; Pathak, J.L.; Yu, S.; Chung, C.Y. Bisphenol A (BPA) the mighty and the mutagenic. *Toxicol. Rep.* **2018**, *5*, 76–84. [CrossRef]
71. Tang, Z.R.; Xu, X.L.; Deng, S.L.; Lian, Z.X.; Yu, K. Oestrogenic Endocrine Disruptors in the Placenta and the Fetus. *Int. J. Mol. Sci.* **2020**, *21*, 1519. [CrossRef] [PubMed]
72. Kang, E.R.; Iqbal, K.; Tran, D.A.; Rivas, G.E.; Singh, P.; Pfeifer, G.P.; Szabo, P.E. Effects of endocrine disruptors on imprinted gene expression in the mouse embryo. *Epigenetics* **2011**, *6*, 937–950. [CrossRef] [PubMed]
73. Susiarjo, M.; Sasson, I.; Mesaros, C.; Bartolomei, M.S. Bisphenol a exposure disrupts genomic imprinting in the mouse. *PLoS Genet.* **2013**, *9*, e1003401. [CrossRef] [PubMed]

Journal of
Clinical Medicine

MDPI

Review

Proteomics and Metabolomics in Varicocele-Associated Male Infertility: Advancing Precision Diagnostics and Therapy

Aris Kaltsas [1], Athanasios Zikopoulos [2], Eleftheria Markou [3], Athanasios Zachariou [4], Marios Stavropoulos [1], Zisis Kratiras [1], Evangelos N. Symeonidis [5], Fotios Dimitriadis [6], Nikolaos Sofikitis [4] and Michael Chrisofos [1,*]

1 Third Department of Urology, Attikon University Hospital, School of Medicine, National and Kapodistrian University of Athens, 12462 Athens, Greece; ares-kaltsas@hotmail.com (A.K.); stamarios@yahoo.gr (M.S.); zkratiras@gmail.com (Z.K.)
2 Department of Obstetrics and Gynecology, Royal Cornwall Hospital, Truro TR1 3LJ, UK; athanasios.zikopoulos1@nhs.net
3 Department of Microbiology, University Hospital of Ioannina, 45500 Ioannina, Greece; eleftheria.markou4@gmail.com
4 Laboratory of Spermatology, Department of Urology, Faculty of Medicine, School of Health Sciences, University of Ioannina, 45110 Ioannina, Greece; azachariou@uoi.gr (A.Z.); nsofikit@uoi.gr (N.S.)
5 Department of Urology II, European Interbalkan Medical Center, 55535 Thessaloniki, Greece; evansimeonidis@gmail.com
6 Department of Urology, Faculty of Medicine, School of Health Sciences, Aristotle University of Thessaloniki, 54124 Thessaloniki, Greece; helabio@yahoo.gr
* Correspondence: mxchris@yahoo.com

Abstract: Background/Objectives: Varicoceles are a common contributor to male infertility, significantly impacting male-factor infertility cases. Traditional diagnostic methods often lack the sensitivity to detect the molecular and cellular disruptions caused by varicoceles, limiting the development of effective, personalized treatments. This narrative review aims to explore the advancements in proteomics and metabolomics as innovative, non-invasive diagnostic tools for varicocele-associated male infertility and their potential in guiding personalized therapeutic strategies. **Methods:** A comprehensive literature search was conducted using databases such as PubMed, Scopus, and Web of Science up to October 2024. Studies focusing on the application of proteomic and metabolomic analyses in varicocele-associated male infertility were selected. The findings were critically analyzed to synthesize current knowledge and identify future research directions. **Results:** Proteomic analyses revealed differentially expressed proteins in the sperm and seminal plasma of varicocele patients, revealing disruptions in pathways related to oxidative stress, mitochondrial dysfunction, apoptosis, and energy metabolism. Key proteins such as heat shock proteins, mitochondrial enzymes, and apoptotic regulators were notably altered. Metabolomic profiling uncovered specific metabolites in seminal plasma—such as decreased levels of lysine, valine, and fructose—that correlate with impaired sperm function and fertility potential. The integration of proteomic and metabolomic data provides a comprehensive molecular fingerprint of varicocele-induced infertility, facilitating the identification of novel biomarkers for early diagnosis and the development of personalized therapeutic interventions. **Conclusions:** Advances in proteomics and metabolomics have significantly enhanced our understanding of the molecular mechanisms underlying varicocele-associated male infertility. These "omics" technologies hold great promise for improving diagnostic accuracy and personalizing treatment, ultimately leading to better outcomes for affected men. Future large-scale clinical trials and validations are essential to confirm these biomarkers and facilitate their integration into routine clinical practice.

Keywords: varicocele; male infertility; proteomics; metabolomics; biomarkers; seminal plasma; spermatozoa; oxidative stress; personalized medicine; diagnostic tools

1. Introduction

Varicoceles, characterized by the abnormal enlargement of the pampiniform plexus veins within the spermatic cord, are among the most prevalent causes of male infertility [1]. Affecting approximately 15% of men globally and contributing to up to 40% of male-factor infertility cases, varicocele formation disrupts the delicate testicular environment [2,3]. Physiological challenges such as elevated scrotal temperatures, increased oxidative stress, and hormonal imbalances collectively impair spermatogenesis [4,5]. Consequently, key sperm parameters including concentration, motility, and morphology are adversely affected, significantly diminishing male fertility potential [6,7]. As illustrated in Figure 1, a varicocele involves complex anatomical abnormalities and molecular disruptions that complicate diagnosis and treatment.

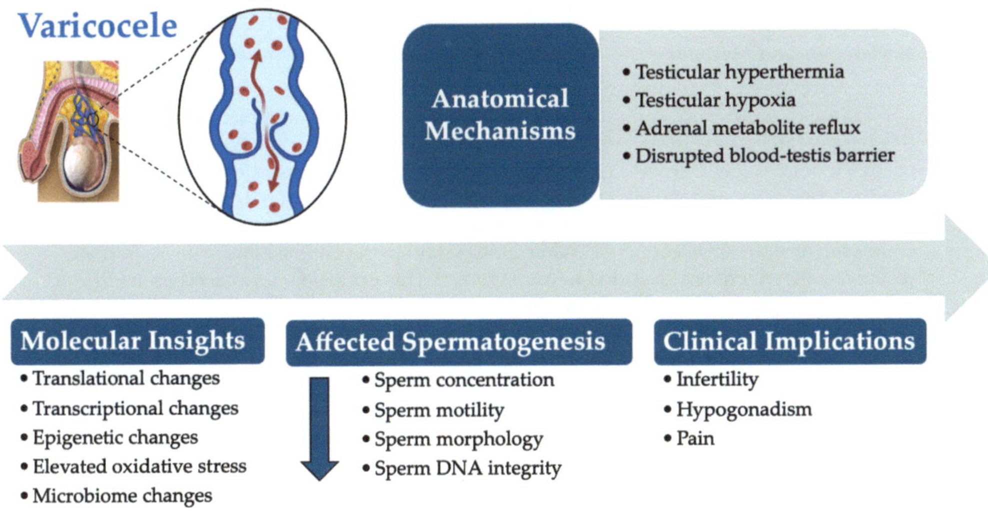

Figure 1. Anatomical, molecular, and diagnostic features associated with varicoceles.

Current clinical diagnostic methods, such as semen analysis and DNA fragmentation tests, provide general insights into sperm health by assessing parameters like sperm count, motility, and morphology. However, these methods lack the sensitivity to detect the subcellular and molecular disruptions induced by varicoceles [8]. While advanced tests for reactive oxygen species (ROS) levels, total antioxidant capacity, and DNA fragmentation offer additional information on oxidative stress and genomic integrity, they still do not capture the full spectrum of biochemical and molecular changes induced by varicoceles [9,10]. Important molecular alterations—such as mitochondrial dysfunction, apoptosis, and post-translational modifications—often remain undetected [11].

To address these limitations, the integration of "omics" technologies—specifically proteomics and metabolomics—offers a promising solution. Proteomics involves the large-scale analysis of proteins, which are crucial for executing cellular functions, while metabolomics examines small molecules or metabolites that represent the final products of cellular processes. By mapping molecular changes at the protein and metabolite levels, these approaches provide a molecular-level perspective on cellular health and function [12,13]. In the context of varicoceles, proteomics can reveal changes in protein expression and post-translational modifications in sperm and seminal plasma, whereas metabolomics offers real-time insights into the physiological state of the reproductive system by analyzing metabolites in seminal plasma. Together, these methods enable the identification of novel biomarkers for more sensitive and personalized diagnostic and therapeutic strategies [14].

Despite some success with treatments like varicocelectomy, outcomes remain inconsistent due to the complex and poorly understood pathophysiology of varicoceles. Without comprehensive tools to detect and analyze these molecular disruptions, clinicians lack crucial insights into the extent of infertility associated with varicoceles, which hinders the development of personalized treatment plans. Consequently, this may contribute to the inconsistent outcomes observed with surgical interventions [15].

This diagnostic gap presents a significant challenge in varicocele management. This manuscript will explore the potential of proteomics and metabolomics in advancing male infertility diagnostics and treatment. By moving beyond traditional semen analysis parameters, these "omics" methods promise the early detection and precise monitoring of varicoceles' impact on fertility. Ultimately, the integration of proteomics and metabolomics could improve management strategies and enable personalized treatment, enhancing outcomes for men affected by this common condition.

2. Materials and Methods

A comprehensive literature search was conducted to gather relevant studies on the application of proteomics and metabolomics in varicocele-associated male infertility. The databases searched included PubMed, Scopus, and Web of Science, selected for their extensive biomedical and scientific coverage and their relevance to studies in reproductive health, proteomics, and metabolomics. These databases were chosen due to their accessibility and the breadth of indexed journals pertinent to our research focus. The literature search spanned up to October 2024. While Embase and the Cochrane Library are important resources, they were not included in our strategy. This exclusion was based on the specific focus of our study and the determination that PubMed, Scopus, and Web of Science would sufficiently capture the relevant literature on proteomics and metabolomics related to varicocele-associated male infertility. Embase primarily covers pharmacological and biomedical literature, and the Cochrane Library specializes in systematic reviews and clinical trials, which were outside the scope of our narrative review. Additionally, only articles published in English were considered, potentially omitting relevant research in other languages.

Keywords and Search Strategy: The search was conducted using keywords such as "varicocele", "male infertility", "proteomics", "metabolomics", "biomarkers", "seminal plasma", "spermatozoa", "oxidative stress", and "personalized medicine". These terms were combined using Boolean operators (AND, OR) to enhance the precision of results. Additionally, Medical Subject Headings (MeSH) terms were employed in PubMed to ensure comprehensive retrieval of relevant articles.

The titles and abstracts of the identified studies were independently evaluated by two reviewers (A.K. and Athanasios Zikopoulos) to determine their eligibility based on the inclusion criteria. Studies not meeting the criteria were excluded at this stage. Full-text versions of potentially eligible articles were subsequently retrieved for a detailed assessment. Discrepancies in study selection were addressed through consensus discussions between the two reviewers. If disagreements persisted, a third reviewer (E.M.) was consulted to ensure methodological accuracy and minimize selection bias. The final list of studies was critically reviewed by all authors to confirm alignment with the research objectives.

Inclusion and Exclusion Criteria: The selection criteria focused on original research articles, reviews, and clinical studies relevant to varicocele-associated male infertility and the use of proteomic and metabolomic analyses. Specific inclusion criteria were as follows:

- Types of Studies: Both clinical and experimental studies were included to encompass a range of research methodologies. Clinical studies provided direct insights into biomarkers and potential diagnostic applications, while experimental studies contributed mechanistic insights into molecular alterations.
- Study Focus: Studies must have addressed either proteomic or metabolomic analyses in relation to varicocele-associated infertility, with a focus on biomarkers, molecular mechanisms, or potential diagnostic or therapeutic applications.

- Population: Studies involving male patients with varicocele or varicocele-associated infertility.
- Publication Date and Language: Studies published in English up to October 2024 were included. Articles with inadequate relevance, low methodological rigor, or insufficiently detailed molecular data were excluded.

Data Extraction and Analysis: Relevant findings were extracted from selected articles, including specific biomarkers, affected molecular pathways, and implications for diagnosis and treatment. The findings were synthesized to identify trends, gaps, and future directions in the application of "omics" technologies for varicocele-associated male infertility. The PRISMA flowchart summarizing the article selection process is presented in Figure 2.

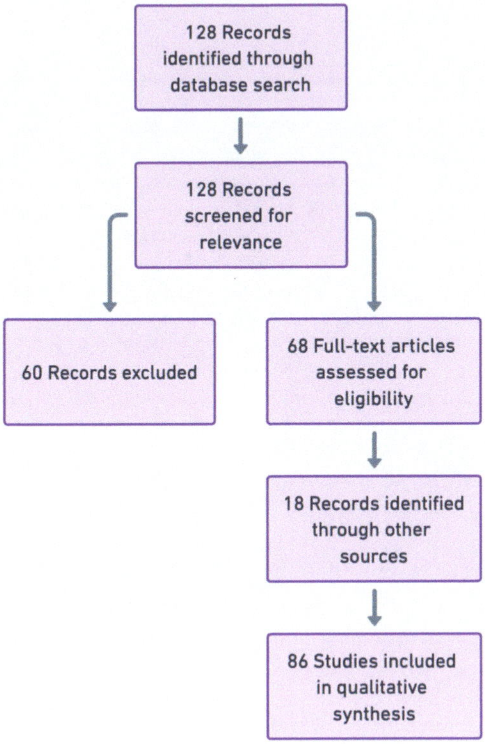

Figure 2. Prisma flow diagram illustrating the article selection process for studies on proteomics and metabolomics in varicocele-associated male infertility.

3. Proteomic Advances in Understanding Varicocele-Associated Male Infertility

Proteomics has emerged as a powerful tool in elucidating the molecular mechanisms underlying male infertility, particularly in conditions like varicoceles. Semen samples are ideal for proteomic studies due to the reliance of spermatozoa on proteins to execute essential physiological functions, given their lack of transcriptional activity. These proteins are involved in various molecular processes, including energy metabolism, post-translational modifications, DNA repair, and responses to oxidative stress [16–18]. Seminal plasma proteins also play a critical role in maintaining sperm function, as they are primarily derived from the testes and accessory sex glands, resulting in a high protein concentration (35–55 g/L), with about 80% being semenogelins [19–21]. Alterations in the expression of these proteins can directly affect sperm health and homeostasis.

Despite the potential of proteomics, several limitations should be acknowledged up front. A major challenge is the detection and quantification of low-abundance proteins that may have significant diagnostic and therapeutic value but are often masked by the high abundance of other proteins in seminal plasma. Current proteomic techniques, such as mass spectrometry and two-dimensional electrophoresis, often require enrichment or fractionation steps to overcome this limitation [22,23]. Advances in methodologies, including the use of targeted proteomics and enhanced bioinformatics tools, are improving sensitivity but remain constrained by sample complexity and variability [24].

3.1. Proteomics in Diagnosing Male Infertility

Proteomic analysis offers significant potential in identifying differential protein expression in semen, serving as a non-invasive biomarker tool for diagnosing male infertility associated with abnormal semen characteristics [25].

3.1.1. Seminal Plasma Protein Markers in General Male Infertility

In azoospermic men, certain seminal plasma proteins are absent, such as acid phosphatase prostate (ACPP), prostate-specific antigen (KLK3), clusterin (CLU), zinc-alpha-2-glycoprotein (AZGP1), and glycodelin (PAEP) [26,27]. Drabovich et al. confirmed testis-expressed protein 101 (TEX101) as a biomarker for azoospermia and extracellular matrix protein 1 (ECM1) to differentiate non-obstructive azoospermia from vasectomy patients [28]. In cases of asthenozoospermia, protein tyrosine phosphatase non-receptor type 14 (PTPN14) shows dysregulation, while cystatin-C (CST3) levels are reduced [29,30]. In contrast, patients with oligoasthenozoospermia exhibit elevated levels of KLK3 and semenogelin-1 (SEMG1) [30]. Key proteins associated with sperm function, such as NPC intracellular cholesterol transporter 2 (NPC2), galectin-3-binding protein (LGALS3BP), lipocalin-1 (LCN1), and prolactin-inducible protein (PIP), show reduced expression in oligoasthenoteratozoospermia (OAT) [31].

3.1.2. Proteomic Insights into Oxidative Stress and DNA Damage

Oxidative stress, a prominent factor in varicocele-associated male infertility, is commonly assessed in clinical settings through markers such as ROS levels, total antioxidant capacity (TAC), and malondialdehyde (MDA) concentrations in semen [32]. These markers help evaluate the extent of oxidative damage but do not provide detailed molecular insights into the affected proteins or pathways that underlie the cellular impairments seen in infertility [33].

Proteomic studies add value by identifying specific differentially expressed proteins (DEPs) involved in stress responses and regulatory pathways in men with elevated seminal ROS levels [30]. For example, Sharma et al. observed that membrane metallo-endopeptidase (MME) was present in the seminal plasma of ROS-positive men but absent in ROS-negative individuals. Conversely, fibronectin 1 (FN1) and macrophage migration inhibitory factor (MIF) were found only in ROS-negative samples, suggesting a complex molecular response to oxidative stress in sperm and seminal plasma [30].

Proteomic insights also provide a deeper understanding of DNA damage beyond what is offered by DNA fragmentation assays alone. A bioinformatic analysis of proteomic data by Intasqui et al. identified several potential markers of sperm nuclear DNA damage, such as solute carrier family 2 member 14 (SLC2A14), phosphoglycerate kinase 2 (PGK2), outer dense fiber protein 1 (ODF1), clusterin (CLU), and voltage-dependent anion-selective channel proteins 2 and 3 (VDAC2 and VDAC3). These proteins are associated with pathways that regulate DNA repair, oxidative stress responses, and cellular stability, offering insights into the molecular mechanisms disrupted by varicocele formation [34,35].

By combining conventional oxidative stress markers with proteomic data, clinicians may better understand the molecular disruptions in varicocele patients, allowing for a more targeted and personalized approach to treatment.

3.2. Proteomic Analysis in Varicocele Patients

While research on sperm proteomics in varicocele patients has been limited, recent studies have provided valuable insights into the molecular alterations associated with this condition.

3.2.1. Sperm Proteomic Alterations in Varicocele Patients

Early protein profiling studies compared normozoospermic men without varicoceles to oligozoospermic men with the condition using techniques like two-dimensional gel electrophoresis (2D-GE), a laboratory method that separates proteins based on their size and electrical charge [36]. These studies identified DEPs mainly related to mitochondrial function, cytoskeletal structure, and heat shock responses [36]. Subsequent research investigated changes in sperm protein expression in varicocele patients before and after varicocelectomy, revealing significant increases in mitochondrial ATP synthase subunit delta (ATP5D), antioxidant enzyme superoxide dismutase 1 (SOD1), and heat shock protein family A member 5 (HSPA5) following surgery [37].

Advanced proteomic approaches like liquid chromatography–tandem mass spectrometry (LC-MS/MS), an advanced laboratory technique used to identify and measure proteins, have uncovered additional molecular mechanisms in varicocele formation [38]. Proteomic analyses have shown that a significant proportion of DEPs related to sperm function and energy metabolism are downregulated in both unilateral and bilateral varicocele cases [39]. Researchers identified 141 mitochondrial proteins in sperm, with 22 associated with mitochondrial structure and function being altered in varicocele patients [40]. Lower expression levels of proteins such as Na^+/K^+ ATPase alpha 4 (ATP1A4), heat shock-related 70 kDa protein 2 (HSPA2), sperm-associated antigen 17 (SPA17), and apolipoprotein A1 (APOA1) were correlated with reduced mitochondrial efficiency [40].

3.2.2. Unilateral vs. Bilateral Varicocele Proteomic Profiles

Unilateral Varicoceles

Unilateral varicoceles predominantly affect the left side in approximately 90% of cases [41]. Comparative proteomic studies between fertile men and unilateral varicocele patients revealed 369 DEPs. Many of these proteins are involved in essential cellular processes such as ion binding, oxidoreductase activity, and pathways like small-molecule metabolism, stress response, and signal transduction [42]. Alterations in these proteins impact the physiological functions of sperm, including post-translational modification, free-radical scavenging, protein ubiquitination, and mitochondrial function. A set of 29 proteins linked to reproductive functions—such as maturation, motility, capacitation, and acrosome reaction—showed significant changes. Notable proteins include calcium-binding tyrosine phosphorylation-regulated protein (CABYR), A-kinase anchor proteins (AKAP), APOA1, semenogelin-1 (SEMG1), and sperm surface protein Sp17 (SPA17), which have been highlighted as potential biomarkers for unilateral varicocele [43].

Bilateral Varicoceles

In bilateral varicocele patients, unique proteomic profiles distinguish them from fertile individuals. The absence of APOA1, reduced expression of translocase of outer mitochondrial membrane 22 (TOM22), and increased expression of transglutaminase-4 (TGM4) correlate with oxidative stress and DNA fragmentation [44]. Proteins related to reproductive functionality, including outer dense fiber protein 2 (ODF2), tektin-3 (TEKT3), t-complex protein 11 homolog (TCP11), and calmegin (CLGN), display altered expression patterns, impairing the sperm's fertilization capacity. Additionally, proteins such as enkurin (ENKUR), semenogelin-1 and -2 (SEMG1/2), sperm adhesion molecule 1 (SPAM1), and CABYR serve as indicators of reduced semen quality in bilateral varicocele patients [42].

Comparative profiling has shown 253 DEPs between unilateral and bilateral varicocele cases. These proteins are involved in pathways related to metabolism, apoptosis, and signal transduction. The dysregulation of sperm functions such as capacitation, hyperactivation, zona pellucida binding, and fertilization-related activities is more pronounced in bilateral varicocele cases due to the differential expression of proteins like glutathione S-transferase Mu 3 (GSTM3), sperm protein associated with the nucleus on the X chromosome B/F (SPANXB/F), cytochrome b5 reductase 2 (CYB5R2), CLGN, and Parkinsonism-associated deglycase (PARK7/DJ-1) [42]. Over half of these DEPs are linked to acetylation, suggesting that the downregulation of proteasome complex proteins could lead to increased DNA damage [45]. Proteins associated with acetylation involved in fertilization and acrosome reaction (transaldolase 1 [TALDO1], histone cluster 1 H2B family member B [HIST1H2B], and glucosamine-6-phosphate deaminase 1 [GNPDA1]), apoptosis and DNA damage (heat shock protein HSP 90-beta [HSP90AB1], serine/threonine-protein phosphatase 5 [PPP5C], and RuvB-like 2 [RUVBL2]), and mitochondrial dysfunction (succinate dehydrogenase complex flavoprotein subunit A [SDHA], peroxiredoxin-1 [PRDX1], and glutathione reductase [GSR]) have been proposed as post-translational protein biomarkers in varicocele patients [45].

3.3. *Seminal Plasma Proteomics in Varicocele Patients*

The proteomic profile of seminal plasma is crucial for enhancing sperm's fertilization capacity [19]. Seminal plasma provides a supportive environment for sperm maturation and reflects overall male reproductive health. Approximately 10% of seminal plasma proteins originate from the testes, offering insights into testicular function [23]. These proteins are involved in critical stages of fertilization, including hyperactivation, capacitation, the acrosome reaction, and sperm–egg interaction [46]. Seminal plasma also contains about 30% of the proteins found in sperm, serving as an indicator of sperm functionality [24].

3.3.1. Proteomic Biomarkers in Adolescents and Adults

Adults with Varicoceles

The initial study on seminal plasma proteomics in adult varicocele patients using two-dimensional sodium dodecyl sulfate–polyacrylamide gel electrophoresis (2D SDS-PAGE) identified 95 proteins with altered expression. Among these, proteins involved in inflammatory response, proteolysis, apoptosis regulation, sperm maturation, and sperm-egg fusion showed notable dysregulation [22]. Pathways related to nitric oxide metabolism and tetratricopeptide repeat domain binding activity were significantly increased, highlighting the adverse effects of varicocele formation on semen quality and sperm functional integrity [47].

Adolescents with Varicoceles

The prevalence of varicoceles shows an age-related increase, affecting approximately 7.9% to 16.2% of adolescents between the ages of 10 and 19, with rates reaching up to 19% by the age of 19 [48,49]. In adolescents with varicoceles and compromised semen quality, seminal plasma proteins essential for normal sperm function exhibit differential expression. Proteins related to sperm motility and capacitation, such as semenogelin I (SEMG1) and prostate-specific antigen (PSA), are overexpressed and underexpressed, respectively [50]. Belardin et al. indicated that the proliferation–apoptosis balance was disrupted in adolescents with varicoceles [51]. Insulin-like growth factor-binding protein 7 (IGFBP7), associated with proliferation, was overexpressed, while deoxyribonuclease-1 (DNASE1), involved in apoptosis regulation, was underexpressed [51]. A high presence of immune response proteins in the seminal plasma indicated a chronic inflammatory state adversely impacting testicular function and semen quality [52].

3.3.2. Proteomic Changes in Seminal Plasma Following Varicocelectomy

Changes in protein expression have been observed in the seminal plasma of patients after varicocelectomy. Post-surgical proteomic analysis identified 38 proteins with unique expression patterns. Pathways associated with oxidative stress response, gluconeogenesis, and protein stability were notably active following varicocelectomy. Key proteins such as

PARK7/DJ-1, S100 calcium-binding protein A9 (S100-A9), superoxide dismutase 1 (SOD1), annexin A1 (ANXA1), glyceraldehyde-3-phosphate dehydrogenase (GAPDH), and malate dehydrogenase (MDH) were overexpressed, suggesting they play a role in re-establishing cellular balance after surgery [47]. Lower levels of negative elongation factor E (NELFE) indicated reduced oxidative stress, while the higher expression of transglutaminase-4 (TGM4) hinted at preserved sperm-binding function after varicocelectomy [50].

Further studies validated certain seminal plasma proteins as potential non-invasive biomarkers for diagnosing varicocele-associated infertility. In varicocele patients, the apoptosis-related protein B-cell lymphoma 2 (BCL2) was downregulated, while BCL2-associated X protein (BAX) was upregulated. An inverse relationship was found between BAX levels and sperm concentration, motility, and normal morphology, underscoring its relevance as a marker of compromised semen quality [53].

Table 1 summarizes key proteins identified in varicocele-associated male infertility, detailing their expression changes, biological functions, and potential as clinical biomarkers.

Table 1. Key proteins identified in varicocele-associated male infertility.

Proteins	Expression Change	Biological Function	Clinical Implication/ Potential as a Biomarker	References
HSPA2	↓	Involved in sperm maturation and capacitation	Marker for impaired sperm function	[40,42,44]
ATP1A4	↓	Sperm motility and ion transport	Indicates reduced mitochondrial efficiency	[40]
APOA1	Ø/↓	Cholesterol transport and lipid metabolism	Marker for oxidative stress and mitochondrial dysfunction	[40,44]
CABYR	↓/↑	Sperm capacitation and motility	Potential biomarker for unilateral varicoceles	[42,44]
SEMG1	↑	Semen coagulation and sperm motility regulation	Indicator of altered semen quality	[42,50]
SEMG2	↓	Semen coagulation and sperm motility regulation	Indicator of altered semen quality	[42,50]
BAX	↑	Promotes apoptosis	Correlates with decreased sperm concentration and motility	[53]
BCL2	↓	Inhibits apoptosis	Reduced levels indicate increased apoptosis in sperm cells	[53]
PARK7/DJ-1	↑	Antioxidant properties, protects against oxidative stress	Marker for recovery after surgery	[45,47]
SOD1	↑	Antioxidant enzyme reducing oxidative stress	Indicates improved oxidative status after surgery	[37,47]

↑: Upregulated or increased expression/levels; ↓: downregulated or decreased expression/levels; Ø: absent (protein or metabolite not detected in the sample); ↑/↓: altered expression, indicates that expression levels can be either upregulated or downregulated depending on individual studies or patient variability; HSPA2: heat shock protein family A member 2; ATP1A4: ATPase Na^+/K^+ transporting subunit alpha 4; APOA1: apolipoprotein A-I; CABYR: calcium-binding tyrosine (Y) phosphorylation-regulated protein; SEMG1: semenogelin 1; SEMG2: semenogelin 2; BAX: BCL2-associated X protein; BCL2: B-cell lymphoma 2; PARK7/DJ-1: Parkinsonism-associated deglycase; SOD1: superoxide dismutase 1.

4. Metabolomics as Diagnostic Tool in Male Infertility

Metabolomics, the comprehensive analysis of small molecules known as metabolites within biological systems, has emerged as a valuable approach to understanding male infertility. Focusing on the non-targeted analysis of small molecules under 1 kDa—including hormones, signaling molecules, and secondary metabolites—metabolomics provides detailed insights into the physiological state of cells and tissues [54]. Unlike proteins and mRNA transcripts, metabolites are simpler in complexity yet represent the final products of cellular processes, exerting immediate influence on biological systems [55].

Both targeted and untargeted metabolomic approaches are employed to explore the metabolome. Targeted metabolomics quantifies specific sets of known metabolites, providing precise measurements of predefined compounds. Untargeted metabolomics aims to detect and quantify as many metabolites as possible without prior selection, offering a global view of the metabolic state. Numerous high-throughput platforms facilitate metabolomic profiling even with small sample volumes. Techniques such as nuclear magnetic resonance (NMR) spectroscopy—particularly ^{1}H NMR—provide detailed structural information without destroying the sample. Mass spectrometry (MS) methods, including electrospray ionization mass spectrometry (ESI-MS) and direct-injection mass spectrometry (DI-MS), offer high sensitivity and specificity. Spectroscopic methods like Raman spectroscopy and near-infrared (NIR) spectroscopy allow for rapid, non-destructive analysis. To preserve sample integrity, biological samples are typically stored at −80 °C to prevent metabolic activity that could alter metabolite concentrations [56].

The metabolome reflects the genome's functional output, making biofluids like seminal plasma ideal for metabolomic studies [57]. Seminal plasma is particularly valuable for assessing reproductive health, as it captures subcellular and molecular changes in sperm [58]. Metabolomic analysis can reveal metabolic signatures linked to semen quality and associated reproductive conditions. Changes in the metabolic composition of seminal plasma are closely related to the underlying causes of male infertility [59]. Comprehensive metabolite profiling in semen—from both sperm and seminal plasma—can detect shifts in molecular composition crucial for managing infertility [60]. Bioinformatics tools aid in mapping pathways connected to sperm pathophysiology, while chemometric analysis effectively distinguishes infertile men from fertile controls [61].

NMR spectroscopy of seminal plasma has identified lysine as a potential biomarker for diagnosing idiopathic male infertility [62]. Other metabolites such as valine, 2-hydroxyisovalerate, hippurate, and fructose are found to be reduced in men with idiopathic infertility [62]. Bonechi et al. utilized NMR spectroscopy combined with principal component analysis (PCA) to classify semen samples based on different infertility conditions, with leukocytospermic patients clustering together [63]. This approach demonstrates the potential of metabolomics in differentiating between various infertility etiologies.

In asthenozoospermia, characterized by reduced sperm motility, metabolomic profiling via Raman spectroscopy has demonstrated the ability to distinguish asthenozoospermic samples from normal samples with an 83% accuracy rate [64]. Elevated levels of metabolites such as 5α-cholesterol and 7-ketocholesterol are associated with oxidative stress in these patients, indicating potential targets for therapeutic intervention [58]. These findings have implications for clinical practices, as oxidative stress biomarkers identified through metabolomics can guide antioxidant therapies aimed at improving sperm motility and overall reproductive outcomes [65].

In cases of non-obstructive azoospermia, Gilany et al. employed gas chromatography–mass spectrometry (GC-MS) paired with advanced chemometric analysis to identify 36 distinctive chemicals in seminal plasma that differentiate between testicular sperm extraction (TESE)-positive and TESE-negative samples. Only five of these metabolites were cataloged in the Human Metabolome Database (version 3.6), including dimethyl-(1S)-bicyclo(3.1.1)hept-2-ene-2-methanol, 2-pyrrolidineacetic acid, and 4,5-dimethoxy-1,2-benzenedicarboxylic acid. These metabolites provide potential biomarkers for differentiating subtypes of azoospermia [66]. This differentiation not only aids in patient counseling but also minimizes unnecessary invasive procedures by identifying candidates more likely to benefit from TESE [67].

In patients with spinal cord injury (SCI), seminal plasma metabolomic analysis of lipids revealed molecules associated with nucleotide synthesis and hydrogen peroxide response pathways. These findings indicate that signal transduction is notably compromised in SCI patients, contributing to infertility [68]. The identification of these disrupted pathways highlights opportunities for targeted therapeutic interventions, such as enhancing nucleotide synthesis or mitigating oxidative stress to improve reproductive outcomes [69].

Overall, metabolomic findings are increasingly being integrated into clinical practices and therapeutic strategies. By combining metabolomic biomarkers with bioinformatics and traditional diagnostic parameters, clinicians can achieve more precise patient stratification and personalized interventions. For example, metabolomic profiles may guide antioxidant supplementation, ART optimization, or minimally invasive sperm retrieval approaches [67]. Such applications underscore the transformative potential of metabolomics in male infertility diagnosis and management.

Table 2 provides an overview of key metabolites associated with varicocele-induced infertility, detailing their roles in cellular function and potential as biomarkers.

Table 2. Key metabolites identified in varicocele-associated male infertility.

Metabolites	Expression Change	Biological Function	Clinical Implication/ Potential as a Biomarker	References
Lysine	↓	Amino acid involved in protein synthesis	Potential biomarker for idiopathic infertility	[62]
Valine	↓	Amino acid involved in energy metabolism	Associated with impaired sperm function	[62]
Fructose	↓	Energy source for spermatozoa	Lower levels correlate with reduced sperm motility	[62]
5α-Cholesterol	↑ *	Steroid involved in membrane fluidity	Marker for oxidative stress in the sperm membrane	[58]
7-Ketocholesterol	↑ *	Oxidized cholesterol derivative	Indicates oxidative damage in sperm cells	[58]
Lactate	↓/↑	Energy metabolism intermediary	Reflects changes in glycolytic pathway activity	[70]
Glycerylphos-phorylcholine	↓/↑	Membrane lipid metabolism	Associated with membrane integrity and sperm viability	[70]

↑: Upregulated or increased expression/levels; ↓: downregulated or decreased expression/levels; ↑/↓: altered expression, indicates that expression levels can be either upregulated or downregulated, depending on individual studies or patient variability; *: in asthenozoospermia.

5. Integration of Proteomics and Metabolomics for Diagnostic Innovation

Proteomics and metabolomics offer complementary perspectives for diagnosing varicocele-associated infertility by targeting different but interconnected molecular elements. Proteomics focuses on the profile and function of proteins in sperm and seminal plasma, revealing changes in protein expression that directly impact cellular function. Metabolomics examines small-molecule metabolites that provide insights into biochemical pathways disrupted by varicoceles, such as oxidative stress and energy metabolism [71]. For instance, a combined analysis of proteomic and metabolomic data identified oxidative stress as a key disruptor in varicocele formation, with proteomics highlighting the underexpression of antioxidant enzymes like superoxide dismutase (SOD1) and metabolomics detecting elevated levels of 7-ketocholesterol, a marker of oxidative damage. These findings have supported clinical decisions to incorporate antioxidant therapies tailored to specific biomarker profiles [58,72]. Integrating data from these two fields allows for a more comprehensive molecular fingerprint, enhancing diagnostic accuracy by identifying specific protein and metabolite biomarkers. This holistic approach paves the way for personalized treatment strategies, tailoring interventions based on each patient's unique molecular profile [73,74].

Proteomic and metabolomic analyses in varicocele patients have identified several critical molecular pathways disrupted by the condition. One major affected pathway is oxidative stress, resulting from an excessive production of ROS that damages sperm DNA and cellular structures, leading to impaired fertility [75]. Additionally, mitochondrial dysfunction has emerged as a key factor, as proteins related to energy production are often underexpressed in varicocele patients, causing reduced ATP synthesis and affecting sperm motility and viability [40]. This interplay is evident in studies where proteomics identified reduced levels of mitochondrial proteins such as COX5B, while metabolomics confirmed decreased levels of citrate and lactate, critical intermediates of mitochondrial respiration and glycolysis, respectively. These findings have informed interventions targeting mitochondrial support to improve sperm viability [40,76]. Metabolomic studies complement this by identifying metabolites such as lactate, which reflects impaired glycolysis, and citrate, which is crucial for mitochondrial respiration. The reduction in these metabolites aligns with proteomic findings of decreased mitochondrial enzyme expression, providing a deeper understanding of how energy metabolism is compromised [40].

Bioinformatic analysis further reveals disruptions in signal transduction pathways and apoptosis, with altered protein expression impacting cellular communication and leading to premature cell death in sperm cells. One study combined proteomics and metabolomics to identify the differential expression of apoptotic regulators, such as Bax and Bcl-2, along with elevated levels of glycerylphosphorylcholine, a metabolite associated with membrane stability and sperm viability. This dual insight has guided personalized therapeutic strategies to mitigate apoptosis and improve membrane integrity in varicocele patients [70,75]. Collectively, these insights provide a framework for understanding the molecular basis of varicoceles' impacts on male infertility.

As proteomics and metabolomics techniques continue to advance, their application to personalized fertility treatments is expected to increase. Molecular profiling could allow clinicians to classify varicocele patients based on specific proteomic and metabolomic markers, enabling more tailored interventions. For example, antioxidant therapies might be optimized for patients showing high oxidative stress biomarkers, while others with significant mitochondrial dysfunction could receive treatments aimed at enhancing energy metabolism [70]. A notable example involves the integration of proteomic and metabolomic data to identify concurrent elevations of oxidative stress proteins (e.g., PRDX2) and metabolites (e.g., 7-ketocholesterol). Patients with these profiles have demonstrated better outcomes with combination therapies targeting both redox balance and mitochondrial function [9].

Ultimately, the integration of these "omics" technologies may facilitate the development of non-invasive diagnostic tools and personalized treatment plans, leading to improved outcomes for patients with varicocele-related infertility. The clinical validation of specific biomarkers will be crucial to translating these molecular insights into standard care, offering infertile men targeted treatments that enhance fertility based on their unique biomolecular profiles [73].

6. Challenges, Limitations, and Future Prospects of 'Omics' Technologies

The application of proteomics and metabolomics to male infertility, particularly varicocele-associated infertility, presents several technical and methodological challenges. A primary obstacle is the complexity of proteins in seminal samples, where high heterogeneity complicates detection and quantification, especially for low-abundance proteins that hold diagnostic value. Current proteomic techniques, like mass spectrometry (MS) and two-dimensional electrophoresis (2DE), require refinement to improve sensitivity for detecting these subtle biomarkers [77]. Advances in proteomic methodologies, including protein enrichment and customized techniques, now allow for the identification of low-abundance proteins and post-translational modifications such as glycosylation, phosphorylation, acetylation, and methylation in sperm and seminal plasma.

Metabolomics also presents challenges in terms of metabolite quantification due to the rapid turnover of small molecules and their sensitivity to environmental factors. High-throughput metabolomic analyses such as NMR and liquid chromatography–mass spectrometry (LC-MS) require advanced analytical methods to accurately distinguish metabolomic profiles. Recent advancements in bioinformatics and data processing have started addressing these issues, allowing for more precise interpretations of complex datasets and enhancing the reproducibility of results [67].

For the successful clinical translation of "omics" technologies, several critical steps must be undertaken. Biomarkers identified through proteomic and metabolomic studies require rigorous validation in large, diverse populations to ensure their reproducibility and reliability across demographic groups. Validation studies should focus on key markers, such as oxidative stress indicators (e.g., 7-ketocholesterol) and mitochondrial dysfunction markers (e.g., citrate), to confirm their diagnostic and prognostic utility in male infertility. Multicenter clinical trials are essential to substantiate these findings and demonstrate their relevance in clinical settings [78].

Regulatory approval processes represent another pivotal challenge in the integration of omics technologies into clinical practice. Omics-based diagnostic tests must comply with stringent regulatory standards, ensuring their safety, accuracy, and clinical relevance. The development of standardized protocols for sample collection, processing, and analysis will be critical to overcoming inter-study variability and facilitating the approval of these diagnostic tools by regulatory bodies such as the Food and Drug Administration (FDA) and the European Medicines Agency (EMA). Adherence to international guidelines for biomarker validation and assay standardization will further streamline the translation of these technologies into widespread clinical use [79].

Cost considerations also play a crucial role in the clinical adoption of omics technologies. The high costs associated with these advanced methodologies currently limit their accessibility in routine diagnostic settings. To address this, ongoing efforts aim to automate workflows and optimize high-throughput assays, which will reduce costs and improve scalability. Integrating omics-based biomarker testing into existing diagnostic frameworks, such as standard semen analyses, represents a practical and economically viable approach to ensuring accessibility for a broader range of patients [80].

Non-invasive diagnostic tools, such as exosome-based panels, represent a promising frontier in translating omics biomarkers into clinical practice. Exosomes, which carry proteins and metabolites reflective of their cell of origin, provide unique insights into sperm health and function. Emerging evidence suggests that exosomal proteins, such as HSP70 and TGF-β, can serve as biomarkers for oxidative stress and inflammation in varicocele-associated infertility. These exosome-based diagnostics could complement traditional semen analysis by offering more granular molecular insights and improving early detection and treatment monitoring [81].

Future developments in omics technologies hold significant promise for advancing the diagnosis and treatment of male infertility. Emerging tools, such as single-cell omics and artificial intelligence (AI)-based algorithms, are expected to revolutionize the field by enabling cell-specific analyses and improving the interpretation of complex datasets. Single-cell omics could provide unprecedented insights into spermatogenesis at the molecular level, while AI-powered models may enhance the predictive accuracy of diagnostic algorithms [82]. Furthermore, integrating microbiome research with proteomics and metabolomics could uncover novel microbial biomarkers that influence spermatogenesis and the integrity of the blood–testicular barrier, presenting new opportunities for therapeutic intervention [83–85].

By addressing these challenges systematically, including biomarker validation, regulatory compliance, cost-effectiveness, and the development of non-invasive diagnostics, omics technologies can transition from research to routine clinical practice. These advancements will enable personalized and precise diagnostic approaches, ultimately improving outcomes for patients with varicocele-associated infertility.

Strengths and Limitations

This review presents a comprehensive examination of advancements in proteomics and metabolomics as diagnostic tools for varicocele-associated male infertility. A significant strength of this review is the integration of advanced "omics" technologies, offering a cutting-edge approach to identifying biomarkers associated with varicocele-induced infertility. These methods surpass conventional semen analysis by providing molecular-level insights that enhance the understanding of underlying pathophysiological mechanisms [70,81].

Another strength lies in the systematic and thorough literature search conducted using robust databases such as PubMed, Scopus, and Web of Science. This approach ensured the inclusion of relevant and high-quality studies, contributing to the reliability of the findings [70]. The emphasis on biomarkers highlights the diagnostic potential of proteomic and metabolomic analyses, paving the way for future advancements in personalized medicine and targeted therapeutic interventions [81].

However, several limitations should be acknowledged. First, the exclusion of non-English studies and certain databases (e.g., Embase and Cochrane) may have led to the omission of potentially relevant research, introducing language bias and limiting the comprehensiveness and generalizability of the findings. This constraint may affect the overall conclusions drawn from the review.

Second, there is significant heterogeneity among the included studies. Variability in methodologies, sample populations, and analytical techniques across different studies may impact the comparability of findings and the reproducibility of identified biomarkers [67,77]. This heterogeneity poses challenges in synthesizing results and drawing definitive conclusions.

Third, the translational application of the identified biomarkers faces challenges. Despite promising findings, the clinical implementation of proteomic and metabolomic biomarkers requires extensive validation and standardization, which remains a barrier to their adoption in routine clinical practice [86]. Large-scale, multicenter clinical trials are necessary to establish the reliability and predictive value of these biomarkers before they can be integrated into standard care.

Additionally, many studies included in this review focus on specific male infertility subtypes, which may not represent the broader population of individuals affected by varicocele-associated infertility [61,75]. This limitation in sample diversity may affect the generalizability of the findings to all varicocele patients.

Furthermore, as a narrative review, this study does not employ the systematic methodology required for a systematic review or meta-analysis. The inclusion of studies was based on relevance rather than a predefined protocol, potentially introducing selection bias. Reliance on published studies without access to raw data restricts the ability to perform quantitative analysis or independently verify the results, as findings are based on the interpretations and conclusions of the original authors.

7. Conclusions

Proteomics and metabolomics offer powerful, non-invasive approaches for diagnosing varicocele-associated infertility. These technologies provide a molecular-level view of cellular processes, enabling the identification of specific protein and metabolite biomarkers associated with oxidative stress, mitochondrial dysfunction, and impaired sperm function. By profiling these biomarkers in sperm and seminal plasma, researchers can elucidate the underlying mechanisms of infertility, offering diagnostic precision beyond traditional semen analysis.

The integration of "omics" approaches into clinical practice has the potential to revolutionize male infertility diagnostics by refining and expanding the parameters that can be assessed. These technologies support a shift toward personalized diagnostics and treatments, tailoring interventions based on each patient's unique molecular profile. Individualized insights can guide clinical decisions, predict responses to treatments like varicocelectomy, and enable the development of targeted therapies that address the specific biological disruptions caused by varicoceles.

Looking ahead, the continued integration of proteomics and metabolomics in male infertility research is poised to deepen our understanding of complex infertility mechanisms and pave the way for novel, non-invasive diagnostic tools. As technology advances, combining proteomics, metabolomics, and emerging fields like exosomal proteomics will allow for the comprehensive profiling of male reproductive health. This convergence of "omics" technologies holds great promise for the future of male infertility diagnostics and treatment, potentially leading to highly effective, individualized care for patients affected by varicocele-associated infertility.

Author Contributions: Conceptualization, A.K., N.S. and A.Z. (Athanasios Zachariou); methodology A.K., A.Z. (Athanasios Zikopoulos), E.M. and M.C.; validation, E.N.S., Z.K., F.D. and N.S.; formal analysis, E.M., M.S., Z.K., E.N.S. and A.Z. (Athanasios Zachariou); investigation, A.K. and M.C.; data curation, A.K., A.Z. (Athanasios Zikopoulos), E.M. and M.S.; writing—original draft preparation, A.K., A.Z. (Athanasios Zikopoulos) and E.M.; writing—review and editing, A.K., F.D., M.C. and N.S.; visualization, F.D.; supervision, M.C. project administration, A.K. and A.Z. (Athanasios Zachariou). All authors have read and agreed to the published version of the manuscript.

Funding: This research received no external funding.

Conflicts of Interest: The authors declare no conflicts of interest.

References

1. Sofikitis, N.; Stavrou, S.; Skouros, S.; Dimitriadis, F.; Tsounapi, P.; Takenaka, A. Mysteries, Facts, and Fiction in Varicocele Pathophysiology and Treatment. *Eur. Urol. Suppl.* **2014**, *13*, 89–99. [CrossRef]
2. Damsgaard, J.; Joensen, U.N.; Carlsen, E.; Erenpreiss, J.; Blomberg Jensen, M.; Matulevicius, V.; Zilaitiene, B.; Olesen, I.A.; Perheentupa, A.; Punab, M.; et al. Varicocele Is Associated with Impaired Semen Quality and Reproductive Hormone Levels: A Study of 7035 Healthy Young Men from Six European Countries. *Eur. Urol.* **2016**, *70*, 1019–1029. [CrossRef] [PubMed]
3. Witt, M.A.; Lipshultz, L.I. Varicocele: A progressive or static lesion? *Urology* **1993**, *42*, 541–543. [CrossRef] [PubMed]
4. Su, J.S.; Farber, N.J.; Vij, S.C. Pathophysiology and treatment options of varicocele: An overview. *Andrologia* **2021**, *53*, e13576. [CrossRef]
5. Kaltsas, A. Oxidative Stress and Male Infertility: The Protective Role of Antioxidants. *Medicina* **2023**, *59*, 1769. [CrossRef]
6. Kang, C.; Punjani, N.; Lee, R.K.; Li, P.S.; Goldstein, M. Effect of varicoceles on spermatogenesis. *Semin. Cell Dev. Biol.* **2022**, *121*, 114–124. [CrossRef]
7. Will, M.A.; Swain, J.; Fode, M.; Sonksen, J.; Christman, G.M.; Ohl, D. The great debate: Varicocele treatment and impact on fertility. *Fertil. Steril.* **2011**, *95*, 841–852. [CrossRef]
8. Kaltsas, A.; Dimitriadis, F.; Zachariou, D.; Zikopoulos, A.; Symeonidis, E.N.; Markou, E.; Tien, D.M.B.; Takenaka, A.; Sofikitis, N.; Zachariou, A. From Diagnosis to Treatment: Comprehensive Care by Reproductive Urologists in Assisted Reproductive Technology. *Medicina* **2023**, *59*, 1835. [CrossRef]
9. Swain, N.; Samanta, L.; Agarwal, A.; Kumar, S.; Dixit, A.; Gopalan, B.; Durairajanayagam, D.; Sharma, R.; Pushparaj, P.N.; Baskaran, S. Aberrant Upregulation of Compensatory Redox Molecular Machines May Contribute to Sperm Dysfunction in Infertile Men with Unilateral Varicocele: A Proteomic Insight. *Antioxid. Redox Signal* **2020**, *32*, 504–521. [CrossRef]
10. Finelli, R.; Darbandi, S.; Pushparaj, P.N.; Henkel, R.; Ko, E.; Agarwal, A. In Silico Sperm Proteome Analysis to Investigate DNA Repair Mechanisms in Varicocele Patients. *Front. Endocrinol.* **2021**, *12*, 757592. [CrossRef]
11. Varnum, A.A.; Shepherd, J.; Campbell, K.; Phan, T.; Velasquez, D.A.; Khodamoradi, K.; Lundy, S.D.; Ramasamy, R. Biomarkers to predict improvement of sperm parameters and hypogonadism after varicocele repair. *F&S Rev.* **2024**, *5*, 100074. [CrossRef]
12. Al-Amrani, S.; Al-Jabri, Z.; Al-Zaabi, A.; Alshekaili, J.; Al-Khabori, M. Proteomics: Concepts and applications in human medicine. *World J. Biol. Chem.* **2021**, *12*, 57–69. [CrossRef]
13. Podgrajsek, R.; Hodzic, A.; Stimpfel, M.; Kunej, T.; Peterlin, B. Insight into the complexity of male infertility: A multi-omics review. *Syst. Biol. Reprod. Med.* **2024**, *70*, 73–90. [CrossRef] [PubMed]
14. Yang, B.; Yang, Y.; Liu, Y.; Li, H.; Ren, S.; Peng, Z.; Fang, K.; Yang, L.; Dong, Q. Molecular characteristics of varicocele: Integration of whole-exome and transcriptome sequencing. *Fertil. Steril.* **2021**, *115*, 363–372. [CrossRef]
15. Franco, A.; Proietti, F.; Palombi, V.; Savarese, G.; Guidotti, M.; Leonardo, C.; Ferro, F.; Manna, C.; Franco, G. Varicocele: To Treat or Not to Treat? *J. Clin. Med.* **2023**, *12*, 4062. [CrossRef]
16. Finelli, R.; Leisegang, K.; Kandil, H.; Agarwal, A. Oxidative Stress: A Comprehensive Review of Biochemical, Molecular, and Genetic Aspects in the Pathogenesis and Management of Varicocele. *World J. Mens Health* **2022**, *40*, 87–103. [CrossRef]
17. Jodar, M.; Sendler, E.; Krawetz, S.A. The protein and transcript profiles of human semen. *Cell Tissue Res.* **2016**, *363*, 85–96. [CrossRef]
18. Amaral, A.; Castillo, J.; Ramalho-Santos, J.; Oliva, R. The combined human sperm proteome: Cellular pathways and implications for basic and clinical science. *Hum. Reprod. Update* **2014**, *20*, 40–62. [CrossRef]
19. Samanta, L.; Parida, R.; Dias, T.R.; Agarwal, A. The enigmatic seminal plasma: A proteomics insight from ejaculation to fertilization. *Reprod. Biol. Endocrinol.* **2018**, *16*, 41. [CrossRef]
20. Panner Selvam, M.K.; Agarwal, A. Update on the proteomics of male infertility: A systematic review. *Arab. J. Urol.* **2018**, *16*, 103–112. [CrossRef]
21. Jodar, M.; Soler-Ventura, A.; Oliva, R.; Molecular Biology of Reproduction and Development Research Group. Semen proteomics and male infertility. *J. Proteom.* **2017**, *162*, 125–134. [CrossRef] [PubMed]
22. Fariello, R.M.; Pariz, J.R.; Spaine, D.M.; Gozzo, F.C.; Pilau, E.J.; Fraietta, R.; Bertolla, R.P.; Andreoni, C.; Cedenho, A.P. Effect of smoking on the functional aspects of sperm and seminal plasma protein profiles in patients with varicocele. *Hum. Reprod.* **2012**, *27*, 3140–3149. [CrossRef] [PubMed]

23. Batruch, I.; Lecker, I.; Kagedan, D.; Smith, C.R.; Mullen, B.J.; Grober, E.; Lo, K.C.; Diamandis, E.P.; Jarvi, K.A. Proteomic analysis of seminal plasma from normal volunteers and post-vasectomy patients identifies over 2000 proteins and candidate biomarkers of the urogenital system. *J. Proteome Res.* **2011**, *10*, 941–953. [CrossRef] [PubMed]
24. Candenas, L.; Chianese, R. Exosome Composition and Seminal Plasma Proteome: A Promising Source of Biomarkers of Male Infertility. *Int. J. Mol. Sci.* **2020**, *21*, 7022. [CrossRef]
25. Panner Selvam, M.K.; Agarwal, A.; Pushparaj, P.N.; Baskaran, S.; Bendou, H. Sperm Proteome Analysis and Identification of Fertility-Associated Biomarkers in Unexplained Male Infertility. *Genes* **2019**, *10*, 522. [CrossRef]
26. Starita-Geribaldi, M.; Roux, F.; Garin, J.; Chevallier, D.; Fenichel, P.; Pointis, G. Development of narrow immobilized pH gradients covering one pH unit for human seminal plasma proteomic analysis. *Proteomics* **2003**, *3*, 1611–1619. [CrossRef]
27. Starita-Geribaldi, M.; Poggioli, S.; Zucchini, M.; Garin, J.; Chevallier, D.; Fenichel, P.; Pointis, G. Mapping of seminal plasma proteins by two-dimensional gel electrophoresis in men with normal and impaired spermatogenesis. *Mol. Hum. Reprod.* **2001**, *7*, 715–722. [CrossRef]
28. Drabovich, A.P.; Dimitromanolakis, A.; Saraon, P.; Soosaipillai, A.; Batruch, I.; Mullen, B.; Jarvi, K.; Diamandis, E.P. Differential diagnosis of azoospermia with proteomic biomarkers ECM1 and TEX101 quantified in seminal plasma. *Sci. Transl. Med.* **2013**, *5*, 212ra160. [CrossRef]
29. Amaral, A.; Paiva, C.; Attardo Parrinello, C.; Estanyol, J.M.; Ballesca, J.L.; Ramalho-Santos, J.; Oliva, R. Identification of proteins involved in human sperm motility using high-throughput differential proteomics. *J. Proteome Res.* **2014**, *13*, 5670–5684. [CrossRef]
30. Sharma, R.; Agarwal, A.; Mohanty, G.; Du Plessis, S.S.; Gopalan, B.; Willard, B.; Yadav, S.P.; Sabanegh, E. Proteomic analysis of seminal fluid from men exhibiting oxidative stress. *Reprod. Biol. Endocrinol.* **2013**, *11*, 85. [CrossRef]
31. Giacomini, E.; Ura, B.; Giolo, E.; Luppi, S.; Martinelli, M.; Garcia, R.C.; Ricci, G. Comparative analysis of the seminal plasma proteomes of oligoasthenozoospermic and normozoospermic men. *Reprod. Biomed. Online* **2015**, *30*, 522–531. [CrossRef] [PubMed]
32. Wood, G.J.A.; Cardoso, J.P.G.; Paluello, D.V.; Nunes, T.F.; Cocuzza, M. Varicocele-Associated Infertility and the Role of Oxidative Stress on Sperm DNA Fragmentation. *Front. Reprod. Health* **2021**, *3*, 695992. [CrossRef] [PubMed]
33. Pavuluri, H.; Bakhtiary, Z.; Panner Selvam, M.K.; Hellstrom, W.J.G. Oxidative Stress-Associated Male Infertility: Current Diagnostic and Therapeutic Approaches. *Medicina* **2024**, *60*, 1008. [CrossRef] [PubMed]
34. Intasqui, P.; Camargo, M.; Del Giudice, P.T.; Spaine, D.M.; Carvalho, V.M.; Cardozo, K.H.; Zylbersztejn, D.S.; Bertolla, R.P. Sperm nuclear DNA fragmentation rate is associated with differential protein expression and enriched functions in human seminal plasma. *BJU Int.* **2013**, *112*, 835–843. [CrossRef]
35. Intasqui, P.; Camargo, M.; Del Giudice, P.T.; Spaine, D.M.; Carvalho, V.M.; Cardozo, K.H.; Cedenho, A.P.; Bertolla, R.P. Unraveling the sperm proteome and post-genomic pathways associated with sperm nuclear DNA fragmentation. *J. Assist. Reprod. Genet.* **2013**, *30*, 1187–1202. [CrossRef]
36. Hosseinifar, H.; Gourabi, H.; Salekdeh, G.H.; Alikhani, M.; Mirshahvaladi, S.; Sabbaghian, M.; Modarresi, T.; Gilani, M.A. Study of sperm protein profile in men with and without varicocele using two-dimensional gel electrophoresis. *Urology* **2013**, *81*, 293–300. [CrossRef]
37. Hosseinifar, H.; Sabbaghian, M.; Nasrabadi, D.; Modarresi, T.; Dizaj, A.V.; Gourabi, H.; Gilani, M.A. Study of the effect of varicocelectomy on sperm proteins expression in patients with varicocele and poor sperm quality by using two-dimensional gel electrophoresis. *J. Assist. Reprod. Genet.* **2014**, *31*, 725–729. [CrossRef]
38. Li, J.; Zhu, H.J. Liquid Chromatography-Tandem Mass Spectrometry (LC-MS/MS)-Based Proteomics of Drug-Metabolizing Enzymes and Transporters. *Molecules* **2020**, *25*, 2718. [CrossRef]
39. Agarwal, A.; Sharma, R.; Samanta, L.; Durairajanayagam, D.; Sabanegh, E. Proteomic signatures of infertile men with clinical varicocele and their validation studies reveal mitochondrial dysfunction leading to infertility. *Asian J. Androl.* **2016**, *18*, 282–291. [CrossRef]
40. Samanta, L.; Agarwal, A.; Swain, N.; Sharma, R.; Gopalan, B.; Esteves, S.C.; Durairajanayagam, D.; Sabanegh, E. Proteomic Signatures of Sperm Mitochondria in Varicocele: Clinical Use as Biomarkers of Varicocele Associated Infertility. *J. Urol.* **2018**, *200*, 414–422. [CrossRef]
41. Baazeem, A.; Belzile, E.; Ciampi, A.; Dohle, G.; Jarvi, K.; Salonia, A.; Weidner, W.; Zini, A. Varicocele and male factor infertility treatment: A new meta-analysis and review of the role of varicocele repair. *Eur. Urol.* **2011**, *60*, 796–808. [CrossRef] [PubMed]
42. Agarwal, A.; Sharma, R.; Durairajanayagam, D.; Cui, Z.; Ayaz, A.; Gupta, S.; Willard, B.; Gopalan, B.; Sabanegh, E. Differential proteomic profiling of spermatozoal proteins of infertile men with unilateral or bilateral varicocele. *Urology* **2015**, *85*, 580–588. [CrossRef] [PubMed]
43. Agarwal, A.; Sharma, R.; Durairajanayagam, D.; Ayaz, A.; Cui, Z.; Willard, B.; Gopalan, B.; Sabanegh, E. Major protein alterations in spermatozoa from infertile men with unilateral varicocele. *Reprod. Biol. Endocrinol.* **2015**, *13*, 8. [CrossRef] [PubMed]
44. Agarwal, A.; Sharma, R.; Durairajanayagam, D.; Cui, Z.; Ayaz, A.; Gupta, S.; Willard, B.; Gopalan, B.; Sabanegh, E. Spermatozoa protein alterations in infertile men with bilateral varicocele. *Asian J. Androl.* **2016**, *18*, 43–53. [CrossRef]
45. Panner Selvam, M.K.; Samanta, L.; Agarwal, A. Functional Analysis of Differentially Expressed Acetylated Spermatozoal Proteins in Infertile Men with Unilateral and Bilateral Varicocele. *Int. J. Mol. Sci.* **2020**, *21*, 3155. [CrossRef]
46. Sun, T.C.; Wang, J.H.; Wang, X.X.; Liu, X.M.; Zhang, C.L.; Hao, C.F.; Ma, W.Z.; Deng, S.L.; Liu, Y.X. Effects of sperm proteins on fertilization in the female reproductive tract. *Front. Biosci.-Landmark* **2019**, *24*, 735–749. [CrossRef]

47. Camargo, M.; Intasqui Lopes, P.; Del Giudice, P.T.; Carvalho, V.M.; Cardozo, K.H.; Andreoni, C.; Fraietta, R.; Bertolla, R.P. Unbiased label-free quantitative proteomic profiling and enriched proteomic pathways in seminal plasma of adult men before and after varicocelectomy. *Hum. Reprod.* **2013**, *28*, 33–46. [CrossRef]
48. Kumanov, P.; Robeva, R.N.; Tomova, A. Adolescent varicocele: Who is at risk? *Pediatrics* **2008**, *121*, e53–e57. [CrossRef]
49. Oster, J. Varicocele in children and adolescents. An investigation of the incidence among Danish school children. *Scand. J. Urol. Nephrol.* **1971**, *5*, 27–32. [CrossRef]
50. Zylbersztejn, D.S.; Andreoni, C.; Del Giudice, P.T.; Spaine, D.M.; Borsari, L.; Souza, G.; Bertolla, R.P.; Fraietta, R. Proteomic analysis of seminal plasma in adolescents with and without varicocele. *Fertil. Steril.* **2013**, *99*, 92–98. [CrossRef]
51. Belardin, L.B.; Del Giudice, P.T.; Camargo, M.; Intasqui, P.; Antoniassi, M.P.; Bertolla, R.P.; Cedenho, A.P. Alterations in the proliferative/apoptotic equilibrium in semen of adolescents with varicocele. *J. Assist. Reprod. Genet.* **2016**, *33*, 1657–1664. [CrossRef] [PubMed]
52. Del Giudice, P.T.; Belardin, L.B.; Camargo, M.; Zylbersztejn, D.S.; Carvalho, V.M.; Cardozo, K.H.; Bertolla, R.P.; Cedenho, A.P. Determination of testicular function in adolescents with varicocoele—A proteomics approach. *Andrology* **2016**, *4*, 447–455. [CrossRef] [PubMed]
53. Mostafa, T.; Rashed, L.; Nabil, N.; Amin, R. Seminal BAX and BCL2 gene and protein expressions in infertile men with varicocele. *Urology* **2014**, *84*, 590–595. [CrossRef]
54. Nicholson, J.K.; Lindon, J.C.; Holmes, E. 'Metabonomics': Understanding the metabolic responses of living systems to pathophysiological stimuli via multivariate statistical analysis of biological NMR spectroscopic data. *Xenobiotica* **1999**, *29*, 1181–1189. [CrossRef]
55. Cuperlovic-Culf, M.; Barnett, D.A.; Culf, A.S.; Chute, I. Cell culture metabolomics: Applications and future directions. *Drug Discov. Today* **2010**, *15*, 610–621. [CrossRef]
56. Cortezzi, S.S.; Cabral, E.C.; Trevisan, M.G.; Ferreira, C.R.; Setti, A.S.; de Almeida Ferreira Braga, D.P.; de Cássia Sávio Figueira, R.; Iaconelli, A., Jr.; Eberlin, M.N.; Borges, E., Jr. Prediction of embryo implantation potential by mass spectrometry fingerprinting of the culture medium. *Reproduction* **2013**, *145*, 453–462. [CrossRef]
57. Baker, M.J.; Hussain, S.R.; Lovergne, L.; Untereiner, V.; Hughes, C.; Lukaszewski, R.A.; Thiefin, G.; Sockalingum, G.D. Developing and understanding biofluid vibrational spectroscopy: A critical review. *Chem. Soc. Rev.* **2016**, *45*, 1803–1818. [CrossRef]
58. Zhang, X.; Diao, R.; Zhu, X.; Li, Z.; Cai, Z. Metabolic characterization of asthenozoospermia using nontargeted seminal plasma metabolomics. *Clin. Chim. Acta* **2015**, *450*, 254–261. [CrossRef]
59. Qiao, S.; Wu, W.; Chen, M.; Tang, Q.; Xia, Y.; Jia, W.; Wang, X. Seminal plasma metabolomics approach for the diagnosis of unexplained male infertility. *PLoS ONE* **2017**, *12*, e0181115. [CrossRef]
60. Deepinder, F.; Chowdary, H.T.; Agarwal, A. Role of metabolomic analysis of biomarkers in the management of male infertility. *Expert Rev. Mol. Diagn.* **2007**, *7*, 351–358. [CrossRef]
61. Zhou, X.; Wang, Y.; Yun, Y.; Xia, Z.; Lu, H.; Luo, J.; Liang, Y. A potential tool for diagnosis of male infertility: Plasma metabolomics based on GC-MS. *Talanta* **2016**, *147*, 82–89. [CrossRef] [PubMed]
62. Jayaraman, V.; Ghosh, S.; Sengupta, A.; Srivastava, S.; Sonawat, H.M.; Narayan, P.K. Identification of biochemical differences between different forms of male infertility by nuclear magnetic resonance (NMR) spectroscopy. *J. Assist. Reprod. Genet.* **2014**, *31*, 1195–1204. [CrossRef] [PubMed]
63. Bonechi, C.; Collodel, G.; Donati, A.; Martini, S.; Moretti, E.; Rossi, C. Discrimination of human semen specimens by NMR data, sperm parameters, and statistical analysis. *Syst. Biol. Reprod. Med.* **2015**, *61*, 353–359. [CrossRef] [PubMed]
64. Gilany, K.; Moazeni-Pourasil, R.S.; Jafarzadeh, N.; Savadi-Shiraz, E. Metabolomics fingerprinting of the human seminal plasma of asthenozoospermic patients. *Mol. Reprod. Dev.* **2014**, *81*, 84–86. [CrossRef]
65. Correnti, S.; Preiano, M.; Fregola, A.; Gamboni, F.; Stephenson, D.; Savino, R.; D'Alessandro, A.; Terracciano, R. Seminal plasma untargeted metabolomic and lipidomic profiling for the identification of a novel panel of biomarkers and therapeutic targets related to male infertility. *Front. Pharmacol.* **2023**, *14*, 1275832. [CrossRef]
66. Jafarzadeh, N.; Mani-Varnosfaderani, A.; Minai-Tehrani, A.; Savadi-Shiraz, E.; Sadeghi, M.R.; Gilany, K. Metabolomics fingerprinting of seminal plasma from unexplained infertile men: A need for novel diagnostic biomarkers. *Mol. Reprod. Dev.* **2015**, *82*, 150. [CrossRef]
67. Minai-Tehrani, A.; Jafarzadeh, N.; Gilany, K. Metabolomics: A state-of-the-art technology for better understanding of male infertility. *Andrologia* **2016**, *48*, 609–616. [CrossRef]
68. Silva, B.; Giudice, P.; Spaine, D.; Gozzo, F.; Turco, E.; Bertolla, R. Metabolomics of male infertility: Characterization of seminal plasma lipid fingerprints in men with spinal cord injury. *Fertil. Steril.* **2011**, *96*, S233. [CrossRef]
69. Majzoub, A.; Esteves, S.C.; Gosalvez, J.; Agarwal, A. Specialized sperm function tests in varicocele and the future of andrology laboratory. *Asian J. Androl.* **2016**, *18*, 205–212. [CrossRef]
70. Agarwal, A.; Panner Selvam, M.K.; Baskaran, S. Proteomic Analyses of Human Sperm Cells: Understanding the Role of Proteins and Molecular Pathways Affecting Male Reproductive Health. *Int. J. Mol. Sci.* **2020**, *21*, 1621. [CrossRef]
71. Panner Selvam, M.K.; Agarwal, A. Proteomic and Metabolomic Profile of Semen and Seminal Plasma in Varicocele. In *Varicocele and Male Infertility*; Springer: Cham, Switzerland, 2019; pp. 73–85.

72. Panner Selvam, M.K.; Agarwal, A.; Sharma, R.; Samanta, L.; Gupta, S.; Dias, T.R.; Martins, A.D. Protein Fingerprinting of Seminal Plasma Reveals Dysregulation of Exosome-Associated Proteins in Infertile Men with Unilateral Varicocele. *World J. Mens Health* **2021**, *39*, 324–337. [CrossRef] [PubMed]
73. Camargo, M.; Intasqui, P.; Belardin, L.B.; Antoniassi, M.P.; Cardozo, K.H.M.; Carvalho, V.M.; Fraietta, R.; Bertolla, R.P. Molecular pathways of varicocele and its repair—A paired labelled shotgun proteomics approach. *J. Proteom.* **2019**, *196*, 22–32. [CrossRef] [PubMed]
74. Kaltsas, A.; Stavros, S.; Kratiras, Z.; Zikopoulos, A.; Machairiotis, N.; Potiris, A.; Dimitriadis, F.; Sofikitis, N.; Chrisofos, M.; Zachariou, A. Predictors of Successful Testicular Sperm Extraction: A New Era for Men with Non-Obstructive Azoospermia. *Biomedicines* **2024**, *12*, 2679. [CrossRef]
75. Neto, F.T.L.; Marques, R.A.; de Freitas Cavalcanti Filho, A.; Araujo, L.C.N.; Lima, S.V.C.; Pinto, L.; Silva, R.O. 1H NMR-based metabonomics for infertility diagnosis in men with varicocele. *J. Assist. Reprod. Genet.* **2020**, *37*, 2233–2247. [CrossRef]
76. Serrano, R.; Garcia-Marin, L.J.; Bragado, M.J. Sperm Phosphoproteome: Unraveling Male Infertility. *Biology* **2022**, *11*, 659. [CrossRef]
77. Huang, X.Y.; Sha, J.H. Proteomics of spermatogenesis: From protein lists to understanding the regulation of male fertility and infertility. *Asian J. Androl.* **2011**, *13*, 18–23. [CrossRef]
78. Wagner, A.O.; Turk, A.; Kunej, T. Towards a Multi-Omics of Male Infertility. *World J. Mens Health* **2023**, *41*, 272–288. [CrossRef]
79. McShane, L.M.; Cavenagh, M.M.; Lively, T.G.; Eberhard, D.A.; Bigbee, W.L.; Williams, P.M.; Mesirov, J.P.; Polley, M.Y.; Kim, K.Y.; Tricoli, J.V.; et al. Criteria for the use of omics-based predictors in clinical trials: Explanation and elaboration. *BMC Med.* **2013**, *11*, 220. [CrossRef]
80. Baskaran, S.; Agarwal, A.; Leisegang, K.; Pushparaj, P.N.; Panner Selvam, M.K.; Henkel, R. An In-Depth Bibliometric Analysis and Current Perspective on Male infertility Research. *World J. Men's Health* **2021**, *39*, 302–314. [CrossRef]
81. Preiano, M.; Correnti, S.; Butt, T.A.; Viglietto, G.; Savino, R.; Terracciano, R. Mass Spectrometry-Based Untargeted Approaches to Reveal Diagnostic Signatures of Male Infertility in Seminal Plasma: A New Laboratory Perspective for the Clinical Management of Infertility? *Int. J. Mol. Sci.* **2023**, *24*, 4429. [CrossRef]
82. Omolaoye, T.S.; Omolaoye, V.A.; Kandasamy, R.K.; Hachim, M.Y.; Du Plessis, S.S. Omics and Male Infertility: Highlighting the Application of Transcriptomic Data. *Life* **2022**, *12*, 280. [CrossRef] [PubMed]
83. Faniev, M.V.; Prokopiev, Y.V.; Faustova, K.V.; Kadyrov, Z.; Vodolazhsky, D.I.; Markelova, M.; Dilyara, K.; Grigoryeva, T.V.; Karslyan, E.M.; Bersanova, M.K.; et al. High-throughput sequencing of the testicular microbiome in patients with non-obstructive azoospermia and varicocele. *Exp. Clinical Urol.* **2023**, *16*, 38–43. [CrossRef]
84. Kaltsas, A.; Zachariou, A.; Markou, E.; Dimitriadis, F.; Sofikitis, N.; Pournaras, S. Microbial Dysbiosis and Male Infertility: Understanding the Impact and Exploring Therapeutic Interventions. *J. Pers. Med.* **2023**, *13*, 1491. [CrossRef] [PubMed]
85. Kaltsas, A.; Markou, E.; Zachariou, A.; Dimitriadis, F.; Mamoulakis, C.; Andreadakis, S.; Giannakis, I.; Tsounapi, P.; Takenaka, A.; Sofikitis, N. Varicoceles in Men with Non-obstructive Azoospermia: The Dilemma to Operate or Not. *Front. Reprod. Health* **2022**, *4*, 811487. [CrossRef] [PubMed]
86. Kovac, J.R.; Pastuszak, A.W.; Lamb, D.J. The use of genomics, proteomics, and metabolomics in identifying biomarkers of male infertility. *Fertil. Steril.* **2013**, *99*, 998–1007. [CrossRef]

Journal of
Clinical Medicine

MDPI

Review

The Roles of GDF-9, BMP-15, BMP-4 and EMMPRIN in Folliculogenesis and In Vitro Fertilization

Serafeim Fountas [1], Efthymia Petinaki [2], Stamatis Bolaris [1], Magdalini Kargakou [1], Stefanos Dafopoulos [3], Athanasios Zikopoulos [4], Efthalia Moustakli [5], Sotirios Sotiriou [6] and Konstantinos Dafopoulos [7,*]

1 Fertility and Sterility Unit, Elena Venizelou General-Maternity District Hospital, 11521 Athens, Greece; serfountas@gmail.com (S.F.); sbolaris@gmail.com (S.B.); magda.kargakou@yahoo.gr (M.K.)
2 Department of Microbiology, University Hospital of Larissa, 41110 Larissa, Greece; petinaki@uth.gr
3 Department of Health Sciences, European University Cyprus, 2404 Nicosia, Cyprus; sn191957@students.euc.ac.cy
4 Royal Devon and Exeter Hospital, Barrack Rd, Exeter EX 25 DW, UK; thanzik92@gmail.com
5 Laboratory of Medical Genetics, Faculty of Medicine, School of Health Sciences, University of Ioannina, 45110 Ioannina, Greece; thaleiamoustakli@gmail.com
6 Department of Embryology, Faculty of Medicine, School of Health Sciences, University of Thessaly, 41110 Larissa, Greece; sotiriousoti@yahoo.gr
7 ART Unit, Department of Obstetrics and Gynecology, Faculty of Medicine, School of Health Sciences, University of Thessaly, 41110 Larissa, Greece
* Correspondence: kdafop@uth.gr

Abstract: Growth differentiation factor 9 (GDF-9) contributes to early ovarian development and oocyte survival. Higher concentrations of GDF-9 in follicular fluid (FF) are associated with oocyte nuclear maturation and optimal embryo development. In in vitro fertilization (IVF), GDF-9 affects the ability of the oocyte to fertilize and subsequent embryonic development. Bone morphogenetic protein 15 (BMP-15) is involved in the regulation of ovarian function and affects oocyte development. During IVF, BMP-15 contributes to the formation of competent blastocysts. BMP-15 may play a role in embryo implantation by affecting endometrial receptivity. Bone morphogenetic protein 4 (BMP-4) is involved in the regulation of follicle growth and development and affects granulosa cell (GC) differentiation. In relation to IVF, BMP-4 is important for embryonic development, influences cell fate and differentiation, and plays a role in facilitating embryo–endometrial interactions during the implantation process. Extracellular matrix metalloproteinase inducer (EMMPRIN) is associated with ovulation and follicle rupture, promotes the release of mature eggs, and affects the modification of the extracellular matrix of the follicular environment. In IVF, EMMPRIN is involved in embryo implantation by modulating the adhesive properties of endometrial cells and promotes trophoblastic invasion, which is essential for pregnancy to occur. The purpose of the current article is to review the studies and recent findings of GDF-9, BMP-15, BMP-4 and EMMPRIN as fundamental factors in normal follicular development and in vitro fertilization.

Keywords: GDF-9; BMP-4; BMP-15; EMMPRIN; normal follicular development; folliculogenesis; in vitro fertilization

1. Introduction

During a normal pregnancy, there are significant physiological adaptations occurring in the uterus, placenta, and maternal circulatory system. The pregnant uterus undergoes growth and expansion to accommodate the developing fetus adequately. Concurrently, the placenta and helical arteries undergo alterations to ensure an ample blood and nutrient supply to support fetal growth. Additionally, notable hemodynamic changes occur in maternal circulation, including increased heart rate, expanded plasma volume and cardiac output, and decreased vascular resistance. These adjustments are orchestrated to optimize blood flow to various organs and reduce strain on the maternal heart. The structural remodeling and functional adjustments in utero-placental tissue and maternal circulation associated with pregnancy represent crucial aspects of gestational physiology [1,2].

The process of embryo selection remains a pivotal consideration in in vitro fertilization (IVF) cycles, particularly in light of legislation mandating single embryo transfer in many countries [3]. The quality of the embryo is intricately linked to the quality of the oocyte, highlighting the significance of oocyte assessment [4]. Traditional approaches have relied on morphological parameters to evaluate oocyte quality; however, studies examining the correlation between oocyte morphology and subsequent embryo quality have yielded conflicting findings, prompting a reevaluation of this paradigm [5–10]. Consequently, recent investigations have shifted focus towards exploring factors within the follicular fluid (FF) that may influence oocyte developmental potential. FF comprises a complex milieu of plasma components, blood-derived factors, and secretory products from oocytes, granulosa cells, and sheath cells [11].

The influence of the follicular microenvironment on oocyte development and embryo quality has been a subject of extensive research since the 1990s [12]. Both oocyte and embryo quality are intricately affected by the hormonal and growth factors present in FF, emphasizing their significant role [13]. However, the precise mechanisms through which these molecules operate remain incompletely understood.

Among the growth factors present in FF, bone morphogenetic proteins (BMPs) and growth differentiation factor 9 (GDF-9), members of the transforming growth factor-β (TGF-β) superfamily, play pivotal roles in oocyte and follicle maturation [14,15] and contribute to various aspects of ovarian function and follicle development, and this is the main reason these proteins were chosen to be reviewed. In particular, growth differentiation factor 9 (GDF-9), bone morphogenetic protein 15 (BMP-15), bone morphogenetic protein 4 (BMP-4) and extracellular matrix metalloproteinase inducer (EMMPRIN) proteins are the subjects of discussion and analysis due to their pivotal roles in ovarian function and female fertility. GDF-9 is particularly essential in the early stages of follicle development, being secreted by oocytes and exerting influence on the proliferation and differentiation of granulosa cells, which are imperative for the establishment of a healthy follicle. Additionally, GDF-9 facilitates communication between the oocyte and surrounding somatic cells, thereby directly impacting oocyte quality and maturation, crucial for successful fertilization and subsequent embryo development. Furthermore, BMP-15 often collaborates with GDF-9 in regulating folliculogenesis, thereby enhancing the efficiency of these processes and underscoring the critical nature of both proteins in proper follicular development [16]. BMP-15 also plays a significant role in regulating granulosa cell function, providing essential support and signaling during oocyte maturation [17]. On the other hand, BMP-4 is involved in the initial phases of follicle development, contributing to cell survival and differentiation, which prepares the follicle for subsequent maturation stages. Moreover, BMP-4 influences the ovarian microenvironment by acting on various somatic cells within the ovary, ensuring an environment conducive to follicle development [18]. Lastly, EMMPRIN is indispensable for extracellular matrix (ECM) remodeling, a process vital for follicle expansion and ovulation. By inducing matrix metalloproteinases (MMPs), EMMPRIN ensures dynamic ECM remodeling to support follicular development. Additionally, it activates intracellular signaling pathways such as MAPK and PI3K/AKT, promoting cell proliferation, survival, and differentiation, thereby further enhancing follicular development and ovulation [19,20].

Mutations impacting the function of these proteins have been associated with decreased fertility in humans, hindering successful conception [21]. The oocyte itself contributes significantly to follicular growth and development through the secretion of its own growth factors, which act paracrinely on the granulosa cells. Mutations in the GDF-9 gene have been identified as causal factors in fertility or infertility in various species, including mice, sheep, and humans. Notably, women with premature ovarian failure (POF) [22–24] and mothers of polyfollicular dizygotic twins [25] have been found to carry numerous GDF-9 mutations [26].

GDF-9 and BMP-15 predominantly govern granulosa cell interaction and oocyte quality, while BMP-4 plays a fundamental role in the initiation of follicle formation. EMMPRIN, on the other hand, orchestrates the structural remodeling necessary for follicle expansion and subsequent ovulation. The proper functioning of these proteins is paramount for female fertility, as disruptions in their pathways can lead to infertility or other reproductive disorders, underscoring their significance as targets for fertility research and therapeutic interventions. These proteins are subjects of extensive study aimed at comprehensively understanding reproductive biology and devising effective treatments for infertility. Their involvement in cell signaling, extracellular matrix remodeling, and follicular development renders them central to discussions regarding ovarian physiology and fertility treatments. The collective analysis of GDF-9, BMP-15, BMP-4, and EMMPRIN offers a holistic perspective on the molecular mechanisms governing ovarian function and female fertility, thereby aiding in the development of advanced reproductive technologies and therapeutic strategies to address infertility [16–20].

Moreover, hormones, particularly those involved in the hypothalamic–pituitary–ovarian (HPO) axis, regulate the entire process of oogenesis. Gonadotropin-releasing hormone (GnRH) from the hypothalamus stimulates the release of FSH and luteinizing hormone from the pituitary gland. FSH promotes follicular development and stimulates the granulosa cells to produce estrogen, which is essential for the growth and maturation of the oocyte. LH triggers ovulation and stimulates the production of progesterone by the corpus luteum, which prepares the uterus for implantation [27]. Additionally, other hormones such as anti-Müllerian hormone (AMH) and inhibin also play roles in regulating folliculogenesis and oocyte maturation. AMH inhibits primordial follicle recruitment, while inhibin suppresses FSH secretion, thereby regulating follicular development and ovulation [28,29]. Age is another crucial factor that affects oogenesis. In females, the number of primordial follicles, which contain immature oocytes, declines with age due to a process called ovarian follicle atresia. This reduction in the ovarian reserve leads to a decline in fertility and an increased risk of chromosomal abnormalities in oocytes, such as aneuploidy. Additionally, aging is associated with changes in hormonal levels, including a decrease in the levels of estrogen and inhibin, which further impact follicular development and ovulation [30]. Therefore, both hormones and age are intricately involved in the process of oogenesis, influencing follicular development, oocyte maturation, and ultimately female fertility.

2. Relevant Sections

2.1. *Growth Differentiation Factor (GDF-9)*

GDF-9 is a member of the TGF-β family and plays a critical role in the early development of the ovaries and the survival of oocytes. It stimulates the proliferation of granulosa cells, facilitates follicle maturation, and contributes to oocyte formation. High levels of mature form of GDF-9 in FF are closely associated with oocyte nuclear maturation and embryo quality of development [21]. Oocyte maturation requires a combination of nuclear and cytoplasmic maturation. Evaluating nuclear maturation is generally considered simpler and more precise than assessing cytoplasmic maturation. Notably, a significant correlation has been identified between nuclear maturation and levels of mature GDF-9, offering strong evidence for the involvement of this paracrine factor in oocyte development [31]. The absence of the GDF-9 gene impedes follicular development to advanced stages, resulting in female infertility. Interestingly, concurrent loss of inhibin, an ovarian hormone, in GDF-9 mutants allows the follicles to resume growth and development [32].

Folliculogenesis is regulated by growth factors produced by oocytes, with numerous growth factors, including GDF-9, identified in mammalian oocytes to date [33]. GDF-9 acts as a paracrine factor within the TGF-β family, facilitating intracellular communication between oocytes and somatic cells, such as granulosa cells, from the early primary follicle stage through to ovulation [34,35].

While the quality of the oocyte is crucial in determining the quality of the embryo, the mechanisms underlying GDF-9 activity are particularly noteworthy. GDF-9 is secreted by the oocyte as an inactive precursor protein and undergoes proteolytic cleavage to form a mature dimer, which then becomes biologically active [36,37]. GDF-9 subsequently binds to type I and type II serine/threonine kinase receptors on granulosa cells, typically involving BMPR-II (type II receptor) and ALK5/ALK6 (type I receptors). Upon ligand binding, a series of events occur: the type II receptor phosphorylates the type I receptor, activating its kinase domain. The activated type I receptor then phosphorylates SMAD2/3 proteins, leading to their activation. Phosphorylated SMAD2/3 forms a complex with SMAD4, which translocates to the nucleus. This complex regulates the transcription of target genes involved in cell proliferation, differentiation, and survival [38–42].

GDF-9 performs various functions, including promoting the proliferation and differentiation of granulosa cells, preventing apoptosis, and supporting cholesterol biosynthesis in cumulus cells [43–45].

Under in vivo conditions, GDF-9 has been shown to stimulate cumulus cell development, inducing the production of a hyaluronic acid-rich matrix during cumulus cell expansion [46]. Moreover, GDF-9 is implicated in the proliferation of granulosa cells in antral follicles before ovulation [47,48]. Studies have reported that recombinant GDF-9 promotes the growth, development, and survival of human follicles, and the injection of exogenous GDF-9 into mouse oocyte maturation culture medium enhances embryo viability and subsequent development [43,49].

An in vivo investigation revealed that the growth factor GDF-9 plays a central role in regulating sheath cell functions. Intraperitoneal injections of GDF-9 in immature rats facilitated the progression of primordial and primary follicles into small preovulatory follicles and led to an upregulation of CYP17 expression in sheath cells [50]. Additionally, GDF-9 stimulates testosterone production in rat preantral follicle cultures. The androgen receptor antagonist flutamide blocks GDF-9-stimulated preantral development, suggesting that GDF-9 acts on both theca cells and granulosa cells to induce the development of preantral follicles at the early antral stage [51].

In the context of in vitro fertilization, GDF-9 plays a crucial role in acquiring oocyte competence and significantly influences the oocyte's ability to fertilize, subsequently impacting embryonic development. GDF-9 is actively engaged in essential follicle–oocyte interactions (maturation, fertilization, embryonic development) required for successful fertilization, affecting both in vitro oocyte maturation and embryo viability [43]. It is necessary for dynamic processes and communication that occur between the oocyte and the surrounding cells and environment as it undergoes maturation and becomes a mature oocyte. These interactions are crucial for successful oocyte development, ovulation, fertilization, and subsequent embryonic development. This role is substantiated by experiments demonstrating that the introduction of exogenous GDF-9 to FSH-cultured mouse granulosa cell–oocyte complexes, prior to in vitro fertilization and subsequent transfer to recipient dams, did not alter the implantation rate or the weight of fetal and placental tissues. However, it did lead to an increase in the number of live embryos [43].

Alterations in the in vitro culture microenvironment can also significantly impact embryonic development. Recent advances have focused on leveraging cumulus granulosa cells and growth factors to enhance the developmental potential of oocytes [52,53]. Zhu et al. (2008) [54] demonstrated that co-culturing immature oocytes with cumulus cells increased the likelihood of polar body exclusion by up to 10% within a 24 h period; however, the embryogenesis rate in these oocytes remained relatively low. Previous studies have investigated the influence of growth factors on embryonic development, with GDF-9 being a key factor secreted by human oocytes during primary follicular development [55]. GDF-9 affects both the early and late stages of follicle growth, primarily by inducing granulosa cell division, suppressing follicle-stimulating hormone (FSH) receptor expression and inducing kit-ligand (KitL) expression in granulosa cells [56–58]. Additionally, GDF-9 induces inhibin-β production and exerts paracrine control over inhibin production in granulosa cells [59].

In vitro studies have shown that GDF-9 can sustain survival, stimulate both oocyte and follicle growth, and activate primordial follicles when cultured in situ. This has been demonstrated with ovarian tissue fragments from women [49] and goats [60]. When preantral follicles were cultured in isolation, GDF-9 effectively promoted the growth of follicles and oocytes in mice [61]. Positive outcomes were observed when a medium containing ascorbic acid was supplemented with 200 ng/mL GDF-9, enhancing the survival of isolated preantral follicles cultured in vitro, particularly in goats [62,63]. However, there is currently a lack of information on the effect of GDF-9 on the in vitro culture of isolated early antral follicles in mammals.

Research on the expression of GDF-9 and its correlation with infertility in individuals with endometriosis is limited. Observations indicate lower GDF-9 expression in women with endometriosis. Recent studies on the granulosa cells of women with endometriosis undergoing controlled ovarian stimulation revealed a significant reduction in GDF-9 mRNA expression in those with moderate to severe endometriosis compared to women without the condition. This reduction results in compromised oocyte maturation and embryo quality [64–66]. GDF-9 levels were found to be lower in the endometriosis group than in the control group, although a direct relationship between individual GDF-9 levels and oocyte quality was not established [67].

The ovarian phenotype characterized by cystic formations is similar to the ovarian morphology observed in women with polycystic ovary syndrome (PCOS). PCOS is the most prevalent cause of anovulation, infertility, and menstrual cycle irregularities in women, affecting approximately 5–10% of women of reproductive age [68]. Analysis of ovarian tissues from women with PCOS revealed a notable delay and decrease in GDF-9 expression during the growth and differentiation phases [69]. In a study comparing oocytes collected from women with and without PCOS after ovarian stimulation, these oocytes gradually matured through in vitro maturation. The results indicated dynamic changes in GDF-9 mRNA expression in the oocytes of women without PCOS [70]. Specifically, the expression of GDF-9 decreased from the germinal vesicle (GV) stage to the metaphase I (MI) stage, contrary to findings by Chen et al. (2009) [71]. Subsequently, GDF-9 expression increased from the MI to the metaphase II (MII) stage, reaching its peak at the final mature stage. In contrast, oocytes from women with PCOS showed no statistically significant changes in GDF-9 expression, and the expression levels in mature oocytes did not reach those observed in normal oocytes.

2.2. Bone Morphogenetic Protein (BMP-15)

BMP-15, a member of the TGF-β family, is crucial in regulating ovarian function and influencing oocyte development. It plays a significant role in controlling ovulation rates and oocyte quality, thereby contributing to the initiation of pregnancy [72]. Additionally, BMP-15 actively promotes follicular growth and exerts significant influence during the initial gonadotrophin-independent phases of folliculogenesis. It regulates the production of follicular granulosa cells, protecting these cells from apoptosis and enhancing their proficiency in supporting oocyte maturation [73]. The involvement of BMP-15 in early follicular development exhibits species-specific characteristics, highlighting distinctions between mono- and poly-ovulatory species [74,75]. Within ovarian follicle development, the BMP-15 gene plays a crucial role in the proliferation and differentiation of granulosa cells [76]. It encourages granulosa cell division while concurrently suppressing the expression of FSH receptors. Due to the significant impact of BMP-15 gene mutations on ovulation rate, litter size, and fertility, this gene is recognized as a key player and a potential marker for breeding in livestock, particularly in sheep [77,78]. BMP-15 exhibits the characteristic cysteine motif found in TGF-β factors, comprising a specific sequence of cysteine amino acids. Notably, BMP-15 diverges from most of these factors by possessing only six of the seven cysteine residues [34,35,79]. Functionally, BMP-15 acts as a potential activator of cell mitosis, contributing significantly to granulosa cell proliferation [31]. As an X-linked gene, its expression spans from the primary stage of oocytes to ovulation [80]. The BMP-15 gene is crucial for promoting granulosa cell growth and regulating folliculogenesis, particularly during the FSH-dependent phase [81].

Researchers have investigated the potential involvement of the BMP-15 gene in premature ovarian insufficiency (POI) [82,83]. The BMP-15 protein consists of an n-terminal pro-domain and a C-terminal mature domain. During the assembly of the BMP-15 molecule, the pro-domain folds to form a mature growth factor dimer [84]. A furinase-like protease, released from the oocyte, subsequently cleaves the BMP-15 protein into several fragments. Unlike many other factors, BMP-15 typically functions as a non-covalent dimer due to the absence of cysteine residues necessary for forming intermolecular disulfide bonds [85]. The rearrangement of the pro-domain allows human BMP-15 (hBMP-15) to be expressed as a type I (ALK6) and type II (BMPRII) receptor group [86]. BMP-15 significantly stimulates mRNA expression of granulosa KitL, a crucial factor in early follicular development [85]. In this capacity, BMP-15 acts as a negative regulator in the interaction between the oocyte and somatic granulosa cells. It promotes the expression of KitL by granulosa cells, which in turn inhibits BMP-15 expression from the oocyte through the binding of KitL to its receptor on the oocyte surface [31,73]. Moreover, BMP-15 is initially secreted as an inactive precursor by the oocyte and subsequently undergoes proteolytic cleavage to form a mature, active dimer. Additionally, BMP-15 binds to both type I and type II serine/threonine kinase receptors located on granulosa cells [41]. Common receptors in this process include BMPR-II (type II receptor) and ALK6/ALK4 (type I receptors). Furthermore, upon ligand binding, the type II receptor phosphorylates the type I receptor, which in turn phosphorylates SMAD1/5/8 proteins. Ultimately, phosphorylated SMAD1/5/8 proteins form a complex with SMAD4, which translocates to the nucleus to regulate the transcription of genes involved in granulosa cell proliferation and differentiation [33,34,82,87–90].

Throughout the development of ovarian follicles, BMP-15, secreted by the oocyte, significantly contributes to follicle development through the paracrine signaling pathway [91]. Its involvement extends from the progression of primordial to primary follicles to the inhibition of early luteinization [92]. BMP-15 exerts regulatory control over the steroidogenesis acute regulatory protein (StAR) and hinders early follicular luteinization by suppressing the luteinizing hormone receptor (LHR). These effects on follicle cell function can ultimately result in the absence of dominant follicles [93]. Following ovulation, the rapid reduction of these oocyte factors in the corpus luteum amplifies StAR expression, thereby regulating follicle maturation by modulating the differentiating effects of FSH [58]. Additionally, BMP-15 has a significant role in governing ovulation rates, oocyte health, and the initiation of pregnancy [72].

In vitro studies on murine granulosa cells reveal that BMP-15 stimulates granulosa cell proliferation and KitL expression while concurrently inhibiting FSH receptor expression [94]. Furthermore, in vitro fertilization studies highlight the significance of BMP-15 in embryonic development, contributing to the formation of competent blastocysts. BMP-15 may also influence embryo implantation by affecting endometrial receptivity. Given the consistent expression of BMP-15 by the oocyte throughout all stages of follicular development, including post-ovulation from cumulus–oocyte complexes, BMP-15 levels in FF are considered predictive of oocyte quality and the subsequent quality and development of corresponding embryos. Research demonstrates a statistically significant association between higher levels of BMP-15 in FF and elevated fertilization rates, increased early hatching rates, and improved quality of embryos with potentially normal development. Additionally, studies reveal a statistically significant positive correlation between BMP-15 levels in the FF of women with a poor response to ovarian stimulation programs. In this context, higher levels of BMP-15 are linked to an improved response in women, manifested by an increased number of produced follicles and, consequently, a heightened rate of fertilization and pregnancy [78,95]. A significant challenge in the in vitro growth of ovarian preantral follicles is the lower rates of oocyte maturation and embryo development compared to in vivo samples. Recognizing this, and in light of various researchers' efforts to enhance follicle development rates in diverse culture systems using different factors, a study was conducted to assess follicular growth and development in mouse ovaries under the influence of BMP-15 [96].

Furthermore, maintaining female fertility fundamentally relies on the normal functioning of BMP-15 in the ovary. Research in sheep has uncovered various mutations in the BMP-15 gene, which correlate with increased folliculogenesis rates in heterozygotes and infertility in homozygotes [21,97,98]. Similarly, human studies underscore the crucial role of BMP-15 in preserving female fertility. Infertile women experiencing early ovarian failure syndrome and PCOS have been found to carry BMP-15 gene mutations [82,83,94]. However, insights from studies involving BMP-15 gene knockout mice suggest that the regulation of folliculogenesis and ovulation does not follow a uniform pattern across species. Homozygous BMP-15-null mice exhibit normal follicular development but experience mild infertility, primarily due to minor dysfunctions in ovulation and fertilization [94]. Among the BMPs, BMP-15 is particularly important for enhancing reproductive performance in female livestock [99]. Its physiological effects are especially pronounced during the early stages of follicle development in sheep [91] and are evident across various livestock species during this stage [58,100]. BMP-15 influences the ovulation rate in livestock through various mechanisms. It actively participates in ovarian follicle formation, and its impact is modulated by the binding protein follistatin, which binds to BMP-15 and blocks its effect on FSH receptor expression in granulosa cells [74,101]. As more follicular lesions synthesize luteinizing hormone receptor (LHR), additional follicles continue developing in the pre-ovulatory phase even as follicle-stimulating hormone receptor (FSHR) levels decrease, resulting in increased oocyte secretion during the anovulatory phase [102]. Mutations in the BMP-15 gene in domestic animals have been linked to higher ovulation rates and a greater proportion of twins in heterozygous animals, while homozygous animals exhibit infertility [74]. This mutation leads to elevated FSHR and LHR levels, increasing granulosa cell density, potentially inhibiting granulosa cell apoptosis, and enhancing ovulation rates [100–102]. Reduced BMP-15 signaling sensitizes granulosa cells to FSH, promoting follicle selection during the follicular phase and leading to improved ovulation in mutant females (ewes) [103]. Conversely, homozygous females (ewes) with BMP-15 mutations exhibit early inhibition of follicle growth and reduced granulosa cell sensitivity to FSH due to inhibited FSH receptor expression [102]. In mutant sheep and cattle with low BMP-15 levels, BMP-15 helps control granulosa cell proliferation by suppressing FSH receptor expression [103–105]. Throughout follicle and oocyte maturation in farm animals, BMP signaling significantly impacts fertility by regulating sex hormone secretion, gonadotropin receptor gene expression, and oocyte quality [58,104]. Additionally, BMP signaling is closely associated with ovulation rates and the estrous cycle [15].

2.3. Bone Morphogenetic Protein (BMP-4)

Ovarian stromal and cumulus cells are known to synthesize BMP-4, which is purported to exert a pivotal role in facilitating the transition from primordial to primary follicles [35]. This protein has been associated with the augmentation of primary and secondary follicles, as well as an increased abundance of primary follicles [106]. As a constituent of the TGF-β family, BMP-4 is intricately involved in gene regulation, exerting influence over gene expression within the oocyte. It is initially synthesized as an inactive precursor protein by various cell types within the ovarian environment. Following proteolytic cleavage, BMP-4 undergoes activation, leading to the formation of a mature dimer [28]. Additionally, BMP-4 interacts with type I and type II serine/threonine kinase receptors present on ovarian somatic cells, including granulosa and theca cells. Key receptors involved in this interaction include BMPR-II (type II receptor) and ALK3/ALK6 (type I receptors). Upon ligand binding, the type II receptor phosphorylates the type I receptor, initiating downstream signaling cascades. Subsequently, the activated type I receptor phosphorylates SMAD1/5/8 proteins, resulting in the formation of a complex with SMAD4. This complex translocates to the nucleus, where it regulates gene transcription processes crucial for early follicular development, cellular survival, and differentiation [33,42,82,88–90].

During the course of typical follicle development, BMP-4 assumes a regulatory role in orchestrating the growth and maturation of follicles, thereby influencing the differentiation of granulosa cells. In the realm of IVF, BMP-4 holds considerable significance for embryonic development, exerting influence over cellular destiny and participating in facilitating interactions between the embryo and the endometrium during the implantation process. The precise mechanistic underpinnings of BMP-4 in the follicle remain incompletely elucidated. Nevertheless, it is hypothesized that BMP-4 likely impedes the apoptosis of human granulosa cells, retards early differentiation, and preserves their steroidogenic properties [107]. In a conducted study [21], increased levels of BMP-4 were noted in women who achieved clinical pregnancy compared to those who did not, verifying the existing literature on the pivotal role of BMP-4 in follicular development. Notably, the inactivation of BMP-4 leads to embryonic lethality, attributed to abnormalities both within and outside the embryo, including aberrations in the formation of the posterior/ventral mesoderm [108].

The significance of BMP-4 in the intricate process of folliculogenesis is notable. Its presence has been consistently detected in the ovaries of female mice throughout all stages of follicular development, indicating a potential involvement in the transition from primordial to primary follicles [109]. Furthermore, BMP-4 is implicated in the regulation of both oocytes and granulosa cells [110,111]. In vitro investigations have revealed a substantial augmentation in cell numbers in oocytes treated with BMP-4 in a dose-dependent manner, with this response being hindered in a dose–response relationship when co-administered with noggin. Administration of BMP-4 into rat ovaries resulted in a notable increase in developing primary follicles and an associated decrease in primordial follicles. Additionally, it was observed that the inclusion of neutralizing BMP-4 antibodies in the culture medium led to diminished ovary size, reduced oocyte and primary follicle counts, and increased cellular apoptosis [112]. Treatment with 100 ng/mL BMP-4 for 6 days in the in vitro culture media has been associated with an enlargement of primary and secondary follicles. However, some animal studies have contested the impact of BMP-4 on the transition process from primordial to primary follicles [14]. Nevertheless, the loss of BMP-4 function leads to the impairment of the formation of primordial germ cells, which serve as the embryonic precursors of gametes (spermatocytes or oocytes) [79]. Furthermore, BMP-4 has been detected in various ovarian compartments, including the ovarian surface epithelium, corpus luteum, and around follicle stromal cells [111,113,114]. Notably, BMP-4 exhibits strong expression in oocyte cumulus cells. Moreover, the influence of BMP-4 on GCs induces substantial alterations in the response of FSH on estradiol and progesterone production in mammalian ovaries [115].

2.4. *Extracellular Matrix Metalloproteinase Inducer (EMMPRIN)*

EMMPRIN, also recognized as Basigin (CD147), is a transmembrane glycoprotein belonging to the immunoglobulin superfamily [116]. Initially denoted as tumor cell-derived collagenase-stimulating factor (TCSF), it underwent renaming to EMMPRIN due to its involvement in inducing extracellular matrix metalloproteinases via both normal and pathological cell–cell interactions [117]. Its ramifications span across tissue remodeling and various pathological conditions such as cancer, rheumatoid arthritis, heart failure, and atherosclerosis. EMMPRIN serves to stimulate MMP-9 production and can modulate MMPs in endothelial cells and tumors [118,119]. A plethora of studies underscore EMMPRIN's involvement in processes including angiogenesis, neuronal signaling, tumorigenesis, wound healing, follicle maturation, and embryo implantation [120–124].

Throughout the course of normal follicle development, EMMPRIN plays a pivotal role in ovulation and follicular rupture, facilitating the release of mature eggs. It exerts influence over the modification of the extracellular matrix within the follicular environment, a critical factor for the proper development of follicles. In the context of a healthy full-term pregnancy, EMMPRIN contributes to maintaining the delicate balance between uterine contraction and relaxation, a regulation pivotal for normal pregnancy. Any disruption in these mechanisms may precipitate preterm labor, with adverse consequences for both the pregnancy and the prematurely born infant. Initial research has explored the levels of EMMPRIN in human FF, highlighting its potential significance in reproductive processes [21]. In the context of the IVF, EMMPRIN emerges as an active participant in embryo implantation, modulating the adhesive properties of endometrial cells and facilitating trophoblastic invasion—processes crucial for successful pregnancy outcomes [21,124].

The precise physiological mechanisms underlying EMMPRIN's involvement in follicle growth and corpus luteum formation remain elusive. Nonetheless, a prevailing hypothesis suggests that EMMPRIN facilitates the activation of matrix metalloproteinases, thereby promoting crucial processes such as follicular development, ovulation rupture, and corpus luteum formation. Studies have reported a significant decrease in fertilization rates in oocytes deficient in EMMPRIN [117]. Actually, EMMPRIN is a transmembrane glycoprotein localized on the surface of various cells within the ovary, including granulosa cells and theca cells. It stimulates the expression and activation of matrix metalloproteinases (MMPs) in neighboring cells. MMPs are enzymes responsible for degrading components of the extracellular matrix (ECM). By inducing MMP expression, EMMPRIN facilitates the remodeling of the ECM, which is essential for follicular expansion and ovulation [125–127]. ECM degradation enables the structural changes necessary for follicle growth and oocyte release. Furthermore, EMMPRIN has the capability to activate intracellular signaling pathways, such as the MAPK and PI3K/AKT pathways. These pathways play crucial roles in cell proliferation, survival, and differentiation [128–130]. Of crucial importance is the noted decline in placental MMP expression during pregnancy, which mirrors a corresponding reduction in placental EMMPRIN expression. This underscores EMMPRIN's significance as a principal stimulator of MMPs in diverse tissues throughout pregnancy. The etiology behind the observed decrease in placental MMPs and EMMPRIN in late pregnancy remains uncertain, potentially linked to the placenta's capacity to generate MMPs or the varying roles of MMPs at different stages of pregnancy.

While EMMPRIN exhibits diverse molecular and cellular properties, its principal function resides in stimulating the synthesis of various matrix metalloproteinases [131]. EMMPRIN molecules are expressed at varying levels across epithelial, endothelial, and leukemic cells [132], as well as in a multitude of other cell types [133]. EMMPRINs are implicated in a variety of fundamental cellular processes, including lymphocyte sensitization and intracellular trafficking [134]. In the context of cancer and inflammatory disorders, EMMPRINs, either directly or indirectly through their interaction with partner molecules, can instigate the activation of matrix metalloproteinases responsible for ECM degradation, cell adhesion, and intercellular communication. Moreover, they have the capacity to induce the differentiation of myofibroblasts associated with ECM deposition and contraction. The precise mechanisms governing the transition between fibrosis and lysis remain elusive; however, EMMPRINs may contribute by up-regulating MMPs secreted by neighboring fibroblasts, thereby assuming a pivotal role in promoting tumor invasion, growth/progression, and metastasis—an assertion supported by existing evidence [124,135].

In rats, an elevation in ovarian EMMPRIN levels during luteinization has been observed, implying its functional significance in this context [16,136]. Disruptions in EMMPRIN have been linked with infertility in both male and female mice [95,109]. EMMPRIN is implicated in various reproductive processes, including oocyte maturation, fertilization, implantation, and early embryonic development [21,117,137], exerting influence over follicle regulation and the degeneration of follicular tissue. While extensive research has delineated the role of EMMPRIN in tumor growth and metastasis, its precise mechanisms in oral squamous cell carcinoma (OSCC) tumorigenesis remain incompletely understood [138]. However, in the realm of reproduction, EMMPRIN emerges as a crucial cell surface molecule involved in early embryogenesis. Experimental findings indicate its significance in development and reproduction, as evidenced by studies involving knockout mice lacking the basigin gene (Bsg), which predominantly succumb before or after implantation, with the few surviving adult mice exhibiting infertility [139]. EMMPRIN's activity in modulating the heightened expression of matrix metalloproteinases (MMPs) induced by sex hormones underscores its role in reproductive physiology. Additionally, EMMPRIN undergoes upregulation in the uterus and aorta of pregnant rats and virgin rats treated with sex hormones [140], suggesting its involvement in hormonal regulation during pregnancy [141].

Despite observations from various animal studies indicating elevated EMMPRIN levels during follicle growth and luteinization, lower EMMPRIN levels were reported in FF samples from women achieving clinical pregnancy. This discrepancy may stem from differences in measurement methods for EMMPRIN; previous studies primarily relied on immunohistologic staining, whereas the present investigation measured EMMPRIN levels in FF samples. Alternatively, the variation could be associated with the correlation between EMMPRIN and luteinization. In a rat model, an increase in EMMPRIN mRNA levels was found during luteinization post-ovulation [136]. Notably, increased EMMPRIN expression during the early corpus luteum (CL) phase in mouse ovaries declines following human chorionic gonadotropin (hCG) stimulation [142]. If increased EMMPRIN levels indeed correlate with follicular luteinization, assessing follicular EMMPRIN levels could serve as an indicator of early luteinization in patients undergoing IVF treatment [117]. The observed reduction in fertility in EMMPRIN-null mutant oocytes, coupled with EMMPRIN's localization in granulosa cells and theca cells during the pre-ovulatory phase, underscores its efficacy in follicle formation and oocyte maturation [117,124].

3. Interaction between Proteins

3.1. Interaction between GDF-9 and BMP-15

GDF-9 and BMP-15, belonging to the TGF-β superfamily, are pivotal in multiple facets of typical follicle development, encompassing oocyte growth, granulosa cell function, and follicle maturation. Their significant contributions to female fertility and infertility have been extensively corroborated in scholarly investigations [37,73,81,142,143]. Both factors are indispensable for normal reproductive processes and may serve as indicators of embryo development. They govern the provision of granulosa cells to the oocyte, serve as a defense against reactive oxygen species, and furnish essential nourishment to the oocyte through mechanisms such as cholesterol biosynthesis and glycolysis [35,143,144].

BMP-15 contributes to granulosa cell proliferation, differentiation, and follicular development, facilitating the transition of follicles from the early to the FSH phase. Conversely, GDF-9 assumes a pivotal role in orchestrating ovarian function and enhancing the developmental competence of oocytes intrinsically. It forms non-covalent heterodimers within the oocyte, exerting synergistic effects on adjacent follicular granulosa cells. This cooperative mechanism implies that BMP-15 and GDF-9 collaborate to promote ovulation, sustain oocyte vitality, and support the occurrence of pregnancy [145]. GDF-9 and BMP-15 frequently collaborate synergistically to regulate folliculogenesis and oocyte development. These proteins are co-expressed within oocytes and exert their influence on surrounding granulosa cells. GDF-9 and BMP-15 bind to specific serine/threonine kinase receptors present on granulosa cells, thereby initiating intracellular signaling cascades. This activation results in the phosphorylation of SMAD proteins, notably SMAD2 and SMAD3, which subsequently form complexes with SMAD4. These complexes translocate to the nucleus, where they regulate the transcription of target genes essential for granulosa cell proliferation, differentiation, and follicle development. The synergistic interplay between GDF-9 and BMP-15 augments the efficiency of these processes, thereby facilitating the proper maturation of follicles and oocytes [34,42,144].

Due to their potential to forecast oocyte quality and quantity, along with their substantial positive correlation with antral follicle count, the secretion of GDF-9 and BMP-15 in FF can serve as markers of ovarian reserve. The concentrations of these factors in FF reflect the quality (maturity) of retrieved oocytes post-stimulation. Investigations have delved into the link between serum levels of BMP-15 and GDF-9 during IVF and the yield of produced oocytes, particularly in women afflicted with genital disorders and polycystic ovary syndrome [146–149]. The evident nexus between mutations/deletions in GDF-9 and BMP-15 genes and their biologically active properties in follicular cells underscores the significance of these factors in female infertility [143,144].

It has been suggested that high BMP-15 levels in FF are associated with enhanced fertilization rates and embryo development [95]. However, these disparate findings may stem from variations in experimental conditions and dimeric structures. Notably, a significant correlation was found between FF levels of mature forms of GDF-9 and BMP-15. In mice, BMP-15 was identified as a multimer consisting of the pro-region and mature protein when bound to GDF-9 [150]. Additionally, the effects of mutations in BMP-15 were only apparent when the mutant BMP-15 protein was co-expressed with GDF-9 [151]. Importantly, this effect was intensified in co-expression scenarios and aligns with the concept that GDF-9 may exert substantial biological activity against BMP-15 in humans [152].

Enhancements in the development of in vitro matured oocytes to the blastocyst stage were observed with the administration of GDF-9 or BMP-15 to oocyte complexes [153]. Furthermore, evidence from human FF supports the idea that IVF outcomes could be improved by supplementing the oocyte culture medium with the mature form of GDF-9 [154].

Dysfunction of these two factors may indicate primary ovarian failure (POF), a condition impacting ovarian function that impedes the production of mature follicles in young women [84]. In cases of GDF-9 deficiency, there is a reduction in granulosa cell proliferation, abnormal oocyte growth, and a failure of follicles to progress beyond the primary stage [16]. GDF-9 also plays a role in inhibiting granulosa cell apoptosis and preventing follicle closure. The mature forms of GDF-9 and BMP-15 can exist as homodimeric or heterodimeric structures [152]. However, the significance of proforms, mature forms, and bilaterals in humans remains uncertain. Mature forms of BMP-15 and GDF-9 were not detected in the FF of 39.5% and 4.9% of infertile women, respectively, suggesting a potential issue in the production of mature forms of these growth factors in these individuals. Possible explanations include mutations in the GDF-9 and BMP-15 genes leading to reduced protein production or incomplete post-transcriptional processing of proforms, contributing to a diminished production of mature forms. A more comprehensive analysis is necessary to elucidate the challenges associated with generating biologically active forms of these growth factors [144,153].

Conversely, BMP-15 induces mitosis and the proliferation of granulosa cells [75]. The identification of homozygous mutations in GDF-9 and BMP-15 in infertile sheep underscores their critical role in these species [154]. Mutations in BMP-15 have also been observed in women with ovaries secreting abnormal levels of gonadotropins [82]. Both GDF-9 and BMP-15 act to inhibit gonadotropin-stimulated progesterone secretion [35,155]. Additionally, these two paracrine factors secreted by oocytes regulate the proliferation, apoptosis, metabolism, and expansion of cumulus cells [37].

A significant correlation has been established between the levels of mature GDF-9 and BMP-15 in FF [156]. In conjunction with GDF-9, mouse BMP-15 is observed to form a polymer of prodomains and mature proteins [150]. Furthermore, the impact of BMP-15 mutants became evident only when the mutant BMP-15 proteins were co-expressed with GDF-9 [151,152]. These findings substantiate the proposition that GDF-9 exerts a substantial influence on BMP-15 in humans [153].

Further studies have indicated that both GDF-9 and BMP-15 influence steroidogenesis and impede premature luteinization [90,156]. Specifically, while GDF-9 alone does not stimulate steroidogenesis, its co-administration suppresses progesterone and estradiol production induced by FSH [127]. A significant discovery is the negative correlation observed between mature forms of GDF-9 and progesterone levels in FF, suggesting the involvement of this paracrine factor in the luteinization process. Therefore, the elevated levels of mature GDF-9 in FF are evidently associated with oocyte nuclear maturation and embryo development [153].

A combination of autocrine/paracrine factors play a crucial role in the growth and differentiation of ovarian follicles [157]. In domestic animals, the expression patterns of BMPs ligands and receptors suggest the significant involvement of the BMPs system and GDF-9 in this intrafollicular network [91]. The BMPs system and GDF-9 jointly regulate granulosa cell proliferation, differentiation, and apoptosis throughout follicle formation [158], acting through autocrine/paracrine mechanisms within the ovary [159]. Oocyte-derived growth factors GDF-9 and BMP-15 are selectively expressed by oocytes from the primordial stage in ruminants and collaboratively influence litter size during follicle development [160]. These oocyte growth factors are essential not only in the early stages but also in the later stages of follicle development [35]. They play a fundamental role in the differentiation of various granulosa cells, regulating crucial granulosa cell functions and influencing gene expression patterns in somatic follicle cells [145]. Additionally, BMP-15 and GDF-9 control the expression of hyaluronan synthase 2, crucial for matrix formation necessary for cumulus cell expansion, thereby participating in the stimulation of cumulus cell expansion [58]. Furthermore, both GDF-9 and BMP-15 significantly contribute to oocyte health and the occurrence of pregnancy, regulating the ovulation rate [34,72].

There is supporting evidence for a combination of BMP-15 and GDF-9 mutations, as demonstrated by females with mutations in both BMP-15 and GDF-9 ovulating more frequently compared to heterozygotes with mutations in only one of them [72]. Consequently, it becomes crucial to consider the interplay between BMP-15 and GDF-9 in follicle development, which subsequently influences the number of births in livestock.

3.2. Interaction between BMP-4 and EMMPRIN

The interaction between BMP-4 and EMMPRIN involves BMP-4's influence on early follicular development and cellular survival, as well as EMMPRIN's role in ECM remodeling by inducing MMP expression and activating intracellular signaling pathways. BMP-4 functions through serine/threonine kinase receptors and SMAD proteins, predominantly influencing early follicular development and cellular survival [34]. EMMPRIN facilitates ECM remodeling by inducing MMP expression and activating intracellular signaling pathways to support cell proliferation and differentiation, which are pivotal for follicular development and ovulation. Grasping these mechanisms is imperative for enhancing reproductive technologies and therapeutic interventions in fertility treatments [28,32,39,44].

Both BMP-4 and EMMPRIN contribute to processes associated with follicular development and pregnancy, albeit in distinct capacities, as integral components of the intricate regulatory network governing the female reproductive process. They are integral to a signaling pathway involving interactions with other growth factors, cytokines, and extracellular matrix components [21].

A correlation was identified between BMP-4 levels and clinical pregnancy, and the combination of BMP-4 with EMMPRIN demonstrated a sensitivity and specificity of 67% each in predicting clinical pregnancy [21]. Cumulative evidence suggests that the quantity of BMP-4 in FF serves as a reliable marker for predicting the outcome of IVF/ICSI. While the existing literature implies a positive impact of these cytokines on follicle maturation and implantation, it merely hints at the potential use of these markers for predicting clinical pregnancy. Consequently, the findings of the aforementioned study do not offer an interpretation of the relationship between the levels of these proteins and embryo development and quality. However, the higher rate of MII (metaphase II) oocytes in the pregnancy group supports the hypothesis that BMP-4 and EMMPRIN might play a role in follicle formation and oocyte maturation [21].

BMP-4 collaborates with EMMPRIN to facilitate follicular development and ovulation. BMP-4 is secreted by various cells within the ovary, including granulosa and theca cells. It interacts with specific serine/threonine kinase receptors on ovarian somatic cells, such as granulosa and theca cells, initiating signaling pathways that promote cell survival, differentiation, and follicular development [36,37]. Concurrently, EMMPRIN, localized on the surface of various ovarian cells, induces the expression and activation of MMPs in neighboring cells. MMPs are enzymes responsible for degrading components of the ECM. Through inducing MMP expression, EMMPRIN facilitates the remodeling of the

ECM, thereby enabling structural changes necessary for follicle expansion and ovulation. Collectively, BMP-4 and EMMPRIN contribute to the dynamic regulation of the ovarian microenvironment, promoting follicular development and ovulation [38–40].

4. Conclusions

In summary, female infertility represents a significant health issue, with genetic factors playing a pivotal role. GDF-9 contributes to early ovarian development and oocyte viability, stimulates granulosa cell proliferation, facilitates follicle maturation, and participates in oocyte formation. Higher concentrations of mature GDF-9 in FF are notably associated with oocyte nuclear maturation and embryo development. BMP-15 regulates ovarian function and impacts oocyte development. During IVF, BMP-15 is essential for embryonic development and aids in the formation of competent blastocysts. BMP-4 is involved in gene regulation within the oocyte, influencing gene expression patterns. In normal follicle development, it governs follicle growth and differentiation and influences granulosa cell maturation. In the context of IVF, BMP-4 is crucial for embryonic development, modulates cell fate and differentiation, and facilitates embryo–endometrial interactions during implantation. EMMPRIN contributes to follicle regulation and degeneration of follicular tissue. During normal follicular development, it is associated with ovulation and follicle rupture, promotes the release of mature eggs, and affects modifications in the extracellular matrix of the follicular environment, which is vital for follicle development. In the context of IVF, EMMPRIN plays a role in embryo implantation by modulating the adhesive properties of endometrial cells and promoting trophoblastic invasion, essential for successful pregnancy establishment.

Conclusively, GDF-9 and BMP-15 exhibit synergistic effects on each other. Their cooperative mechanism implies that these variables collaborate to promote ovulation, sustain oocyte vitality, and support the occurrence of pregnancy. Therefore, their interaction suggests a synergistic effect, where the combined action of both GDF-9 and BMP-15 enhances the efficiency of folliculogenesis and oocyte development. Moreover, the relationship between BMP-4 and EMMPRIN appears to be more synergistic than antagonistic. Although they have distinct roles, their actions seem to complement each other in promoting follicular development and tissue remodeling. Therefore, their interaction suggests a synergistic effect, where the combined action of both BMP-4 and EMMPRIN contributes to the overall regulation of folliculogenesis and ECM dynamics.

Funding: This research received no external funding.

Conflicts of Interest: The authors declare no conflicts of interest.

References

1. Valdes, G.; Corthorn, J. Review: The angiogenic and vasodilatory utero-placental network. *Placenta* **2011**, *32* (Suppl. 2), S170–S175. [CrossRef] [PubMed]
2. Mandala, M.; Osol, G. Physiological Remodeling of the Maternal Uterine Circulation during Pregnancy. *Basic. Clin. Pharmacol. Toxicol.* **2012**, *110*, 12–18. [CrossRef] [PubMed]
3. Lan, K.C.; Huang, F.J.; Lin, Y.C.; Kung, F.T.; Hsieh, C.H.; Huang, H.W.; Tan, P.H.; Chang, S.Y. The predictive value of using a combined Z-score and day 3 embryo morphology score in the assessment of embryo survival on day 5. *Hum. Reprod.* **2003**, *18*, 1299–1306. [CrossRef] [PubMed]
4. Wang, Q.; Sun, Q.Y. Evaluation of oocyte quality: Morphological, cellular and molecular predictors. *Reprod. Fertil. Dev.* **2007**, *19*, 1–12. [CrossRef] [PubMed]
5. Rienzi, L.; Ubaldi, F.M.; Iacobelli, M.; Minasi, M.G.; Romano, S.; Ferrero, S.; Sapienza, F.; Baroni, E.; Litwicka, K.; Greco, E. Significance of metaphase II human oocyte morphology on ICSI outcome. *Fertil. Steril.* **2008**, *90*, 1692–1700. [CrossRef]
6. de Sutter, P.; Dozortsev, D.; Qian, C.; Dhont, M. Oocyte morphology does not correlate with fertilization rate and embryo quality after intracytoplasmic sperm injection. *Hum. Reprod.* **1996**, *11*, 595–597. [CrossRef]
7. Xia, P. Intracytoplasmic sperm injection: Correlation of oocyte grade based on polar body, perivitelline space and cytoplasmic inclusions with fertilization rate and embryo quality. *Hum. Reprod.* **1997**, *12*, 1750–1755. [CrossRef] [PubMed]
8. Mikkelsen, A.L.; Lindenberg, S. Morphology of in-vitro matured oocytes: Impact on fertility potential and embryo quality. *Hum. Reprod.* **2001**, *16*, 1714–1718. [CrossRef] [PubMed]

9. Balaban, B.; Urman, B.; Sertac, A.; Alatas, C.; Aksoy, S.; Mercan, R. Oocyte morphology does not affect fertilization rate, embryo quality and implantation rate after intracytoplasmic sperm injection. *Hum. Reprod.* **1998**, *13*, 3431–3433. [CrossRef]
10. Balaban, B.; Urman, B. Effect of oocyte morphology on embryo development and implantation. *Reprod. Biomed. Online* **2006**, *12*, 608–615. [CrossRef]
11. Revelli, A.; delle Piane, L.; Casano, S.; Molinari, E.; Massobrio, M.; Rinaudo, P. Follicular fluid content and oocyte quality: From single biochemical markers to metabolomics. *Reprod. Biol. Endocrinol.* **2009**, *4*, 7–40. [CrossRef]
12. Burge, G.C.; Hanson, M.A.; Slater-Jefferies, J.L.; Lillycrop, K.A. Epigenetic regulation of transcription: A mechanism for inducing variations in phenotype (fetal programming) by differences in nutrition during early life? *Br. J. Nutr.* **2007**, *97*, 1036–1046. [CrossRef] [PubMed]
13. Leroy, J.L.M.R.; Vanholder, T.; Delanghe, J.R.; Opsomer, G.; Van Soom, A.; Bols, P.E.J.; Dewulf, J.; de Kruif, A. Metabolic changes in follicular fluid of the dominant follicle in high-yielding dairy cows early postpartum. *Theriogenology* **2004**, *62*, 1131–1143. [CrossRef]
14. Tong, Z.; Guo, J.; Glen, R.C.; Morrell, N.W.; Li, W. A Bone Morphogenetic Protein (BMP)-derived Peptide Based on the Type I Receptor-binding Site Modifies Cell-type Dependent BMP Signalling. *Sci. Rep.* **2019**, *9*, 13446. [CrossRef] [PubMed]
15. Lochab, A.K.; Extavour, C.G. Bone Morphogenetic Protein (BMP) signaling in animal reproductive system development and function. *Dev. Biol.* **2017**, *427*, 258–269. [CrossRef]
16. Dong, J.; Albertini, D.F.; Nishimori, K.; Kumar, T.R.; Lu, N. Growth differentiation factor-9 is required during early ovarian folliculogenesis. *Nature* **1996**, *383*, 531–535. [CrossRef]
17. Yan, C.; Wang, P.; DeMayo, J.; DeMayo, F.J.; Elvin, J.A.; Carino, C.; Prasad, S.V.; Skinner, S.S.; Dunbar, B.S.; Dube, J.L.; et al. Synergistic roles of bone morphogenetic protein 15 and growth differentiation factor 9 in ovarian function. *Mol. Endocrinol.* **2001**, *15*, 854–866. [CrossRef]
18. Nilsson, E.E.; Skinner, M.K. Bone Morphogenetic Protein-4 (BMP-4). Signaling pathways regulating gene expression that mediate oogenesis and ovulation. *Mol. Cell. Endocrinol.* **2004**, *225*, 19–24. [CrossRef] [PubMed]
19. Ogren, L.; Tani, T.; Marikawa, Y. Wt1 and Sf1 are regulators of the switch between fetal and adult adrenal development. *Mol. Cell. Biol.* **2006**, *26*, 9482–9491.
20. Kameda, T.; Shintani, Y.; Nakayama, Y.; Tani, M. CD147-induced cell proliferation is associated with Smad4 signal inhibition. *J. Biol. Chem.* **2009**, *284*, 29170–29179.
21. Takmaz, O.; Yozgatli, D.; Ozaltin, S.; Ozbasli, E.; Kocyigit, Y.; Kuran, S.B.; Bulut, H.; Gungor, M.; Buyru, F.; Bastu, E. Can follicular Emmprin and BMP 4 levels predict ICSI outcome? *J. Assist. Reprod. Genet.* **2019**, *36*, 1127–1133. [CrossRef] [PubMed]
22. Dixit, H.; Rao, L.K.; Padmalatha, V.V.; Kanakavalli, M.; Deenadayal, M.; Gupta, N.; Chakrabarty, B.; Singh, L. Missense mutations in the BMP15 gene are associated with ovarian failure. *Hum. Genet.* **2006**, *119*, 408–415. [CrossRef] [PubMed]
23. Laissue, P.; Christin-Maitre, S.; Touraine, P.; Kuttenn, F.; Ritvos, O.; Aittomaki, K.; Bourcigaux, N.; Jacquesson, L.; Bouchard, P.; Frydman, R.; et al. Mutations and sequence variants in GDF9 and BMP15 in patients with premature ovarian failure. *Eur. J. Endocrinol.* **2006**, *154*, 739–744. [CrossRef]
24. Zhao, H.; Qin, Y.; Kovanci, E.; Simpson, J.L.; Chen, Z.-J.; Rajkovic, A. Analyses of GDF9 mutation in 100 Chinese women with premature ovarian failure. *Fertil. Steril.* **2007**, *88*, 1474–1476. [CrossRef] [PubMed]
25. Palmer, J.S.; Zhen, Z.Z.; Hoekstra, C.; Hayward, N.K.; Webb, P.M.; Whiteman, D.C.; Martin, N.G.; Boomsma, D.I.; Duffy, D.L.; Montgomery, G.W. Novel variants in growth differentiation factor 9 in mothers of dizygotic twins. *J. Clin. Endocrinol. Metab.* **2006**, *91*, 4713–4716. [CrossRef] [PubMed]
26. Otsuka, F.; McTavish, K.J.; Shimasaki, S. Integral role of GDF-9 and BMP-15 in ovarian function. *Mol. Reprod. Dev.* **2011**, *78*, 9–21. [CrossRef]
27. Knight, P.G. Roles of inhibins, activins, and follistatin in the female reproductive system. *Front. Neuroendocrinol.* **2000**, *21*, 199–215. [CrossRef] [PubMed]
28. Visser, J.A.; de Jong, F.H.; Laven, J.S. Follicle-stimulating hormone and advanced follicle development in the human. *Arch. Med. Res.* **2003**, *34*, 565–571.
29. La Marca, A.; Volpe, A. Anti-Müllerian hormone (AMH) in female reproduction: Is measurement of circulating AMH a useful tool? *Clin. Endocrinol.* **2006**, *64*, 603–610. [CrossRef]
30. Broekmans, F.J.; Knauff, E.A.; te Velde, E.R.; Macklon, N.S.; Fauser, B.C. Female reproductive ageing: Current knowledge and future trends. *Trends Endocrinol. Metab.* **2007**, *18*, 58–65. [CrossRef]
31. Otsuka, F.; Yao, Z.; Lee, T.; Yamamoto, S.; Erickson, G.F.; Shimasaki, S. Bone morphogenetic protein-15. Identification of target cells and biological functions. *J. Biol. Chem.* **2000**, *275*, 39523–39528. [CrossRef]
32. Chen, Y.; Zhang, H.; Gou, X. The role of matrix metalloproteinase-2 in the remodeling of the extracellular matrix during mouse follicular development and ovulation. *Reprod. Biol. Endocrinol.* **2014**, *12*, 73.
33. Juengel, J.L.; Hudson, N.L.; Whiting, L.; McNatty, K.P. Effects of immunization against BMP15 and GDF9 on ovulation rate, fertilization, and pregnancy in ewes. *Biol. Reprod.* **2004**, *70*, 557–561. [CrossRef]
34. Elvin, J.A.; Yan, C.; Matzuk, M.M. Oocyte-expressed TGF-beta superfamily members in female fertility. *Mol. Cell. Endocrinol.* **2000**, *159*, 1–5. [CrossRef]
35. Knight, P.G.; Glister, C. TGF-β superfamily members and ovarian follicle development. *Reproduction* **2006**, *132*, 191–206. [CrossRef]

36. Vitt, U.A.; Hsueh, A.J.; Hsueh, A.J. Stage-dependent role of growth differentiation factor-9 in ovarian follicle development. *Mol. Endocrinol.* **2001**, *15*, 1218–1228. [CrossRef] [PubMed]
37. Gilchrist, R.B.; Lane, M.; Thompson, J.G. Oocyte-secreted factors: Regulators of cumulus cell function and oocyte quality. *Hum. Reprod. Update* **2008**, *14*, 159–177. [CrossRef]
38. Mazerbourg, S.; Hsueh, A.J. Growth differentiation factor-9 signaling in the ovary: Insights into the molecular basis of ovarian physiology. *Reproduction* **2006**, *132*, 191–206.
39. Peng, J.; Li, Q.; Wigglesworth, K.; Rangarajan, A.; Kattamuri, C.; Peterson, R.T.; Eppig, J.J.; Thompson, T.B.; Matzuk, M.M. Growth differentiation factor 9: Bone morphogenetic protein 15 heterodimers are potent regulators of ovarian functions. *Proc. Natl. Acad. Sci. USA* **2013**, *110*, E776–E785. [CrossRef]
40. Orisaka, M.; Orisaka, S.; Jiang, J.Y.; Craig, J.; Wang, Y.; Kotsuji, F.; Tsang, B.K. Growth differentiation factor 9 is antiapoptotic during follicular development from preantral to early antral stage. *Mol. Endocrinol.* **2006**, *20*, 2456–2468. [CrossRef]
41. Uyar, A.; Torrealday, S.; Seli, E. Cumulus and granulosa cell markers of oocyte and embryo quality. *Fertil. Steril.* **2013**, *99*, 979–997. [CrossRef] [PubMed]
42. Yamamoto, N.; Christenson, L.K.; McAllister, J.M.; Strauss, J.F. Growth differentiation factor-9 inhibits 3050-adenosine monophosphate–stimulated steroidogenesis in human granulosa and theca cells. *J. Clin. Endocrinol. Metab.* **2002**, *87*, 2849–2856. [PubMed]
43. Pangas, S.A.; Jorgez, C.J.; Matzuk, M.M. Growth differentiation factor 9 regulates expression of the bone morphogenetic protein antagonist gremlin. *J. Biol. Chem.* **2004**, *279*, 32281–32286. [CrossRef]
44. Belli, M.; Shimasaki, S. Molecular aspects and clinical relevance of GDF9 and BMP15 in ovarian function. *Vitam. Horm.* **2018**, *107*, 317–348. [PubMed]
45. Chatroudi, M.H.; Khalili, M.A.; Ashourzadeh, S.; Anbari, F.; Shahedi, A.; Safari, S. Growth differentiation factor 9 and cumulus cell supplementation in in vitro maturation culture media enhances the viability of human blastocysts. *Clin. Exp. Reprod. Med.* **2019**, *46*, 166–172. [CrossRef] [PubMed]
46. Hreinsson, J.G.; Scott, J.E.; Rasmussen, C.; Swahn, M.L.; Hsueh, A.J.; Hovatta, O. Growth differentiation factor-9 promotes the growth, development, and survival of human ovarian follicles in organ culture. *J. Clin. Endocrinol. Metab.* **2002**, *87*, 316–321. [CrossRef] [PubMed]
47. Vitt, U.A.; Hayashi, M.; Klein, C.; Hsueh, A.J. Growth differentiation factor-9 stimulates proliferation but suppresses the follicle-stimulating hormone-induced differentiation of cultured granulosa cells from small antral and preovulatory rat follicles. *Biol. Reprod.* **2000**, *62*, 370–377. [CrossRef] [PubMed]
48. Orisaka, M.; Tajima, K.; Tsang, B.K.; Kotsuji, F. Oocyte-granulosa-theca cell interactions during preantral follicular development. *J. Ovarian Res.* **2009**, *2*, 9. [CrossRef] [PubMed]
49. Sanchez, F.; Lolicato, F.; Romero, S.; De Vos, M.; Van Ranst, H.; Verheyen, G.; Anckaert, E.; Smitz, J.E. An improved IVM method for cumulus-oocyte complexes from small follicles in polycystic ovary syndrome patients enhances oocyte competence and embryo yield. *Hum. Reprod.* **2017**, *32*, 2056–2068. [CrossRef]
50. Diaz, F.J.; Wigglesworth, K.; Eppig, J.J. Oocytes determine cumulus cell lineage in mouse ovarian follicles. *J. Cell Sci.* **2007**, *120*, 1330–1340. [CrossRef]
51. Zhu, X.M.; Zhu, Y.M.; Xu, C.M.; Qian, Y.L.; Jin, F.; Huang, H.F. Autologous mature follicular fluid: Its role in in vitro maturation of human cumulus-removed oocytes. *Fertil. Steril.* **2008**, *90*, 1094–1102. [CrossRef] [PubMed]
52. Li, Y.; Li, R.Q.; Ou, S.B.; Zhang, N.F.; Ren, L.; Wei, L.N.; Zhang, Q.X.; Yang, D.Z. Increased GDF9 and BMP15 mRNA levels in cumulus granulosa cells correlate with oocyte maturation, fertilization, and embryo quality in humans. *Reprod. Biol. Endocrinol.* **2014**, *12*, 81. [CrossRef]
53. Juengel, J.L.; Hudson, N.L.; Heath, D.A.; Smith, P.; Reader, K.L.; Lawrence, S.B.; O'Connell, A.R.; Laitinen, M.P.; Cranfield, M.; Groome, N.P.; et al. Growth differentiation factor 9 and bone morphogenetic protein 15 are essential for ovarian follicular development in sheep. *Biol. Reprod.* **2002**, *67*, 1777–1789. [CrossRef] [PubMed]
54. Chu, Y.L.; Xu, Y.R.; Yang, W.X.; Sun, Y. The role of FSH and TGF-β superfamily in follicle atresia. *Aging* **2018**, *10*, 305. [CrossRef] [PubMed]
55. Sanfins, A.; Rodrigues, P.; Albertini, D.F. GDF-9 and BMP-15 direct the follicle symphony. *J. Assist. Reprod. Genet.* **2018**, *35*, 1741–1750. [CrossRef] [PubMed]
56. Mazerbourg, S.; Hsueh, A.J. Genomic analyses facilitate identification of receptors and signaling pathways for growth differentiation factor 9 and related orphan bone morphogenetic protein/growth differentiation factor ligands. *Hum. Reprod. Update* **2006**, *12*, 373–383. [CrossRef] [PubMed]
57. Martins, F.S.; Celestino, J.J.H.; Saraiva, M.V.A.; Matos, M.H.T.; Bruno, J.B.; Rocha, C.M.C.; Lima-Verde, I.B.; Lucci, C.M.; Báo, S.N.; Figueiredo, J.R. Growth and differentiation factor-9 stimulates activation of goat primordial follicles in vitro and their progression to secondary follicles. *Reprod. Fertil. Dev.* **2008**, *20*, 916–924. [CrossRef] [PubMed]
58. Cook-Andersen, H.; Curnow, K.J.; Su, H.I.; Chang, R.J.; Shimasaki, S. Growth and differentiation factor 9 promotes oocyte growth at the primary but not the early secondary stage in three-dimensional follicle culture. *J. Assist. Reprod. Genet.* **2016**, *33*, 1067–1077. [CrossRef] [PubMed]
59. Santos, A.; Ferreira, A.; Sa, N.; Silva, R.; Palomino, G.; Pimentel, E.; Cadenas, J.; Alves, B.G.; Celestino, J.J.; Rodrigues, A.P.; et al. Growth and differentiation factor-9 (GDF-9) increases the in vitro growth rates of isolated goat early antral follicles. *Ciência Anim. Bras.* **2023**, *24*, e-74980E.

60. Almeida, A.P.; Saraiva, M.V.A.; Araújo, V.R.; Magalhães, D.M.; Duarte, A.B.G.; Frota, I.M.A.; Lopes, C.A.; Campello, C.C.; Silva, J.R.; Figueiredo, J.R. Expression of growth and differentiation factor 9 (GDF-9) and its effect on the in vitro culture of caprine preantral ovarian follicles. *Small Rumin. Res.* **2011**, *100*, 169–176. [CrossRef]
61. Hendarto, H.; Prabowo, P.; Moeloek, F.A.; Soetjipto, S. Growth differentiation factor 9 concentration in the follicular fluid of infertile women with endometriosis. *Fertil. Steril.* **2010**, *94*, 758–760. [CrossRef]
62. Kawabe, S.; Yamashita, Y.; Saito, N.; Kokunai, K.; Kayashi, A.; Hayashi, M.; Terai, Y.; Miyazaki, K.; Ohmichi, M. The effect of moderate to severe endometriosis on expression of growth differentiation factor-9 mRNA in human granulosa cells under controlled ovarian hyperstimulation. *Reprod. Biomed.* **2015**, *14*, 179–184. [CrossRef] [PubMed]
63. Evkuran Dal, G.; Baykal, A.; Toydemir Karabulut, T.S.F.; Dokuzeylul Gungor, N.; Turna, O. Preliminary results of blood growth differentiation factor-9 (GDF-9) measurement in cats: Future aspects of GDF-9 on stage of the cycle and spaying history. *Pol. J. Vet. Sci.* **2022**, *25*, 149–154. [CrossRef] [PubMed]
64. Wiweko, B.; Natadisastra, M.; Situmorang, H.; Rectifa, Z.; Mutia, K.; Amelia, P.; Muna, N. Expressions of growth differentiation factor-9 on granulosa cells of infertile women with endometriosis undergoing in vitro fertilization. *J. Phys. Conf. Ser.* **2018**, *1073*, 3. [CrossRef]
65. Knochenhauer, E.S.; Key, T.J.; Kahsar-Miller, M.; Waggoner, W.; Boots, L.R.; Azziz, R. Prevalence of the polycystic ovary syndrome in unselected black and white women of the southeastern United States: A prospective study. *J. Clin. Endocrinol. Metab.* **1998**, *83*, 3078–3082. [CrossRef] [PubMed]
66. Teixeira Filho, F.L.; Baracat, E.C.; Lee, T.H.; Suh, C.S.; Matsui, M.; Chang, R.J.; Shimasaki, S.; Erickson, G.F. Aberrant expression of growth differentiation factor-9 in oocytes of women with polycystic ovary syndrome. *J. Clin. Endocrinol. Metab.* **2002**, *87*, 1337–1344. [CrossRef] [PubMed]
67. Wei, L.N.; Liang, X.Y.; Fang, C.; Zhang, M.F. Abnormal expression of growth differentiation factor 9 and bone morphogenetic protein 15 in stimulated oocytes during maturation from women with polycystic ovary syndrome. *Fertil. Steril.* **2011**, *96*, 464–468. [CrossRef] [PubMed]
68. Chen, W.; Zhai, Y.; Zhu, B.; Wu, K.; Fan, Y.; Zhou, X.; Liu, L.; Ge, W. Loss of growth differentiation factor 9 causes an arrest of early folliculogenesis in zebrafish—A novel insight into its action mechanism. *PLoS Genet.* **2022**, *18*, e1010318. [CrossRef]
69. Ghoreishi, H.; Fathi-Yosefabad, S.; Shayegh, J.; Barzegari, A. Identification of mutations in BMP15 and GDF9 genes associated with prolificacy of Markhoz goats. *Arch. Anim. Breed.* **2019**, *62*, 565–570. [CrossRef]
70. Persani, L.; Rossetti, R.; Di Pasquale, E.; Cacciatore, C.; Fabre, S. The fundamental role of bone morphogenetic protein 15 in ovarian function and its involvement in female fertility disorders. *Hum. Reprod. Update* **2014**, *20*, 869–883. [CrossRef]
71. Silva, J.R.V.; Van Den Hurk, R.; Van Tol, A.T.H.; Roelen, J.A.B.; Figueiredo, R.J. Expression of growth differentiation factor 9 (GDF9), bone morphogenetic protein 15 (BMP15), and BMP receptors in the ovaries of goats. *Mol. Reprod. Dev.* **2004**, *70*, 11–19. [CrossRef]
72. Moore, R.K.; Shimasaki, S. Molecular biology and physiological role of the oocyte factor, BMP-15. *Mol. Cell. Endocrinol.* **2005**, *234*, 67–73. [CrossRef] [PubMed]
73. Crawford, J.L.; Heath, D.A.; Reader, K.L.; Quirke, L.D.; Hudson, N.L.; Juengel, J.L.; McNatty, K.P. Oocytes in sheep homozygous for a mutation in bone morphogenetic protein receptor 1B express lower mRNA levels of bone morphogenetic protein 15 but not growth differentiation factor 9. *Reproduction* **2011**, *142*, 53–61. [CrossRef] [PubMed]
74. Nagdy, H.; Mahmoud, K.G.M.; Kandiel, M.M.; Helmy, N.A.; Ibrahim, S.S.; Nawito, M.F.; Othman, O.E. PCR-RFLP of bone morphogenetic protein 15 (BMP15/FecX) gene as a candidate for prolificacy in sheep. *Int. J. Vet. Sci. Med.* **2018**, *6*, S68–S72. [CrossRef] [PubMed]
75. Taheri, M.M.; Moghadam, S.; Saki, G.; Nikbakht, R.; Eftekhari, A.R. Moghadam. Bone morphogenetic protein 15 induces differentiation of mesenchymal stem cells derived from human follicular fluid to oocyte-like cell. *Cell Biol. Int.* **2021**, *45*, 127–139. [CrossRef]
76. Dube, J.L.; Wang, P.; Elvin, J.; Lyons, K.M.; Celeste, A.J.; Matzuk, M.M. The bone morphogenetic protein 15 gene is X-linked and expressed in oocytes. *Mol. Endocrinol.* **1998**, *12*, 1809–1817. [CrossRef] [PubMed]
77. Otsuka, F.; Yamamoto, S.; Erickson, G.F.; Shimasaki, S. Bone morphogenetic protein-15 inhibits follicle-stimulating hormone (FSH) action by suppressing FSH receptor expression. *J. Biol. Chem.* **2001**, *276*, 11387–11392. [CrossRef] [PubMed]
78. Kumar, R.; Alwani, M.; Kosta, S. BMP15 and GDF9 gene mutations in premature ovarian failure. *J. Reprod. Infertil.* **2017**, *18*, 185–189. [PubMed]
79. Di Pasquale, E.; Beck-Peccoz, P.; Persani, L. Hypergonadotropic ovarian failure associated with an inherited mutation of human bone morphogenetic protein-15 (BMP15) gene. *Am. J. Hum. Genet.* **2004**, *75*, 106–111. [CrossRef] [PubMed]
80. Tiotiu, D.; Alvaro Mercadal, B.; Imbert, R.; Verbist, J.; Demeestere, I.; De Leener, A.; Englert, Y.; Vassart, G.; Costagliola, S.; Delbaere, A. Variants of the BMP15 gene in a cohort of patients with premature ovarian failure. *Hum. Reprod.* **2010**, *25*, 1581–1587. [CrossRef]
81. Shi, M.; Zhu, J.; Wang, R.; Chen, X.; Mi, L.; Walz, T.; Springer, T.A. Latent TGF-bstructure and activation. *Nature* **2011**, *474*, 343–349. [CrossRef]
82. Mottershead, D.G.; Harrison, C.A.; Mueller, T.D.; Stanton, P.G.; Gilchrist, R.B.; McNatty, K.P. Growth differentiation factor 9: Bone morphogenetic protein 15 (GDF9: BMP15) synergism and protein heterodimerization. *Proc. Natl. Acad. Sci. USA* **2013**, *110*, E2257. [CrossRef] [PubMed]

83. Faiza, H.; Khan, M.; Rafiq, M.; Khan, A.A.; Rind, N.A.; Naqvi, S.H.A. Two novel mutations in exon 2 of bone morphogenetic protein (BMP) 15 gene in Pakistani infertile females. *Saudi J. Biol. Sci.* **2021**, *28*, 5364–5370. [CrossRef] [PubMed]
84. Otsuka, F.; Shimasaki, S. A novel function of bone morphogenetic protein-15 in the pituitary: Selective synthesis and secretion of FSH by gonadotropes. *Endocrinology* **2002**, *143*, 4938–4941. [CrossRef] [PubMed]
85. Moore, R.K.; Otsuka, F.; Shimasaki, S. Molecular basis of bone morphogenetic protein-15 signaling in granulosa cells. *J. Biol. Chem.* **2003**, *278*, 304–310. [CrossRef] [PubMed]
86. Otsuka, F.; Shimasaki, S. A negative feedback system between oocyte bone morphogenetic protein 15 and granulosa cell kit ligand: Its role in regulating granulosa cell mitosis. *Proc. Natl. Acad. Sci. USA* **2002**, *99*, 8060–8065. [CrossRef]
87. Shimasaki, S.; Moore, R.K.; Erickson, G.F.; Otsuka, F. The role of bone morphogenetic proteins in ovarian function. *Reprod. Biol. Endocrinol.* **2004**, *2*, 58. [CrossRef]
88. Rossi, R.O.D.S.; Portela, A.M.L.R.; Passos, J.R.S.; Cunha, E.V.; Silva, A.W.B.; Costa, J.J.N.; Silva, J.R.V. Effects of BMP-4 and FSH on growth, morphology and mRNA expression of oocyte-secreted factors in cultured bovine secondary follicles. *Anim. Reprod.* **2015**, *12*, 910–919.
89. Juárez-Rodríguez, P.; Palma-Flores, C.; Téllez-Valencia, A. BMP-4 is a key signal in murine fetal testis development. *J. Dev. Biol.* **2016**, *4*, 5.
90. Dalbies-Tran, R.; Cadoret, V.; Desmarchais, A.; Elis, S.; Maillard, V.; Monget, P.; Uzbekova, S. A comparative analysis of oocyte development in mammals. *Cells* **2020**, *9*, 1002. [CrossRef]
91. Liu, J.; Wang, B.; Wei, Z.; Zhou, P.; Zu, Y.; Zhou, S.; Wen, Q.; Wang, J.; Cao, Y.; Ma, X. Mutational analysis of human bone morphogenetic protein 15 in Chinese women with polycystic ovary syndrome. *Metabolism* **2011**, *60*, 1511–1514. [CrossRef]
92. Wu, Y.T.; Tang, L.; Cai, J.; Lu, X.E.; Xu, J.; Zhu, X.M.; Luo, Q.; Huang, H.F. High bone morphogenetic protein-15 level in follicular fluid is associated with high quality oocyte and subsequent embryonic development. *Hum. Reprod.* **2007**, *22*, 1526–1531. [CrossRef]
93. Shekarian, A.; Nadia Sharifi, Z.; Nazarnejad, M.M.; Saeinia, A.; Abdi, S. In Vitro Culture of Mouse Preantral Follicle in Supplemented Medium with Bone Morphogenetic Protein 15 (BMP15). *J. Otorhinolaryngol. Facial Plast. Surg.* **2021**, *6*, 1–7.
94. Galloway, S.M.; Gregan, S.M.; Wilson, T.; McNatty, K.P.; Juengel, J.L.; Ritvos, O.; Davis, G.H. Bmp15 mutations and ovarian function. *Mol. Cell. Endocrinol.* **2002**, *191*, 15–18. [CrossRef]
95. Hanrahan, J.P.; Gregan, S.M.; Mulsant, P.; Mullen, M.; Davis, G.H.; Powell, R.; Galloway, S.M. Mutations in the genes for oocyte-derived growth factors GDF9 and BMP15 are associated with both increased ovulation rate and sterility in Cambridge and Belclare sheep (*Ovis aries*). *Biol. Reprod.* **2004**, *70*, 900–909. [CrossRef]
96. Hernández-Montiel, W.; Martínez-Núñez, M.A.; Ramón-Ugalde, J.P.; Román-Ponce, S.I.; Calderón-Chagoya, R.; Zamora-Bustillos, R. Genome-Wide Association Study Reveals Candidate Genes for Litter Size Traits in Pelibuey Sheep. *Animals* **2020**, *10*, 434. [CrossRef]
97. Ferrarini, E.; De Marco, G.; Orsolini, F.; Gianetti, E.; Benelli, E.; Fruzzetti, F.; Simoncini, T.; Agretti, P.; Tonacchera, M. Characterization of a novel mutation V136L in bone morphogenetic protein 15 identified in a woman affected by POI. *J. Ovarian Res.* **2021**, *14*, 85. [CrossRef]
98. Yang, Y.; Zhao, L.; Lei, L.; Zhang, J.; Zhou, Q.; Han, J.; Zou, S. Effects of BMP-4 on the expression of type I collagen and MMP-1 in human skin fibroblasts. *J. Dermatol. Sci.* **2013**, *71*, 187–195.
99. Wang, F.; Chu, M.; Pan, L.; Wang, X.; He, X.; Zhang, R.; Di, R. Polymorphism detection of GDF9 gene and its association with litter size in Luzhong mutton sheep (*Ovis aries*). *Animals* **2021**, *11*, 571. [CrossRef]
100. Estienne, A.; Lahoz, B.; Jarrier-Gaillard, P.; Bodin, L.; Folch, J.; Alabart, J.L.; Monniaux, D. BMP15 regulates the inhibin/activin system independently of ovulation rate control in sheep. *Reproduction* **2017**, *153*, 395–404. [CrossRef]
101. Zhang, H.; Klausen, C.; Zhu, H.; Chang, H.M.; Leung, P.C. BMP4 and BMP7 suppress StAR and progesterone production via ALK3 and SMAD1/5/8-SMAD4 in human granulosa-lutein cells. *Endocrinology* **2015**, *156*, 4269–4280. [CrossRef]
102. Haas, C.S.; Rovani, M.T.; Ilha, G.F.; Bertolin, K.; Ferst, J.G.; Bridi, A.; Gasperin, B.G. Transforming growth factor-beta family members are regulated during induced luteolysis in cattle. *Anim. Reprod.* **2019**, *16*, 829–837. [CrossRef]
103. da Cunha, E.V.; de Souza, G.B.; Passos, J.R.S.; Silva, A.W.B.; Dau, A.M.; Saraiva, M.V.A.; Dau, A.M.; Saraiva, M.V.; Lobo, R.N.; Silva, J.R. Effects of bone morphogenetic protein 4 (BMP4) on in vitro development and survival of bovine preantral follicles enclosed in fragments ovarian tissue. *Zygote* **2017**, *25*, 256–264. [CrossRef]
104. Childs, A.J.; Kinnell, H.L.; Collins, C.S.; Hogg, K.; Bayne, R.A.; Green, S.J.; McNeilly, A.S.; Anderson, R.A. BMP signaling in the human fetal ovary is developmentally regulated and promotes primordial germ cell apoptosis. *Stem Cells* **2010**, *28*, 1368–1378. [CrossRef]
105. Winnier, G.; Blessing, M.; Labosky, P.A.; Hogan, B.L. Bone morphogenetic protein-4 is required for mesoderm formation and patterning in the mouse. *Genes Dev.* **1995**, *9*, 2105–2116. [CrossRef]
106. Tanwar, P.S.; McFarlane, J.R. Dynamic expression of bone morphogenetic protein 4 in reproductive organs of female mice. *Reproduction* **2011**, *142*, 573–579. [CrossRef]
107. Kobayashi, A.; Kwan, K.-M.; Carroll, T.J.; McMahon, A.P.; Mendelsohn, C.L.; Behringer, R.R. Distinct and sequential tissue-specific activities of the LIM-class homeobox gene Lim1 for tubular morphogenesis during kidney development. *Development* **2005**, *132*, 2809–2823. [CrossRef]
108. Koch, L. BMPR-2 signalling is essential for maintenance of pregnancy. *Nat. Rev. Endocrinol.* **2013**, *9*, 380. [CrossRef]

109. Nilsson, E.E.; Skinner, M.K. Bone morphogenetic protein-4 acts as an ovarian follicle survival factor and promotes primordial follicle development. *Biol. Reprod.* **2003**, *69*, 1265–1272. [CrossRef]
110. Kumar, S.; Punetha, M.; Jose, B.; Bharati, J.; Khanna, S.; Sonwane, A.; Green, J.A.; Whitworth, K.; Sarkar, M. Modulation of granulosa cell function via CRISPR-Cas fueled editing of BMPR-IB gene in goats (*Capra hircus*). *Sci. Rep.* **2020**, *10*, 20446. [CrossRef]
111. Lawson, K.A.; Dunn, N.R.; Roelen, B.A.J.; Zeinstra, L.M.; Davis, A.M.; Wright, C.V.E.; Korving, J.P.W.F.M.; Hogan, B.L.M. Bmp4 is required for the generation of primordial germ cells in the mouse embryo. *Genes Dev.* **1999**, *13*, 424–436. [CrossRef]
112. Magro-Lopez, E.; Muñoz-Fernández, M.Á. The Role of BMP Signaling in Female Reproductive System Development and Function. *Int. J. Mol. Sci.* **2021**, *22*, 11927. [CrossRef] [PubMed]
113. Ramirez-Carracedo, R.; Tesoro, L.; Hernandez, I.; Diez-Mata, J.; Filice, M.; Toro, R.; Rodriguez-Piñero, M.; Zamorano, J.L.; Saura, M.; Zaragoza, C. Non-Invasive Detection of Extracellular Matrix Metalloproteinase Inducer EMMPRIN, a New Therapeutic Target against Atherosclerosis, Inhibited by Endothelial Nitric Oxide. *Int. J. Mol. Sci.* **2018**, *19*, 3248. [CrossRef] [PubMed]
114. Nabeshima, K.; Iwasaki, H.; Koga, K.; Hojo, H.; Suzumiya, J.; Kikuchi, M. Emmprin (basigin/CD147): Matrix metalloproteinase modulator and multifunctional cell recognition molecule that plays a critical role in cancer progression. *Pathol. Int.* **2006**, *56*, 359–367. [CrossRef] [PubMed]
115. Sheu, B.-C.; Chang, W.C.; Cheng, C.Y.; Wang, P.H.; Lin, S.; Huang, S.C. Extracellular Matrix Proteases—Cytokine Regulation Role in Cancer and Pregnancy. *Front. Biosci.* **2009**, *14*, 1571–1588.
116. Yang, J.; Wu, J.; Guo, F.; Wang, D.; Chen, K.; Li, J.; Du, L.; Yin, A. Maternal serum disintegrin and metalloprotease protein-12 in early pregnancy as a potential marker of adverse pregnancy outcomes. *PLoS ONE* **2014**, *9*, e97284. [CrossRef] [PubMed]
117. Davidson, B.; Goldberg, I.; Berner, A.; Kristensen, G.B.; Reich, R. EMMPRIN (extracellular matrix metalloproteinase inducer) is a novel marker of poor outcome in serous ovarian carcinoma. *Clin. Exp. Metastasis* **2003**, *20*, 161–169. [CrossRef] [PubMed]
118. Muramatsu, T.; Miyauchi, T. Basigin (CD147): A multifunctional transmembrane protein involved in reproduction, neural function, inflammation and tumor invasion. *Histol. Histopathol.* **2003**, *18*, 981–987. [PubMed]
119. Biswas, C.; Zhang, Y.; DeCastro, R.; Guo, H.; Nakamura, T.; Kataoka, H.; Nabeshima, K. The human tumor cell-derived collagenase stimulatory factor (renamed EMMPRIN) is a member of the immunoglobulin superfamily. *Cancer Res.* **1995**, *55*, 434–439. [PubMed]
120. Fan, Q.W.; Yuasa, S.; Kuno, N.; Senda, T.; Kobayashi, M.; Muramatsu, T.; Kadomatsu, K. Expression of basigin, a member of the immunoglobulin superfamily, in the mouse central nervous system. *Neurosci. Res.* **1998**, *30*, 53–63. [CrossRef]
121. Nabha, S.M.; Bonfil, R.D.; Aboukameel, A. Extracellular matrix metalloproteinase inducer (EMMPRIN) in cancer and inflammation. *Cancer Metastasis Rev.* **2008**, *27*, 303–315.
122. Muramatsu, T.; Miyauchi, T. Extracellular matrix metalloproteinase inducer (EMMPRIN/CD147): Unique glycoprotein modulator of matrix metalloproteinases in the pathogenesis of cancer. *J. Biochem.* **2003**, *134*, 657–661.
123. Curry, T.E.; Osteen, K.G. The matrix metalloproteinase system: Changes, regulation, and impact throughout the ovarian and uterine reproductive cycle. *Endocr. Rev.* **2003**, *24*, 428–465. [CrossRef]
124. Fingleton, B. Matrix metalloproteinases as valid clinical targets. *Curr. Pharm. Des.* **2007**, *13*, 333–346. [CrossRef]
125. Bourguignon, L.Y.W.; Gilad, E.; Brightman, A.; Diedrich, F. Hyaluronan-CD44 interaction with EMMPRIN (CD147) regulates MMP-9 expression and cell migration in ovarian tumor cells. *J. Biol. Chem.* **2006**, *281*, 25893–25908.
126. Huang, L.; Zhang, L.; Liu, X.; Zhang, Y.; Li, Y.; Xu, Y.; Sun, S. EMMPRIN promotes angiogenesis, proliferation, invasion and resistance to sunitinib in renal cell carcinoma, and its level predicts patient outcome. *PLoS ONE* **2019**, *14*, e0218439.
127. Yan, L.; Zucker, S.; Toole, B.P. Roles of the multifunctional glycoprotein, emmprin (basigin; CD147), in tumour progression. *Thromb. Haemost.* **2005**, *93*, 199–204. [CrossRef]
128. Pata, S.; Surinkaew, S.; Takheaw, N.; Laopajon, W.; Chuensirikulchai, K.; Kasinrerk, W. Differential CD147 functional epitopes on distinct leukocyte subsets. *Front. Immunol.* **2021**, *12*, 3157. [CrossRef]
129. Huang, Z.; Tan, N.; Guo, W.; Wang, L.; Li, H.; Zhang, T.; Liu, X.; Xu, Q.; Li, J.; Guo, Z. Overexpression of EMMPRIN isoform 2 is associated with head and neck cancer metastasis. *PLoS ONE* **2014**, *9*, e91596. [CrossRef]
130. Guindolet, D.; Gabison, E.E. Role of CD147 (EMMPRIN/Basigin) in tissue remodeling. *Anatom. Rec.* **2020**, *303*, 1584–1589. [CrossRef]
131. Yang, M.; Yuan, Y.; Zhang, H.; Yan, M.; Wang, S.; Feng, F.; Ji, P.; Li, Y.; Li, B.; Gao, G.; et al. Prognostic significance of CD147 in patients with glioblastoma. *J. Neurooncol.* **2013**, *115*, 19–26. [CrossRef]
132. Smedts, A.M.; Lele, S.M.; Modesitt, S.C.; Curry, T.E. Expression of an extracellular matrix metalloproteinase inducer (basigin) in the human ovary and ovarian endometriosis. *Fertil. Steril.* **2006**, *86*, 535–542. [CrossRef] [PubMed]
133. Chang, H.; Ni, H.; Ma, X.H.; Xu, L.B.; Kadomatsu, K.; Muramatsu, T.; Yang, Z.M. Basigin expression and regulation in mouse ovary during the sexual maturation and development of corpus luteum. *Mol. Reprod. Dev.* **2004**, *68*, 135–141. [CrossRef] [PubMed]
134. Lescaille, G.; Menashi, S.; Cavelier-Balloy, B.; Khayati, F.; Quemener, C.; Podgorniak, M.P.; Naïmi, B.; Calvo, F.; Lebbe, C.; Mourah, S. EMMPRIN/CD147 up-regulates urokinase-type plasminogen activator: Implications in oral tumor progression. *BMC Cancer* **2012**, *12*, 115. [CrossRef] [PubMed]
135. Igakura, T.; Kadomatsu, K.; Kaname, T.; Muramatsu, H.; Fan, Q.W.; Miyauchi, T.; Toyama, Y.; Kuno, N.; Yuasa, S.; Takahashi, M.; et al. A null mutation in basigin, an immunoglobulin superfamily member, indicates its important roles in periimplantation development and spermatogenesis. *Dev. Biol.* **1998**, *194*, 152–165. [CrossRef] [PubMed]

136. Dang, Y.; Li, W.; Tran, V.; Khalil, R.A. EMMPRIN-mediated induction of uterine and vascular matrix metalloproteinases during pregnancy and in response to estrogen and progesterone. *Biochem. Pharmacol.* **2013**, *86*, 734–747. [CrossRef] [PubMed]
137. Mazzuca, M.Q.; Wlodek, M.E.; Dragomir, N.M.; Parkington, H.C.; Tare, M. Uteroplacental insufficiency programs regional vascular dysfunction and alters arterial stiffness in female offspring. *J. Physiol.* **2010**, *588*, 1997–2010. [CrossRef] [PubMed]
138. Chang, H.; Cheng, J.C.; Klausen, C.; Leung, P.C. BMP15 suppresses progesterone production by down-regulating StAR via ALK3 in human granulosa cells. *Mol. Endocrinol.* **2016**, *27*, 2093–2104. [CrossRef] [PubMed]
139. Gupta, S.D.; Dhar, B.; Kundu, S.; Das, N.; Choudhury, A.P.; Deb, M.; Das, A.; Das, A.; Das, N.; Choudhury, B.; et al. Association between gene expression levels of GDF9 and BMP15 and clinicopathological factors in the prognosis of female infertility in northeast Indian populations. *Meta Gene* **2021**, *30*, 100964. [CrossRef]
140. Alam, M.H.; Miyano, T. Interaction between growing oocytes and granulosa cells in vitro. *Reprod. Med. Biol.* **2019**, *19*, 13–23. [CrossRef]
141. Riepsamen, A.H.; Chan, K.; Lien, S.; Sweeten, P.; Donoghoe, M.W.; Walker, G.; Fraison, E.H.; Stocker, W.A.; Walton, K.L.; Harrison, C.A.; et al. Serum concentrations of oocyte-secreted factors BMP15 and GDF9 during IVF and in women with reproductive pathologies. *Endocrinology* **2019**, *160*, 2298–2313. [CrossRef]
142. Riepsamen, A.H.; Donoghoe, M.W.; Indran, I.R.; Hechtman, L.; Robertson, D.M.; Gilchrist, R.B.; Ledger, W.L.; Yong, E.L. Serum GDF9 and BMP15 as potential markers of ovarian function in women with and without polycystic ovary syndrome. *Clin. Endocrinol.* **2023**, *98*, 567–577. [CrossRef]
143. Juengel, J.L.; Bodensteiner, K.J.; Heath, D.A.; Hudson, N.L.; Moeller, C.L.; Smith, P.; Galloway, S.M.; Davis, G.H.; Sawyer, H.R.; McNatty, K.P. Physiology of GDF9 and BMP15 Signalling Molecules. *Anim. Reprod. Sci.* **2004**, *82–83*, 447–460. [CrossRef]
144. Abdulhameed, W.; Hassan, F. Serum Follicular Fluid Growth Differentiation Factor 9 (GDF-9) and Bone Morphogenic Protein 15 (BMP-15) as Markers of Ovarian Reserve. *Al-Anbar Med. J.* **2024**, *20*, 25–30. [CrossRef]
145. McIntosh, C.J.; Lun, S.; Lawrence, S.; Western, A.H.; McNatty, K.P.; Juengel, J.L. The Proregion of Mouse BMP15 Regulates the Cooperative Interactions of BMP15 and GDF9. *Biol. Reprod.* **2008**, *79*, 889–896. [CrossRef]
146. Hashimoto, O.; Moore, R.K.; Shimasaki, S. Posttranslational Processing of Mouse and Human BMP15: Potential Implication in the Determination of Ovulation Quota. *Proc. Natl. Acad. Sci. USA* **2005**, *102*, 5426–5431. [CrossRef]
147. McNatty, K.P.; Juengel, J.L.; Reader, K.L.; Lun, S.; Myllymaa, S.; Lawrence, S.B. Bone Morphogenetic Protein 15 and Growth Differentiation Factor 9 Co-operate to Regulate Granulosa Cell Function. *Reproduction* **2005**, *129*, 473–480. [CrossRef]
148. Hussein, T.S.; Thompson, J.G.; Gilchrist, R.B. Oocyte Secreted Factors Enhance Oocyte Developmental Competence. *Dev. Biol.* **2006**, *296*, 514–521. [CrossRef]
149. Gode, F.; Gulekli, B.; Dogan, E.; Korhan, P.; Dogan, S.; Bige, O.; Cimrin, D.; Atabey, N. Influence of Follicular Fluid GDF9 and BMP15 on Embryo Quality. *Fertil. Steril.* **2011**, *95*, 2274–2278. [CrossRef]
150. Aaltonen, J.; Laitinen, M.P.; Vujolainen, K.; Jaatinen, R.; Kuitunen, N.; Seppa, L.; Louhio, H.; Tuuri, T.; Sjoberg, J.; Butzow, R.; et al. Human growth differentiation factor 9 (GDF-9) and its novel homolog GDF-9B are expressed in oocytes during early folliculogenesis. *J. Clin. Endocrinol. Metab.* **1999**, *84*, 2744–2750. [CrossRef]
151. Spicer, L.J.; Aad, P.Y.; Allen, D.T.; Mazerbourg, S.; Hsueh, A.J. Growth differentiation factor-9 has divergent effects on proliferation and steroidogenesis of bovine granulosa cells. *J. Endocrinol.* **2006**, *189*, 329–339. [CrossRef]
152. Kawashima, I.; Kawamura, K. Regulation of follicle growth through hormonal factors and mechanical cues mediated by Hippo signaling pathway. *Syst. Biol. Reprod. Med.* **2018**, *64*, 3–11. [CrossRef] [PubMed]
153. Shimasaki, S.; Moore, R.K.; Otsuka, F.; Erickson, G.F. The bone morphogenetic protein system in mammalian reproduction. *Endocr. Rev.* **2004**, *25*, 72–101. [CrossRef] [PubMed]
154. Liu, T.; Qin, Q.Y.; Qu, J.X.; Wang, H.Y.; Yan, J. Where are the theca cells from: The mechanism of theca cells derivation and differentiation. *Chin. Med. J.* **2020**, *133*, 1711. [CrossRef] [PubMed]
155. Heath, D.A.; Pitman, J.L.; McNatty, K.P. Molecular forms of ruminant BMP15 and GDF9 and putative interactions with receptors. *Reproduction* **2017**, *154*, 521–534. [CrossRef] [PubMed]
156. Shi, Y.; Massagué, J. Mechanisms of TGF-β signaling from cell membrane to the nucleus. *Cell* **2003**, *113*, 685–700. [CrossRef] [PubMed]
157. Chang, H.; Brown, C.W.; Matzuk, M.M. Genetic analysis of the mammalian transforming growth factor-β superfamily. *Endocr. Rev.* **2002**, *23*, 787–823. [CrossRef] [PubMed]
158. Moore, R.K.; Erickson, G.F.; Shimasaki, S. Are BMP-15 and GDF-9 primary determinants of ovulation quota in mammals? *Trends Endocrinol. Metab.* **2004**, *15*, 356–361. [CrossRef] [PubMed]
159. Fujii, M.; Takeda, K.; Imamura, T.; Aoki, H.; Sampath, T.K.; Enomoto, S.; Kawabata, M.; Kato, M.; Ichijo, H.; Miyazono, K. Roles of bone morphogenetic protein type I receptors and Smad proteins in osteoblast and chondroblast differentiation. *Mol. Biol. Cell* **1999**, *10*, 3801–3813. [CrossRef]
160. Yu, P.; Guo, J.; Liu, Y.; Zhang, C.; Qian, W.; Wang, Y. Expression of extracellular matrix metalloproteinase inducer glycosylation and its effect on angiogenesis in non-small cell lung cancer. *Oncol. Lett.* **2017**, *14*, 2769–2774.

Journal of
Clinical Medicine

MDPI

Review

Advanced Paternal Age in Focus: Unraveling Its Influence on Assisted Reproductive Technology Outcomes

Aris Kaltsas [1,2], Athanasios Zikopoulos [3], Dionysios Vrachnis [4], Chara Skentou [5], Evangelos N. Symeonidis [6], Fotios Dimitriadis [6], Sofoklis Stavros [7], Michael Chrisofos [1], Nikolaos Sofikitis [2], Nikolaos Vrachnis [7,8] and Athanasios Zachariou [2,*]

1 Third Department of Urology, Attikon University Hospital, School of Medicine, National and Kapodistrian University of Athens, 12462 Athens, Greece; a.kaltsas@uoi.gr (A.K.); mxchris@yahoo.com (M.C.)
2 Laboratory of Spermatology, Department of Urology, Faculty of Medicine, School of Health Sciences, University of Ioannina, 45110 Ioannina, Greece; nsofikit@uoi.gr
3 Department of Obstetrics and Gynecology, Royal Cornwall Hospital, Truro TR1 3LJ, UK; athanasios.zikopoulos1@nhs.net
4 Medical School, National and Kapodistrian University of Athens, 12462 Athens, Greece; dionisisvrachnis@gmail.com
5 Department of Obstetrics and Gynaecology, Faculty of Medicine, School of Health Sciences, University of Ioannina, 45110 Ioannina, Greece; haraskentou@uoi.gr
6 Department of Urology, Faculty of Medicine, School of Health Sciences, Aristotle University of Thessaloniki, 54124 Thessaloniki, Greece; evansimeonidis@gmail.com (E.N.S.); difotios@auth.gr (F.D.)
7 Third Department of Obstetrics and Gynecology, Attikon University Hospital, School of Medicine, National and Kapodistrian University of Athens, 12462 Athens, Greece; sfstavrou@med.uoa.gr (S.S.)
8 Vascular Biology, Molecular and Clinical Sciences Research Institute, St George's University of London, London SW17 0RE, UK
* Correspondence: azachariou@uoi.gr

Abstract: As global demographics shift toward increasing paternal age, the realm of assisted reproductive technologies (ARTs), particularly in vitro fertilization (IVF) and intracytoplasmic sperm injection (ICSI), faces new challenges and opportunities. This study provides a comprehensive exploration of the implications of advanced paternal age on ART outcomes. Background research highlights the social, cultural, and economic factors driving men toward later fatherhood, with a focus on the impact of delayed paternity on reproductive outcomes. Methods involve a thorough review of existing literature, centering on changes in testicular function, semen quality, and genetic and epigenetic shifts associated with advancing age. Study results point to intricate associations between the father's age and ART outcomes, with older age being linked to diminished semen quality, potential genetic risks, and varied impacts on embryo quality, implantation rates, and birth outcomes. The conclusions drawn from the current study suggest that while advanced paternal age presents certain risks and challenges, understanding and mitigating these through strategies such as sperm cryopreservation, lifestyle modifications, and preimplantation genetic testing can optimize ART outcomes. Future research directions are identified to further comprehend the epigenetic mechanisms and long-term effects of the older father on offspring health. This study underscores the need for a comprehensive approach in navigating the intricacies of delayed fatherhood within the context of ART, aiming for the best possible outcomes for couples and their children.

Keywords: advanced paternal age; assisted reproductive technologies; sperm quality; genetic risks; epigenetic shifts; embryo quality; preimplantation genetic testing; delayed fatherhood

1. Introduction

In recent decades, a significant demographic shift has been observed globally, with an increasing number of men choosing to embrace fatherhood later in life [1]. This trend towards deferred paternity, caused and/or influenced by an array of social, cultural, and economic factors, has profound implications for the realm of assisted reproductive technologies (ARTs), particularly in vitro fertilization (IVF) and intracytoplasmic sperm injection (ICSI) [2]. Moreover, the rising prevalence of obesity among reproductive-age men has emerged as a critical factor influencing male fertility, exacerbating issues related to age and reproductive outcomes [3,4]. As couples seek ART services at older ages, the effects of advancing paternal age on reproductive outcomes have become a focal point of intense research and discussion.

This article aims to elucidate the multifaceted landscape of increasing paternal age and its ramifications within the context of ART. It delves into the driving forces behind this demographic shift, such as delayed marriage, extended life expectancies, and the enhanced efficacy of ART [5]. It also critically examines the burgeoning body of research that seeks to unravel the complex biological, psychological, and sociocultural dimensions of this phenomenon. In many countries, there has been a marked increase in the proportion of older fathers involved in live births, reflecting, as mentioned, a broader trend towards delayed childbearing [6]. While the ramifications of increased maternal age on fertility and pregnancy outcomes are well-documented, the implications of advancing paternal age are less clear and present unique challenges [7,8]. It is important to note that the intersection of advancing age and obesity introduces additional complications, such as hormonal changes, oxidative stress, and temperature stress, which are particularly exacerbated by the common occurrence of varicocele in older males, further impairing fertility [9–11]. The present work navigates through these complexities, exploring the decline in testicular function and semen quality as well as the potential genetic and epigenetic shifts that accompany advancing paternal age.

This study further investigates the consequential impacts of these changes on ART outcomes, including fertilization rates, embryo quality, implantation success, and the risks of miscarriages and birth complications [12]. It underscores the need for a comprehensive approach that considers both the biological and psychological aspects of delayed fatherhood. The geopolitical, cultural, and psychological dimensions that lead to delayed parenthood are also dissected, elucidating their roles in shaping contemporary paternity trends and the associated mental health considerations [2].

As the landscape of reproductive medicine evolves with these demographic shifts, understanding the intricacies of advanced paternal age becomes crucial. The present paper not only provides a detailed investigation into the current state of knowledge but also discusses strategies for mitigating risks associated with delayed fatherhood and outlines future research directions that can enhance our insight into and management of the effects of advanced paternal age on ART outcomes [13]. The current article comprises a wide-ranging narrative 'voyage' covering the cellular, molecular, and anatomical aspects of aging of the male reproductive system all the way to the wider ramifications extending to reproductive health and well-being.

2. Trends in Increasing Paternal Age and ART

Increasing paternal age in the context of ART is influenced by a myriad of social, cultural, and economic factors, the increase being variously attributed to delayed marriage, extended life expectancies, and the enhanced efficacy of ART [14]. Recent demographic studies have indicated a noticeable shift in family planning, with both men and women opting to put off parenthood. In England and Wales, the proportion of fathers aged 35–54 years contributing to live births increased from 25% in 1993 to 40% in 2003, illustrating a broader trend towards postponement of childbearing [6]. In the USA, paternal age at the time of childbirth has seen a notable upward trend over the past four decades, with the average age at which men become fathers having risen from 27.4 years in the early 70s to 30.9 in recent times [15].

In numerous nations, guidelines recommend restricting access to ART for men who are younger than 60 years due to the potential impacts on offspring health and ART outcomes. This threshold is based on the general observation of increasing risk with advancing age, although the rationale behind this specific age is not always clearly articulated [16]. However, in order to minimize the potential risks associated with couples using a sperm donation program, various countries have implemented age restrictions for sperm donors. In Great Britain, the age limit is set at 46 years [17], while in the USA it is 40 years [18]. Australia and France have set the age limit at 45 years [19,20], and the European Society of Human Reproduction and Embryology recommends a limit of 50 years [21]. The absence of a true drop in male fertility until the age of 45 is evident from the lack of consensus among these different guidelines.

Meanwhile, although there is much documentation of the unfavorable consequences of higher maternal age on fertility, including reduced conception rates and higher risks of complications during pregnancy and childbirth [22], the impact of paternal age is less well understood [23]. To underscore the increasing relevance of this demographic shift, it is critical to recognize the corresponding rise in the utilization of IVF, reflecting changes in reproductive strategies. Over the past 30 years, there has been a significant increase in the number of IVF cycles initiated, driven by greater societal acceptance and advancements in reproductive technologies. This trend correlates with the expanding body of research emphasizing the influence of paternal factors on ART outcomes. Notably, the data from the Society of Assisted Reproductive Technology (SART) indicate that the average number of embryos transferred per cycle has been significantly reduced since the late 1990s, paralleled by a steady increase in the number of pregnancies and live births per cycle, highlighting the evolving efficiency of ART practices [24].

A systematic review indicated that paternal age did not affect ART outcomes significantly up to the age of 45, but beyond this age, there seems to be a decline in pregnancy and live birth rates. This suggests that 45 could be considered a cautionary threshold for evaluating ART outcomes [25]. Studies show that increasing paternal age is linked to diminished testicular function [26], leading to decreased sperm concentration and motility [27,28]. This decline in semen quality, particularly evident in men over 40, has been associated with reduced fecundity and higher miscarriage rates [29]. In the context of ART, these changes have significant repercussions. Research studies have shown that among couples who opt for in vitro fertilization (IVF), the chances of a couple getting pregnant are smaller in males aged over 40 [29], a trend that is similarly reflected in lower fertilization rates [30], live birth rates [31], and embryo quality scores [32]. This age-related decline in male fertility factors underlines the need for scrupulous consideration of paternal age in fertility treatments and family planning.

Furthermore, the implications of these changes extend beyond reproductive success in ART. The reduction in semen quality and fertility rates in older men can lead to increased psychological stress and anxiety related to infertility and the ART process. As such, the integral role of paternal factors in ART outcomes cannot be understated, necessitating a holistic approach that takes into account both the biological and the psychological aspects of late fatherhood [33].

Geopolitical and cultural dynamics also play a role, often leading to delayed parenthood and signifying a shift in societal norms and expectations regarding fatherhood [34]. Additionally, postponing fatherhood extends beyond mere physical implications. Studies have shown an increase in depressive symptoms among men who defer fatherhood, highlighting potential mental health consequences [35]. The use of gestational carriers has also risen, driven by increased awareness, broader access to ART services for various patient groups, and evolving surrogacy laws, all of which impact paternity trends [36].

The gradual increase in the age at which men become fathers for the first time reflects changing social and cultural norms [37]. Fatherhood significantly impacts men's cognitive and emotional well-being, often leading to unease and uncertainty [38]. Additionally, the challenges young fathers face in balancing work and parenting further reinforce the decision to postpone fatherhood [39,40].

In essence, the use of ART among men is dictated by a complex interplay of social, cultural, and economic influences, ranging from shifts in societal standards and cultural expectations to the psychological impact of fatherhood on employment, as well as biological aspects. A comprehensive understanding of these factors is crucial in effectively managing the consequences of delayed fatherhood and optimizing the use of ART.

3. Aging and Its Impact on Male Reproductive Health: Anatomical, Cellular, and Molecular Perspectives

Aging in men brings about notable anatomical changes in the reproductive system, particularly within the testes, which are critical for maintaining healthy spermatogenesis [41]. Figure 1 below illustrates the comprehensive effects of aging, including anatomical alterations, decreases in semen parameters, hormonal changes, oxidative stress, and DNA fragmentation, highlighting the multifaceted nature of age-related decline in male fertility.

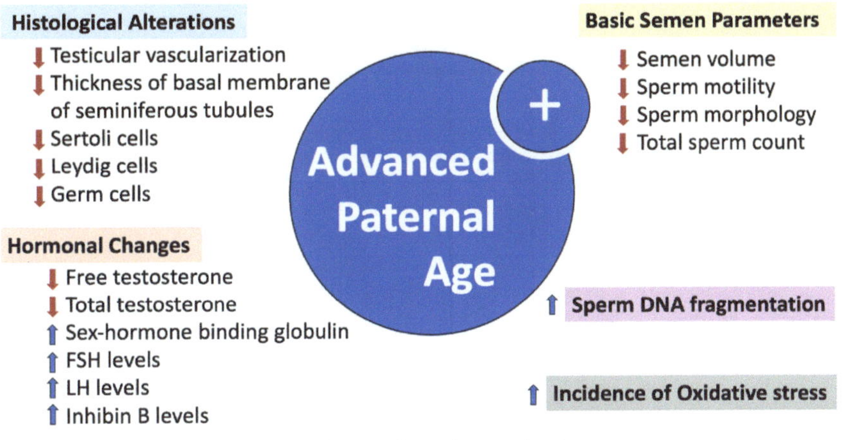

Figure 1. Effects of advanced paternal age on the male reproductive system.

As men age, there is a reduction in the number of Sertoli cells, possibly due to compromised blood flow to the testes. This decline is often accompanied by a drop in proteins that are secreted by Sertoli cells, loss of germ cells, and heightened cell apoptosis; moreover, the number of Leydig cells responsible for testosterone production also diminishes with age [42]. This leads to a disruption in hormonal balance, specifically in the levels of testosterone, luteinizing hormone (LH), and follicle-stimulating hormone (FSH), altering the hormonal milieu essential for spermatogenesis [43]. In older men, the amount of FSH increases in response to elevated inhibin B levels, a regulatory mechanism for activity in the testes [7].

These cellular changes are compounded by a general decline in the structural integrity of the testicular tissue. With age, the testes may exhibit signs of fibrosis and increased deposition of extracellular matrix, contributing to a thicker basement membrane [44]. These histological alterations can impact the overall functionality of the testes, including reduced efficiency in sperm production and a potential decrease in overall sperm quality. Additionally, the testicular vasculature undergoes changes, often leading to compromised blood flow, which can further affect the health and function of testicular cells [45].

The relationship between traditional semen quality measures (count, motility, and morphology) and age remains a topic of debate, with various studies yielding inconsistent findings [46–50]. To quote one example, Frattarelli et al. noted a drop in semen volume and motility in males aged over 45 [51], and Bellver et al. reported a strong negative association between father's sperm motility and concentration [52].

Likewise, Girsh et al. and Duran et al. observed a considerable reduction in a number of sperm parameters among males over 50 years of age as compared to those under 40 [53,54]. In contrast to these results, studies by Beguería et al. and Ferreira et al. presented varying findings, with Beguería et al. noting a decrease in semen amount and motile sperm count but an unexpected increase in sperm concentration and Ferreira et al. observing no noteworthy link between sperm parameters and paternal age in normozoospermic and oligozoospermic individuals [55,56].

The inconsistent findings may be attributed to the perplexing influence of variations in ejaculatory frequency that often occur with male aging [57]. These inconsistencies may also indicate variations across research in the level of detail in the basic semen analysis. Studies have consistently demonstrated a decrease in key sperm parameters such as semen volume, sperm count, motility, morphology, and viability as paternal age advances [14,16,58,59]. Notably, a marked reduction in semen volume, which starts at 45 years old, has been reported, this being expected to diminish by 0.22 mL every 5 years ($p < 0.001$) [55]. Sperm motility has also been reported to decrease annually by 0.6% to 0.5% starting from the age of 40 ($p < 0.001$) [60].

The application of Computer-Assisted Sperm Analysis (CASA) for detailed evaluation of sperm movement characteristics consistently reveals a marked decrease in sperm motility quality as paternal age increases, a finding that has been recurrently observed across various studies [61–63]. Aging can impact aspects of sperm function that are not typically evaluated in standard semen analyses. Studies have shown that advanced paternal age leads to significant changes in sperm ultrastructure [64] and alterations in the sperm proteome [65–67]. These variations can impact the integrity of structures and proteins that play a crucial role in sperm motility and fertilization. In addition, a comprehensive examination of the sperm's metabolome and proteome revealed that paternal age affects certain proteins involved in energy metabolism and oxidative stress [67]. This observation is significant because it aligns with other findings indicating that oxidative stress plays a crucial role in the reduction of male fertility as individuals age, as predicted by the free radical theory of aging [68].

4. Paternal Aging: Effects on Sperm Integrity, Epigenetics, and Reproductive Health Implications

In addition to traditional semen parameters, there has been an examination of the genetic traits of sperm as related to paternal age. With advancing age in males, there is an increased vulnerability of the germ line to oxidative damage, characterized by lipid peroxidation, a reduction in the effectiveness of DNA repair processes, and a significant augmentation in DNA fragmentation [69].

This rise in oxidative damage to the germ line could be attributable to a diminishment in the levels of antioxidant protection that these cells have accumulated over the years [70]. This oxidative-induced damage to sperm DNA predominantly takes place during the postmeiotic phase of the male gamete's development [71–74]. Several research studies have observed a striking link between the father's age and sperm chromatin packing, indicating a decline in the integrity of sperm chromatin with age [75]. Meanwhile, other research has reported a rise in sperm DNA fragmentation in males aged 50 years and above, correlating with lower rates of blastocyst formation, although not with the proportion of high-quality blastocysts [76]. Additionally, some studies have highlighted the fact that, beyond DNA fragmentation and oxidative stress, advanced paternal age adversely affects sperm chromatin integrity, encompassing not only the integrity of DNA strands but also the higher-order structural and epigenetic organization of chromatin. This includes modifications of histones, changes in the ratio of histones to protamines, and alterations in the spatial conformation of chromatin. These factors are crucial in determining the success of ART procedures as they influence the functional capacity of sperm to successfully fertilize an oocyte and support normal embryonic development [14,77,78]. Moreover, increased concentrations of sperm reactive oxygen species (ROS) linked to the older age of fathers may be lessened through the addition of antioxidants. The latter intervention could potentially enhance both the rates of fertilization and implantation, as well as embryo quality [79,80].

As men age, their testes are increasingly subjected to oxidative stress, which activates telomerase activity and consequently leads to an increase in sperm telomere length

(STL) within the germ line. This change in STL, which is crucial for chromosome stability and cellular division, is a notable aspect of how paternal age affects sperm characteristics. Regarding male fertility, several studies have observed a clear correlation between telomere length and oxidative stress. More specifically, heightened levels of oxidative stress have been correlated with reduced sperm telomere length, while moderate oxidative stress appears to increase telomere length [81]. Longer telomeres extend the replication capacity of cell lineages before reaching the Hayflick limit and apoptosis. This increased replication might raise the risk of mutations and prolonged exposure to environmental hazards. Recent research suggests a connection between longer telomeres and increased cancer risks, including melanoma and lung adenocarcinoma [82]. Some research studies have demonstrated a positive connection between embryo quality and STL without this necessarily being associated with pregnancy rates [83]. The longer STL in older men may result from elevated testicular telomerase activity or the selective depletion of spermatogonial stem cells with shorter telomeres, a phenomenon known as 'selfish spermatogonial selection' [84].

Intriguingly, while paternal age does not significantly affect overall sperm aneuploidy rates, with research showing no major differences in chromosomal aberrations between older and younger men [85], among older men, observations have been made of a higher prevalence of chromosomal deletions, duplications, and balanced translocations in their sperm. This may be attributable to accumulated mutations during spermatogenesis and sperm transit [86,87]. Significantly, approximately 75% of new mutations in the human species stem from male reproductive cells and are tightly linked to paternal age [88]. These mutations are diverse and may result from replication errors and insufficient repair of DNA damage within male reproductive cells, which is exacerbated by age. It is important to note that mainly single-strand DNA breaks are repaired and less often double-stranded ones, predominantly involving the base excision repair (BER) DNA repair system. Moreover, up to 8% of sperm nuclear DNA damage can be repaired by the oocyte post-fertilization. The sperm is equipped with the OGG1 enzyme, which detects and initiates the repair of oxidative DNA damage. As a result of its action, abasic (AP) sites are created, which, if not properly repaired after fertilization, may lead to mutations [89]. DNA damage in sperm increases exponentially with paternal age [90], contributing to issues observed in ART outcomes and early pregnancy loss [91,92]. Post-fertilization, any imprecise repair of sperm DNA damage can lead to mutations affecting offspring health. This 'post-meiotic oocyte collusion theory' suggests a collaborative influence of both male and female germ lines in mutation formation, with older age impacting DNA integrity in spermatozoa and the DNA repair capacity of the oocyte [90,93–95].

Furthermore, oxidative stress in sperm due to aging particularly affects chromosome 15, which is known to be linked with various neuropathological conditions and sensitive to oxidative damage [95,96]. Such susceptibility to oxidative stress, especially within the interlinker regions of sperm chromatin, may lead to mutations associated with a range of disorders often associated with the older age of the father, emphasizing the complex interplay between oxidative stress, the father's age, and the risk for genetic disorders in offspring [97–100].

Epigenetic modifications in older males, specifically in DNA methylation patterns and chromatin structure, are garnering significant research interest due to their potential impact on offspring phenotypes, embryo development, and embryonic transcription [33,34]. With advancing paternal age, sperm DNA methylation signatures undergo notable changes affecting gene function [16,101]. Aging male spermatozoa exhibit several DNA methylation changes, particularly in CpG regions that regulate genes associated with neurological, psychiatric, and behavioral disorders. Such disorders, with a higher incidence in children of older fathers, include spontaneous schizophrenia, bipolar disease, mood disorders, and autism [86,102]. Recent studies suggest that sperm cell epigenetic profile alterations are linked to autism-related changes in offspring, indicating a critical mechanism by which paternal age influences child health and well-being [103].

The exact molecular processes behind the latter epigenetic alterations in the male germ line remain under investigation but may be related to oxidative stress, a common aspect of male reproductive aging. Oxidative stress can alter various epigenetic components in spermatozoa, including DNA methylation, non-coding RNA species, and the amount and methylation status of histones [104–106]. The effect of age-related oxidative stress on the epigenetic state of men's reproductive cells and its subsequent effects on offspring health is a burgeoning area of study that promises to significantly enhance our understanding of paternal influences on development [107].

5. Impact of Advanced Paternal Age on ART Outcomes

Although the adverse effects of the mother's age on ART outcomes have been richly documented, the effect of older paternal age comprises a more complex and less understood landscape. This section delves into the nuanced impacts of paternal age on several features of ART, including fertilization rates, embryo quality, implantation, miscarriages, and live birth rates. Table 1 below summarizes the impacts of advanced paternal age on ART outcomes and potential mitigation strategies, providing a concise overview of the challenges and solutions identified in this study.

Table 1. Impact and mitigation of paternal aging on ART outcomes.

Aspects of Paternal Aging	Impact on ART Outcomes	Mitigation Strategies
Semen Quality	- Decline in sperm concentration and motility, affecting fertilization rates and embryo development. Increased sperm DNA fragmentation, affecting fertilization and embryo viability.	- Lifestyle changes (e.g., diet, exercise) - Sperm cryopreservation
Genetic Risks	- Increased DNA fragmentation, leading to higher miscarriage rates and potential chromosomal abnormalities in offspring. Increased risk of gene mutations.	- Preimplantation genetic testing - Genetic counseling
Epigenetic Shifts	- Changes in sperm DNA methylation patterns, impacting embryo development and risks of neurological disorders in offspring.	- Ongoing research into epigenetic interventions and their effects
Psychological Aspects	- Increased stress and anxiety related to infertility and the ART process.	- Psychological support and counseling for prospective fathers
Impact on Embryo and Birth Outcomes	- Lower blastocyst development rates and increased risk of adverse birth outcomes (e.g., low birth weight, preterm birth).	- Long-term follow-up studies of offspring health - Genetic screening and counseling
Long-Term Offspring Health	- Higher risk of genetic and neurodevelopmental disorders in children of older fathers.	- Long-term follow-up studies of offspring health. - Genetic screening and counseling

Despite conflicting results and limited data, emerging trends highlight the intricate links between paternal age and ART outcomes [53,108–111].

5.1. Impact of Paternal Age on Fertilization Rates

Numerous studies have examined the impact of paternal age on fertilization rates, particularly within the context of ART, revealing a pattern of decline in older male cohorts. Luna et al. noted a significant decrease in conception rates using IVF among men aged 50 and above, considering the age of egg recipients [27]. Kaarouch et al. similarly observed reduced fertilization rates in males over 40 compared to younger men. However, in cases employing intracytoplasmic sperm injection (ICSI) [108], no unfavorable impact of paternal age was reported on rates of fertilization ($p = 0.008$) [53]. Tiegs et al. additionally observed a drop in fertilization rates as paternal age increased, even after adjusting for the age of egg donors [112]. Moreover, Duran et al. [53] saw a considerable diminishment in fertilization rates that correlated with paternal age in the ICSI subgroup, in particular when a comparison was made between men aged 25–38 and those aged >50.

By contrast with the above findings, other studies present a varied perspective. Johnson et al. pointed to a trade-off between aging in males and early offspring fitness, suggesting a potential influence on fertilization [113]. Hassan & Killick argued that standard sperm evaluations might not fully capture the fertilizing capacity in the context of aging [114]. Meanwhile, Wu et al. reported no significant impact of paternal age on fertilization rates. Collectively, the latter studies point to intricate links between the father's age and ART outcomes, with evidence indicating a decline in fertilization ability in older males, though some results showed no clear effect [115]. This underscores the need for further research to unravel the enigma concerning how advanced paternal age influences ART success.

The effects of advanced paternal age on fertilization rates using ART are complex and multifaceted, stemming from various biological mechanisms. As men age, their risk of de novo mutations of sperm increases, potentially altering its genetic integrity and impairing its fertilizing power [116,117]. Changes to genetic imprinting due to aging may alter gene expression patterns critical for early embryonic development, potentially decreasing fertilization success and leading to difficulties during fertilization [118]. Advanced paternal age has also been linked to an increased risk of genetic diseases that could reduce sperm's effectiveness at fertilizing an egg effectively, as well as declining quality due to DNA fragmentation and chromosomal anomalies [107]. Age-related changes to sperm contribute to both decreased quantity and quality, further decreasing fertilization rates. Genetic and epigenetic alterations suggest a complex but clear pathway through which advanced paternal age influences fertilization outcomes in ART.

5.2. Effect of Paternal Age on Embryo Quality

There has been an ever-increasing focus in recent research on the impact of older paternal age on embryo development and quality in ART. A variety of studies have shown that as men age, there are discernible changes in embryo development rates and quality. A study by Luna et al. reported a drop in the quantity of embryos, having over seven cells on day 3, while a slower pace of blastulation with increasing paternal age [27]. In a study using an egg donation model for ICSI, Girsh et al. found a significant age difference between males in the pregnant group (average age 43.2 ± 8.1 years) and the non-pregnant group (average age 46.8 ± 7.8 years), with a lower proportion of high-quality embryos on day 3 in the non-pregnant group [54]. Frattarelli et al. reported a decline in blastocyst development in males over 55 years, noting a reduction in blastulation rates starting from age 50 [51]. Similarly, Chapuis et al. identified a decrease in blastocyst development rates in couples where the male partner was over 50 years old during IVF procedures [119].

Complementing these findings, García-Ferreyra et al. associated older paternal age with higher aneuploidy rates in embryos coming from donated oocytes, signifying a potential impact on chromosomal abnormalities and embryo quality [120]. Wu et al. provided further insights when analyzing the effect of paternal age on various aspects of embryo quality, such as fertilized oocytes and viable embryos [121]. García-Ferreyra et al. also underlined the correlation between advanced father's age and aneuploidy rates [76].

Adding to this, a recent meta-analysis reported increased rates of blastocyst formation and a higher number of cleavage-stage embryos when the paternal age was under 50 years, again highlighting the controlled maternal age as a significant factor [122]. These findings underscore the nuanced impact of paternal age, suggesting that its negative effects may be mitigated in contexts where maternal factors are standardized.

These studies collectively highlight a potential relationship between higher paternal age and various facets of embryo quality, including aneuploidy rates, blastocyst development, and the overall quality of embryos. They suggest that advanced paternal age could well be related to impaired embryo development and a heightened risk of chromosomal abnormalities, thus impacting reproductive outcomes in ART. The need for further research to elucidate the mechanisms behind these observations and to develop strategies to enhance embryo quality in ART is evident from these diverse and insightful studies.

Advanced paternal age leads to significant genetic and epigenetic changes that adversely affect embryo development and quality. As men age, the structural integrity of sperm DNA diminishes, resulting in increased fragmentation. This fragmentation can impair early embryonic development, compromising both the quality and viability of embryos [86]. Additionally, sperm from older males are more prone to chromosomal anomalies, such as aneuploidies and Y chromosome microdeletions. These abnormalities can disrupt chromosomal segregation during embryo development, increasing the likelihood of miscarriages and diminishing embryo quality [78].

Epigenetic alterations, including changes in DNA methylation and histone configurations, also significantly influence development by altering gene expression in sperm. These modifications can be inherited by embryos, disrupting normal developmental processes and potentially leading to delays or abnormalities [7]. Moreover, these genetic defects and epigenetic changes contribute to what is termed 'sperm genome decay', where the overall genomic integrity of sperm is compromised. Research has shown that this decay negatively affects the sperm's fertilization capability, thereby reducing the quality of embryos and the success rates of ART outcomes [108].

Considering these factors is crucial when assessing embryo quality in ART settings. Implementing genetic screening for egg donor cycles using sperm from older men is recommended to identify and mitigate the risks associated with these genomic and epigenetic changes [123].

5.3. *Effect of Paternal Age on Implantation*

The influence of paternal age on implantation rates in ART has been the subject of several significant studies, each contributing unique insights into this complex relationship. Khandwala et al. conducted a comprehensive cohort study which, while not directly focused on implantation rates, revealed that higher paternal age is related to higher rates of premature birth, low birth weight, and lower Apgar scores [124]. These findings, though indirect, provide valuable context for an enhanced understanding of the broader implications of paternal age on pregnancy outcomes.

Luna et al. examined ART outcomes in ovum recipients, uncovering a possible impact of paternal age on pregnancy outcomes and blastocyst formation rates [27]. Though their research did not explicitly target implantation rates, it pointed to a potential link between paternal age and overall success in ART procedures. In contrast to the above results, Wu et al. explored the reproductive outcomes of in vitro fertilization while reporting a range of differing findings and proposing that paternal age does not appreciably affect implantation rates [115]. This highlights the complexities and variabilities involved in determining the specific effects of paternal age on implantation.

Further adding to the conversation, Meijerink et al. observed that embryo implantation rates tend to decrease as paternal age increases [125]. However, this study also noted inconsistencies regarding overall pregnancy outcomes and did not account for the age of the recipient, indicating the need for a more nuanced understanding of these dynamics [125]. Setti et al. offered a more comprehensive view, reporting that paternal age adversely affects several key factors in ART, including fertilization rates, the quality of embryos on day 3, blastocyst formation, and implantation rates [126]. The latter study additionally identified correlations between advanced paternal age and lower rates of pregnancy and live births.

Collectively, the aforementioned studies point to a nuanced association between advanced paternal age and implantation rates in ART procedures. While some research indicates a potential detrimental effect of increased paternal age on implantation and subsequent pregnancy outcomes, other findings present a more complex and less definitive picture. This diversity in research outcomes underscores the necessity for further studies in this area in order to more accurately decipher the part played by paternal age in implantation success and, overall, ART outcomes. In summary, although evidence exists indicating a correlation between advanced paternal age and implantation rates in ART, the exact nature and scope of this impact still remain areas of active investigation and debate.

The impact of advanced paternal age on embryo implantation in ART involves various factors that have been investigated in several studies. It has been observed that the transfer of euploid embryos resulted in an implantation rate of approximately 60%, while almost 40% of embryos remained unaccounted for, indicating a potential impact of paternal age on implantation rates [127]. Ferreira et al. documented that paternal age could adversely impact implantation and pregnancy rates, particularly in cases of oligozoospermia [56]. Furthermore, a decrease was reported in implantation and pregnancy rates with paternal age in specific maternal age groups, suggesting a potential influence of paternal age on implantation outcomes [121].

Advanced paternal age has been associated with an increase in sperm DNA fragmentation, contributing to blastocyst formation failure and poor clinical outcomes, which could impede embryo implantation [76]. This age-related genetic degradation can compromise embryo integrity by interfering with the early stages of embryo development, leading to lower implantation rates [108]. Furthermore, increased ROS concentrations in sperm associated with older paternal ages may damage sperm and embryo DNA. However, interventions like the addition of idebenone have been shown to lower ROS levels, thereby potentially enhancing embryo quality and improving implantation rates after IVF [79].

Moreover, embryos from older fathers often exhibit decreased quality, evident from higher miscarriage rates and reduced implantation and live birth rates, likely due to increased genetic anomalies and epigenetic modifications prevalent in older males [78]. Despite these findings, Dain et al. report no clear correlation between advanced paternal age and ART outcomes, underscoring the variability and complexity inherent to these procedures and emphasizing the need for further research to fully understand these dynamics [35].

5.4. Effect of Paternal Age on Miscarriages

The extensive discussion surrounding the risks of miscarriage and other negative reproductive outcomes in older men who undergo ART is complex and nuanced. Although several studies tend to suggest that there is no major link between paternal age and the rates of miscarriage or live births, the situation changes slightly when men reach the age of 50 or above [51,110,115,128,129]. After reaching a certain age, a noticeable pattern appears wherein the number of live births tends to decline while the likelihood of miscarriage increases. The risk of miscarriage notably rises, especially beyond the age of 50 [130], and continues to climb even after men reach 40 years old [131]. In addition, offspring of males above 45 are more likely to experience premature birth, with a reported 14% increase in risk [124].

However, a recent meta-analysis has shown that paternal age under 50 years significantly reduces the miscarriage rate in donor oocyte cycles, where maternal age is controlled [122]. This introduces a critical perspective into the ongoing debate about the effects of paternal age, particularly under controlled maternal age conditions.

Nevertheless, there is, at present, no consensus in the literature, and the interpretation of these results is susceptible to various biases. Maternal age often serves as a confounding variable that may influence results [52,55,109,112,132–135]. In order to elucidate this issue, researchers have used IVF data obtained from oocyte donation programs as a means of partly circumventing the danger associated with maternal age. However, the age of the pregnant woman is still a risk factor for giving birth prematurely [136]. Besides age, several variables such as paternal smoking, the type/cause of infertility, the number of previous efforts to achieve ART, maternal smoking habits, and alcohol consumption may significantly impact ART results, hence contributing to the intricacy of risk assessment [129,131].

While the results vary, the overall pattern indicates that a careful approach should be used when contemplating ART for older males. Although 12 studies did not discover a substantial connection between the age of fathers and either miscarriage or live births, other research has shown a decline in the percentage of successful live births and an increase in spontaneous miscarriages as men age. These results emphasize the need for meticulous preimplantation genetic screening as well as the necessity to take into account all possible factors that might affect the evaluation of risks related to advanced paternal age in assisted reproductive technology procedures.

Research has consistently demonstrated that paternal age plays a significant role in miscarriage rates. Men, as they age, experience increased sperm DNA fragmentation rates that compromise embryo development and raise miscarriage risk [108]. Furthermore, studies indicate these age-related changes may lead to an accumulation of chromosomal abnormalities within sperm that, when fertilizing an egg, may result in embryos with genetic defects predisposing them to miscarriage [86,137].

Additionally, advanced paternal age has been found to negatively impact sperm quality overall, manifesting as increased abnormal sperm cells and reduced motility; such changes reduce both successful conception rates as well as increasing risks for poor embryonic outcomes once conception does take place [138,139]. Such findings highlight the intimate link between paternal age and increased miscarriage rates, thus emphasizing the necessity for comprehensive genetic screening, as well as carefully considering all paternal factors when assessing ART risks and outcomes.

5.5. *Effect of Advanced Paternal Age and Perinatal Risks*

The effect of advanced paternal age on certain birth complications, namely, the risk of premature birth, low birth weight, and stillbirth, constitute a crucial area of study in the context of ART procedures. Indeed, a wealth of research has identified a clear association between advanced father's age and a number of unfavorable perinatal outcomes.

Risk of Premature Birth: Advanced paternal age has been associated with a higher risk of premature birth. Studies suggest that fathers aged 40 to 45 years and above may contribute to a higher incidence of preterm births, with infants also facing increased risks of low Apgar scores, a measure of the physical condition of a newborn [124]. A population-based cohort analysis found that 13.2% of premature births were associated with older fathers, indicating a notable correlation between advanced paternal age and the risk for preterm delivery in ART outcomes [124]. Additionally, the same study revealed that higher paternal age is associated with an elevated risk of preterm delivery, gestational diabetes, and neonatal convulsions [124]. After accounting for many confounders, it was shown that the odds ratios of birth abnormalities such as cleft lip, diaphragmatic hernia, right ventricular outflow tract blockage, and pulmonary stenosis increased dramatically with each additional year of paternal age [140].

However, some studies indicate that the father's older age may not be independently linked to any risk of very early preterm delivery [141]. Moreover, another study suggests that in ART-treated and subfertile couples, no association can be identified between older paternal age and a higher risk of prematurity, low birth weight, or small for gestational age, highlighting the variability of findings and the need for further research [133]. This underscores the complexity of assessing risks and the importance of considering individual circumstances and a range of contributing factors when evaluating the potential impacts of advanced paternal age on birth outcomes.

Risk of Low Birth Weight: Advanced paternal age has been linked to a higher risk of low birth weight in neonates, indicating that there is a greater possibility of infants born to fathers of an older age weighing less than what is considered normal for their gestational age at birth. This association holds even when accounting for the age of the mother, a traditionally recognized factor in birth weight [142]. Advanced paternal age is also associated with an increased risk of low birth weight in ART outcomes. The study by Khandwala et al. further reported gestational diabetes in 18.2% of births associated with older fathers, which can be a contributing factor to low birth weight [124]. This underlines the importance of taking paternal age into account in the context of ART treatments and potential birth outcomes, highlighting the multifaceted implications of older paternal age on infant health.

Stillbirth Concerns: Advanced paternal age has been associated with a higher rate of stillbirths, particularly in the case of fathers aged above 40. This suggests a link between the father's age and the viability of the pregnancy, with older paternal age contributing to increased risk during the gestational period [143,144]. It has been observed that fathers of ages 40–45 have a 24% higher risk of their partner suffering stillbirth; this, however, is accompanied by a lower risk of small for gestational age (SGA) infants [145]. The association between older fathers and a higher rate of stillbirths is a significant concern in ART outcomes [145]. This underscores the need for careful consideration and potentially additional monitoring in pregnancies via ART involving older fathers, emphasizing the delicate balance and the complex implications of advanced paternal age on pregnancy outcomes.

Of note, the above adverse outcomes may be influenced by various confounding factors such as maternal age, lifestyle factors (smoking, alcohol consumption), and the type of infertility being treated. An association has also been noted between advanced paternal age and higher risk of gestational diabetes among mothers and infants, complicating the perinatal period [146]. While important associations have been noted between advanced father's age and a number of adverse birth outcomes in the framework of ART, it is essential to consider that these outcomes may additionally stem from other factors, such as the specific ART methods used and individual health conditions.

While the research indicates a clear trend towards increased risks with advancing paternal age, the extent and nature of these risks can vary greatly, with individual outcomes depending on a multitude of factors. The findings also highlight the variability and complexity of the impacts of advanced paternal age on ART outcomes, suggesting that a personalized approach might be necessary for the management of pregnancies involving older fathers. This evidence forms a crucial component of the current article discussing the effects of advanced paternal age on ART outcomes.

In conclusion, it is clear that advanced paternal age has, in many cases, been associated with a higher risk of complications in ART, including premature birth, low birth weight, and stillbirth. These findings should be integrated into clinical practice to optimize the care and counseling provided to couples undergoing ART, especially where the paternal factor is a concern.

Research into the biological mechanisms underlying the association between advanced paternal age and higher perinatal risks has provided us with important insight into how genetic and epigenetic changes within sperm may influence these outcomes. As men age, their sperm becomes subject to genetic mutations and epigenetic modifications that may significantly compromise the health and development of an embryo. Studies have documented an accumulation of DNA mutations in sperm from older fathers that can lead to developmental abnormalities and compromise pregnancies [7,8]. Epigenetic changes often exacerbate genetic modifications, as changes to DNA methylation patterns can influence gene expression within an embryo and impact its survival and development [86].

Age also diminishes the quality of semen, leading to decreased motility and increasing incidences of abnormal sperm. These changes reduce the probability of successful fertilization while simultaneously increasing miscarriages and low birthweight births [108]. Furthermore, advanced paternal age could serve as a proxy for other risk factors that accumulate with age, such as health conditions or environmental exposures that impact offspring's health and further complicate perinatal risks associated with older fathers [147].

Understanding these mechanisms is vital in order to effectively assess risks in ART treatments, and it stresses the significance of paternal age as a significant factor in prenatal care and counseling. With this knowledge comes an ability to create targeted interventions that may reduce risks and improve perinatal outcomes.

5.6. Effect of Paternal Age on Live Birth Rate

Campos et al. discovered a detrimental impact of increased paternal age on clinical pregnancy within the context of oocyte donation [111]. However, the authors noted that maternal age might potentially be a confounding factor. Specifically, the negative association between pregnancy and age became insignificant when one of the parents was below the age of 39. Wu et al. conducted a research study that found a decline in clinical pregnancy rates among males over the age of 36 compared to those under the age of 32 [115]. The latter was demonstrated among couples of whom the mother was aged 30–34 years. In a similar manner, Ferreira et al. assessed the results of ICSI based on the age of the father in men with normal sperm count and men with low sperm count [56]. Upon adjusting for mother's age, number of oocytes extracted, sperm concentration, and rate of fertilization, the authors observed a drop in implantation and pregnancy rates, particularly among older fathers with oligozoospermia. The researchers reached the conclusion that the likelihood of successful pregnancy decreases by 5% for every additional year of paternal age in individuals with oligozoospermia [56]. Various studies have established a connection between greater paternal age and a longer duration needed for conception after the age of 34 [12], as well as a reduced success rate in ARTs [14].

In a study conducted by Park et al. on males with azoospermia, it was shown that couples with male partners beyond the age of 46 had lower clinical pregnancy rates, regardless of the etiology of azoospermia [148]. Frattarelli et al. observed a direct correlation between higher rates of pregnancy loss and older paternal age [51]. The study revealed a notable disparity in the rates of pregnancy loss between males under the age of 50 (41.5%) and those above the age of 50 (24.4%; relative risk 0.61, 95% confidence interval: 0.45–0.84; $p < 0.01$) [51]. Additional research indicated a tendency towards higher rates of pregnancy loss among dads of advanced age; however, the findings did not achieve statistical significance [119].

A number of studies have investigated the effect of paternal age on the frequency of successful live births [51,128]. McPherson et al. observed a decline in LBR in couples with advanced maternal age (>35) and paternal age (>40) [128]. The authors postulated that the detrimental impact of advancing age on SDF (sperm DNA fragmentation), the oocyte's cytoplasmic DNA repair systems, and endometrial receptivity could account for the suboptimal reproductive results observed in couples of older age. Nevertheless, the authors of the above study cautioned that the damaging effect of paternal age on ART results is, in fact, a good deal less significant than the influence of the mother's age [128]. Subsequent to artificial insemination, the pregnancy rate declined by half among males aged 35 and over [149], while following IVF, the pregnancy rate was considerably altered among men aged 50 and over [30].

In contrast, other groups did not demonstrate any influence of paternal age on ART outcomes. In a research study conducted by Bellver et al., it was shown that there were no statistically significant variations in pregnancy rates and miscarriage rates across various paternal age categories [52]. Within the subset of egg donors, the researchers observed a rise in embryo fragmentation linked to paternal age. However, the association was minimal, casting doubt on its clinical relevance [52]. In a separate research study including 278 couples, Nijs et al. noted no discernible variations in fertilization rates, pregnancy rates, and live birth rates when the age of the mother was taken into account [75]. However, this research work excluded males with severe oligoasthenoteratozoospermia (OAT), men using testicular sperm for ICSI, and instances that included preimplantation genetic testing.

It is of note that most studies that indicated no impact of paternal age on ART results had limited sample sizes and a smaller number of males over the age of 40 [52,150,151]. However, other research work included large groups of participants and considered such factors as the age of the mother and the quantity of embryos transplanted in each reproductive cycle. Meijerink et al. carried out a study in which they assessed the effect of paternal age on the first attempt at ART in 7051 couples [125]. The authors additionally evaluated the influence of paternal age based on the origin of sperm used for ICSI, specifically, ejaculated sperm and sperm obtained by procedures such as percutaneous epididymal sperm aspiration (PESA), microsurgical epididymal sperm aspiration (MESA), and testicular sperm extraction (TESE). The latter wide-ranging research study reported no association between paternal age and continued pregnancy rates achieved via ART. Furthermore, the source of sperm did not have any impact on the outcomes of pregnancy. In contrast, Whitcomb et al. noted no negative effect of paternal age in a study comprising 1083 couples who used an oocyte donor [152]. This finding remained consistent even after accounting for the female partner's age.

A study by Begueria et al., which examined an egg donation model using ICSI as the only fertilization method, reported that male age did not have any impact on pregnancy outcomes [55]. The latter method includes the rates of biochemical pregnancy (RR: 1.0; 95% CI: 0.96–1.05), miscarriage (RR: 1.06; 95% CI: 0.94–1.03), ongoing pregnancy (RR: 0.98; 95% CI: 0.94–1.033), and live birth (RR: 0.98; 95% CI: 0.94–1.03) [55]. Ghuman et al., who carried out a study on the effect of advanced paternal age (i.e., 40–45 years of age) in a sperm donation method, reported analogous results. After considering female age, treatment technique, and the impact of prior treatment cycles, no correlation was noted between the father's age and miscarriage or LBR. Despite these findings, the authors warned that it may not be feasible to apply their conclusions to a wider population since the sperm used in the study came from a specific group of donors, even though most men seeking assisted reproductive technology had abnormal sperm characteristics [109].

In summary, while there are minimal data indicating a potential detrimental effect of greater paternal age on ART outcomes, the possible association between these two factors remains uncertain. Among all of the research studies, it is evident that maternal age is the primary determinant of pregnancy success in IVF and ICSI.

Advanced paternal age profoundly impacts reproductive outcomes, primarily due to increased SDF. As men age, there is an increase in DNA mutations and chromosomal aneuploidies, which are linked to reduced fertilization rates, higher miscarriage rates, and an increase in congenital anomalies. Such genetic risks significantly compromise embryo quality, reducing implantation rates and live birth rates from IVF/ICSI treatments, especially notable in fathers over 40 years of age [7,153].

Moreover, the combined effects of paternal and maternal ages intensify these risks, with advanced age in both parents exacerbating the decline in live birth rates. Interestingly, the negative impacts of older paternal age on live birth outcomes are somewhat mitigated when the female partner is under 35, suggesting that younger maternal age can buffer the adverse effects of aged sperm [128]. Furthermore, advanced paternal age is linked to a higher risk of adverse birth outcomes such as low birth weight, preterm birth, and stillbirth, which indirectly affect the live birth rate by compromising pregnancy viability [154,155].

The negative impacts of advanced paternal age on live birth rates arise from a complex interaction among decreased sperm quality, genetic risks, and combined maternal age effects. These findings underscore the necessity of reproductive counseling and ART protocols that take paternal age into account to optimize care and increase the chances of successful pregnancy outcomes. Further research must be conducted in order to fully comprehend these dynamics and tailor treatment plans appropriately.

6. Strategies for Deferred Fatherhood and Future Research Directions

ART has revolutionized the treatment of infertility. However, the influence of advanced paternal age presents unique challenges that impact the success and outcomes of ART procedures. Understanding these challenges is crucial for the development of strategies to mitigate risks and improve outcomes. Meanwhile, the exact connection between paternal age and ART results is highly complex and, thus, at present, remains beyond our understanding. While a considerable amount of research often suggests a detrimental impact, particularly for men aged 40 or above [110,128], pinpointing a specific age threshold where risks significantly increase remains challenging [111,115]. This ambiguity arises from the diverse methodologies and demographics employed in studies, along with a diversity of outcome measures, making qualitative comparisons and meta-analyses difficult. Guidelines from the Society of Obstetricians and Gynecologists of Canada (SOGC) and the American College of Obstetricians and Gynecologists (ACOG) suggest considering men aged 40 and above as "older fathers" in ART contexts [156,157] and recommend counseling regarding the risks of postponing parenthood, which entails probable diminishing success in ART procedures, as well as a number of health challenges for the offspring.

Despite the expanding corpus of research on ART in older males, numerous questions remain unresolved. At present, a definitive counseling guideline expressly designed for older men seeking reproductive assistance is notably absent. In practice, counseling is predicated on the clinical condition of the patient, the possible existence of comorbidities, and his social and cultural background. This approach underscores the necessity for a nuanced and individualized framework to address the unique needs and circumstances of this demographic.

Oral antioxidants have been extensively used, though with varied outcomes, to mitigate the adverse effects of oxidative stress on sperm in men with infertility [158]. This approach might also be considered for older males, whose sperm are more susceptible to oxidative harm. Similarly, in the broader community of men with infertility, there is as yet no knowledge concerning which could be the most efficacious combination(s) of antioxidants nor what their dose and duration should be. While antioxidant supplements could be efficacious for the enhancement of male productive health in older-aged men, it is crucial to be aware of 'the antioxidant paradox'. This term, introduced by Halliwell et al., highlights the potential downsides to the excessive use of antioxidants [159]. Overexposure to these reducing agents can lead to reductive stress, a condition similar to oxidative stress, which might impair the fertilizing potential of the spermatozoa in a manner akin to oxidative stress itself [160].

In counseling prospective fathers, it is imperative to engage in a comprehensive discourse regarding the merits and demerits of deferring paternity. Young men contemplating postponed fatherhood might consider sperm cryopreservation as a strategic intervention to ameliorate the age-related decline in fertility. Nonetheless, the decision to opt for elective sperm freezing necessitates a careful evaluation of several pivotal factors, particularly as the thawed sperm will require utilization in conjunction with assisted reproductive techniques [161].

While the utilization of semen from a younger patient may theoretically diminish the incidence of such conditions as Down syndrome, schizophrenia, and autism spectrum disorders, the potential compromise to sperm quality and DNA integrity due to the freeze–thaw process warrants serious consideration [162]. Moreover, beyond these biological risks, it is critical to meticulously address and evaluate the associated ethical, legal, and financial implications when counseling potential fathers about sperm cryopreservation [162].

While there are established protocols for sperm storage among patients with conditions such as nonobstructive azoospermia (NOA) or those undergoing chemotherapy, the absence of explicit guidelines for sperm freezing solely for the purpose of delayed fatherhood presents a challenge [163]. Consequently, it is vital to conduct personalized discussions with each patient, thoroughly weighing the potential benefits against the inherent risks and uncertainties. This tailored approach ensures informed decision-making, aligning with each patient's unique circumstances and aspirations [163].

When providing counseling to older males who are about to undergo ART, it is important to address the topic of preimplantation genetic testing (PGT). Preimplantation genetic testing for aneuploidy screening (PGT-a) is often used to identify abnormalities in embryos and choose healthy embryos for transfer to the uterus. This technique is especially beneficial for women of advanced age and those who have had repeated pregnancy loss. The latter approach is also applied to conduct tests for particular genetic diseases, such as monogenic and single gene abnormalities (PGT-m), as well as chromosomal structural rearrangements (PGT-Sr). The use of PGT may result in an 18% improvement in implantation rates for older women as compared to using unscreened ICSI embryos [164,165].

Furthermore, it is equally crucial to provide counseling to infertile patients, particularly those who are aging, on the potential detrimental effects of smoking, exposure to gonadotoxins, and alcohol usage since all of these factors may significantly affect fertility [166]. While couples undergoing ART frequently overlook the need for detection and treatment of underlying disorders linked to infertility, it is crucial to prioritize these features in the care of males seeking fertility, regardless of their age group. This approach has the potential to enhance the results of ART procedures [167].

The adoption of antioxidant supplementation, the pursuit of a health-conscious lifestyle, the management of underlying conditions associated with infertility, and the preservation of sperm through cryobanking constitute viable strategies for younger individuals contemplating deferred parenthood. Older persons who are considering ART, particularly those beyond the age of 50, should contemplate the incorporation of PGT-A as a prudent aid to mitigate potential genetic risks. This multifaceted approach represents a proactive stance towards reproductive planning, aligning with contemporary advancements in reproductive health and technology.

Future research directions in the setting of advanced paternal age and ART are crucial to deepening our understanding and improving outcomes. One critical area demanding further exploration is the epigenetic mechanisms that accompany advancing paternal age. In-depth research is needed to elucidate how changes in DNA methylation and histone modifications, as well as the influence of non-coding RNAs, contribute to paternal age-related reproductive outcomes. Gaining greater insight into these epigenetic alterations is essential in order to better comprehend their potential impact on ART outcomes and offspring health. Investigations into these mechanisms promise to reveal significant findings regarding potential therapeutic targets and interventions that can profoundly influence the field [107].

Another vital future direction involves the implementation of longitudinal studies, which are essential to monitor and, thereby, increase our knowledge about the long-term health trajectories of offspring conceived through ART from older fathers. By tracking these individuals over extended periods, researchers can gather invaluable data on the prevalence and nature of genetic, neurodevelopmental, and psychiatric disorders. Such long-term follow-up studies are crucial for a comprehensive understanding of the multifaceted impact that advanced paternal age has on the health and well-being of progeny [168].

Also, with regard to crucial future directions, employing sophisticated genetic and epigenetic profiling techniques enabling assessment of the impact of advanced paternal age on sperm quality, embryo development, and offspring health constitutes yet another vital area of research. Utilizing these methodologies can provide critical data for identification of biomarkers and predictive indicators essential for ART success and offspring health [169].

Simultaneously, the design and execution of interventional studies are crucial to evaluate the effectiveness of lifestyle and health interventions in mitigating the risks associated with advanced paternal age in ART. Such studies are invaluable for developing evidence-based strategies aimed at optimizing reproductive outcomes and reducing the incidence of genetic and neurodevelopmental disorders in offspring [170].

In summary, effectively addressing the challenges posed by advanced paternal age in ART requires a comprehensive and integrative approach involving clinical interventions, advancements in research, and multidisciplinary collaboration. By focusing on these research directions and potential solutions, the field of reproductive medicine is well positioned to enhance ART outcomes and improve the health and well-being of offspring conceived through ART with older fathers.

7. Conclusions

In conclusion, today's growing trend towards advanced paternal age poses challenges in ART, involving declining sperm quality, genetic risks, and psychological impacts. Men aged 40 or older face increased genetic risks and sperm quality decline, though the impact of these on ART results is smaller than those arising from maternal age. Meanwhile, the offspring of older fathers are exposed to a greater risk of developing a number of health issues. In view of all the latter considerations, reproductive medicine must adapt. Strategies for men considering delayed fatherhood include early disease detection, sperm freezing, and antioxidants. Preimplantation genetic testing is an option for men over 50 using ART. A wide-ranging approach is certainly required to plot a course through the numerous complexities pertaining to advanced paternal age in order to guarantee optimal outcomes both for couples and for their children in the context of ART.

Author Contributions: A.K. was involved in the conceptualization and writing of the major part of the original draft, providing a strong foundation for the study. A.Z. (Athanasios Zikopoulos), D.V., and C.S. were instrumental in searching the relevant literature and contributed significantly to writing various parts of the manuscript, ensuring a comprehensive review of existing knowledge. N.V. and S.S. contributed their expertise through critical review and editing of the manuscript, enhancing its academic rigor. E.N.S. and F.D. also engaged in the critical review process, offering valuable insights that refined the manuscript further. M.C., N.S. and A.Z. (Athanasios Zachariou), the corresponding author, were involved in the overarching conceptualization of the study and provided the final editing and review of the manuscript, ensuring its readiness for publication. All authors have read and agreed to the published version of the manuscript.

Funding: This research received no external funding.

Institutional Review Board Statement: Not applicable.

Informed Consent Statement: Not applicable.

Data Availability Statement: Not applicable.

Conflicts of Interest: The authors declare no conflicts of interest.

References

1. Sartorius, G.A.; Nieschlag, E. Paternal age and reproduction. *Hum. Reprod. Update* **2010**, *16*, 65–79. [CrossRef] [PubMed]
2. Schmidt, L.; Sobotka, T.; Bentzen, J.G.; Nyboe Andersen, A.; Reproduction, E.; Society Task, F. Demographic and medical consequences of the postponement of parenthood. *Hum. Reprod. Update* **2012**, *18*, 29–43. [CrossRef] [PubMed]
3. Craig, J.R.; Jenkins, T.G.; Carrell, D.T.; Hotaling, J.M. Obesity, male infertility, and the sperm epigenome. *Fertil. Steril.* **2017**, *107*, 848–859. [CrossRef] [PubMed]
4. Campbell, J.M.; Lane, M.; Owens, J.A.; Bakos, H.W. Paternal obesity negatively affects male fertility and assisted reproduction outcomes: A systematic review and meta-analysis. *Reprod. Biomed. Online* **2015**, *31*, 593–604. [CrossRef] [PubMed]
5. Mills, M.; Rindfuss, R.R.; McDonald, P.; te Velde, E.; Reproduction, E.; Society Task, F. Why do people postpone parenthood? Reasons and social policy incentives. *Hum. Reprod. Update* **2011**, *17*, 848–860. [CrossRef] [PubMed]
6. Bray, I.; Gunnell, D.; Davey Smith, G. Advanced paternal age: How old is too old? *J. Epidemiol. Community Health* **2006**, *60*, 851–853. [CrossRef] [PubMed]
7. Sharma, R.; Agarwal, A.; Rohra, V.K.; Assidi, M.; Abu-Elmagd, M.; Turki, R.F. Effects of increased paternal age on sperm quality, reproductive outcome and associated epigenetic risks to offspring. *Reprod. Biol. Endocrinol.* **2015**, *13*, 35. [CrossRef] [PubMed]
8. Kaltsas, A.; Moustakli, E.; Zikopoulos, A.; Georgiou, I.; Dimitriadis, F.; Symeonidis, E.N.; Markou, E.; Michaelidis, T.M.; Tien, D.M.B.; Giannakis, I.; et al. Impact of Advanced Paternal Age on Fertility and Risks of Genetic Disorders in Offspring. *Genes* **2023**, *14*, 486. [CrossRef] [PubMed]
9. Santi, D.; Lotti, F.; Sparano, C.; Rastrelli, G.; Isidori, A.M.; Pivonello, R.; Barbonetti, A.; Salonia, A.; Minhas, S.; Krausz, C.; et al. Does an increase in adipose tissue 'weight' affect male fertility? A systematic review and meta-analysis based on semen analysis performed using the WHO 2010 criteria. *Andrology* **2024**, *12*, 123–136. [CrossRef] [PubMed]
10. Du Plessis, S.S.; Cabler, S.; McAlister, D.A.; Sabanegh, E.; Agarwal, A. The effect of obesity on sperm disorders and male infertility. *Nat. Rev. Urol.* **2010**, *7*, 153–161. [CrossRef]
11. Kaltsas, A.; Markou, E.; Zachariou, A.; Dimitriadis, F.; Mamoulakis, C.; Andreadakis, S.; Giannakis, I.; Tsounapi, P.; Takenaka, A.; Sofikitis, N. Varicoceles in Men With Non-obstructive Azoospermia: The Dilemma to Operate or Not. *Front. Reprod. Health* **2022**, *4*, 811487. [CrossRef] [PubMed]

12. Stone, B.A.; Alex, A.; Werlin, L.B.; Marrs, R.P. Age thresholds for changes in semen parameters in men. *Fertil. Steril.* **2013**, *100*, 952–958. [CrossRef] [PubMed]
13. D'Onofrio, B.M.; Rickert, M.E.; Frans, E.; Kuja-Halkola, R.; Almqvist, C.; Sjolander, A.; Larsson, H.; Lichtenstein, P. Paternal age at childbearing and offspring psychiatric and academic morbidity. *JAMA Psychiatry* **2014**, *71*, 432–438. [CrossRef] [PubMed]
14. Halvaei, I.; Litzky, J.; Esfandiari, N. Advanced paternal age: Effects on sperm parameters, assisted reproduction outcomes and offspring health. *Reprod. Biol. Endocrinol.* **2020**, *18*, 110. [CrossRef] [PubMed]
15. Khandwala, Y.S.; Zhang, C.A.; Lu, Y.; Eisenberg, M.L. The age of fathers in the USA is rising: An analysis of 168 867 480 births from 1972 to 2015. *Hum. Reprod.* **2017**, *32*, 2110–2116. [CrossRef] [PubMed]
16. Gourinat, A.; Mazeaud, C.; Hubert, J.; Eschwege, P.; Koscinski, I. Impact of paternal age on assisted reproductive technology outcomes and offspring health: A systematic review. *Andrology* **2023**, *11*, 973–986. [CrossRef] [PubMed]
17. Human, F.; Embryology, A. *Code of Practice*, 9th ed.; HM Revenue & Customs: Belfast, Ireland, 2023.
18. Practice Committee of the American Society for Reproductive Medicine; The Practice Committee for the Society for Assisted Reproductive Technology. Guidance regarding gamete and embryo donation. *Fertil. Steril.* **2021**, *115*, 1395–1410. [CrossRef] [PubMed]
19. Fertility Society of Australia & New Zealand. RTAC Code of Practice. Available online: https://www.fertilitysociety.com.au/rtac-australia-new-zealand/ (accessed on 12 April 2021).
20. Agence de la biomédecine. Avis du Conseil D'orientation émis à L'initiative de Son Président et Concernant L'âge de Procréer. Available online: https://www.agence-biomedecine.fr/Avis-du-conseil-d-orientation-emis,880 (accessed on 5 July 2017).
21. European Society of Human Reproduction and Embryology. Statements by the Task Force Ethics and Law. Available online: https://www.eshre.eu/Specialty-groups/Special-Interest-Groups/Ethics-and-Law/Documents-of-the-Task-Force-Ethics-Law (accessed on 27 April 2021).
22. Cavazos-Rehg, P.A.; Krauss, M.J.; Spitznagel, E.L.; Bommarito, K.; Madden, T.; Olsen, M.A.; Subramaniam, H.; Peipert, J.F.; Bierut, L.J. Maternal age and risk of labor and delivery complications. *Matern. Child Health J.* **2015**, *19*, 1202–1211. [CrossRef] [PubMed]
23. Phillips, N.; Taylor, L.; Bachmann, G. Maternal, infant and childhood risks associated with advanced paternal age: The need for comprehensive counseling for men. *Maturitas* **2019**, *125*, 81–84. [CrossRef]
24. Jain, T.; Grainger, D.A.; Ball, G.D.; Gibbons, W.E.; Rebar, R.W.; Robins, J.C.; Leach, R.E. 30 years of data: Impact of the United States in vitro fertilization data registry on advancing fertility care. *Fertil. Steril.* **2019**, *111*, 477–488. [CrossRef]
25. Marsidi, A.M.; Kipling, L.M.; Kawwass, J.F.; Mehta, A. Influence of paternal age on assisted reproductive technology cycles and perinatal outcomes. *Fertil. Steril.* **2021**, *116*, 380–387. [CrossRef] [PubMed]
26. Sampson, N.; Untergasser, G.; Plas, E.; Berger, P. The ageing male reproductive tract. *J. Pathol.* **2007**, *211*, 206–218. [CrossRef] [PubMed]
27. Luna, M.; Finkler, E.; Barritt, J.; Bar-Chama, N.; Sandler, B.; Copperman, A.B.; Grunfeld, L. Paternal age and assisted reproductive technology outcome in ovum recipients. *Fertil. Steril.* **2009**, *92*, 1772–1775. [CrossRef] [PubMed]
28. Bartolacci, A.; Pagliardini, L.; Makieva, S.; Salonia, A.; Papaleo, E.; Vigano, P. Abnormal sperm concentration and motility as well as advanced paternal age compromise early embryonic development but not pregnancy outcomes: A retrospective study of 1266 ICSI cycles. *J. Assist. Reprod. Genet.* **2018**, *35*, 1897–1903. [CrossRef] [PubMed]
29. De La Rochebrochard, E.; Thonneau, P. Paternal age: Are the risks of infecundity and miscarriage higher when the man is aged 40 years or over? *Rev. D'épidémiologie Et Santé Publique* **2005**, *53*, 47–55. [CrossRef]
30. Aboulghar, M.; Mansour, R.; Al-Inany, H.; Abou-Setta, A.M.; Aboulghar, M.; Mourad, L.; Serour, G. Paternal age and outcome of intracytoplasmic sperm injection. *Reprod. Biomed. Online* **2007**, *14*, 588–592. [CrossRef] [PubMed]
31. Horta, F.; Vollenhoven, B.; Healey, M.; Busija, L.; Catt, S.; Temple-Smith, P. Male ageing is negatively associated with the chance of live birth in IVF/ICSI cycles for idiopathic infertility. *Hum. Reprod.* **2019**, *34*, 2523–2532. [CrossRef]
32. Van Opstal, J.; Fieuws, S.; Spiessens, C.; Soubry, A. Male age interferes with embryo growth in IVF treatment. *Hum. Reprod.* **2021**, *36*, 107–115. [CrossRef]
33. Ilacqua, A.; Izzo, G.; Emerenziani, G.P.; Baldari, C.; Aversa, A. Lifestyle and fertility: The influence of stress and quality of life on male fertility. *Reprod. Biol. Endocrinol.* **2018**, *16*, 115. [CrossRef]
34. Laurentino, S.; Cremers, J.F.; Horsthemke, B.; Tuttelmann, F.; Czeloth, K.; Zitzmann, M.; Pohl, E.; Rahmann, S.; Schroder, C.; Berres, S.; et al. A germ cell-specific ageing pattern in otherwise healthy men. *Aging Cell* **2020**, *19*, e13242. [CrossRef]
35. Dain, L.; Auslander, R.; Dirnfeld, M. The effect of paternal age on assisted reproduction outcome. *Fertil. Steril.* **2011**, *95*, 1–8. [CrossRef] [PubMed]
36. Shandley, L.M.; DeSantis, C.E.; Lee, J.C.; Kawwass, J.F.; Hipp, H.S. Trends and Outcomes of Assisted Reproductive Technology Cycles Using a Gestational Carrier Between 2014 and 2020. *JAMA* **2023**, *330*, 1691–1694. [CrossRef] [PubMed]
37. Paavilainen, M.; Bloigu, A.; Hemminki, E.; Gissler, M.; Klemetti, R. Aging fatherhood in Finland—First-time fathers in Finland from 1987 to 2009. *Scand. J. Public Health* **2016**, *44*, 423–430. [CrossRef] [PubMed]
38. Lewington, L.; Lee, J.; Sebar, B. "I'm not Just a Babysitter": Masculinity and Men's Experiences of First-Time Fatherhood. *Men Masculinities* **2021**, *24*, 571–589. [CrossRef]
39. Wang, Z.; Liu, X.; Xu, J.; Yang, Q.; Niu, W.; Dai, S.; Hu, L.; Guo, Y. Paternal age, body mass index, and semen volume are associated with chromosomal aberrations-related miscarriages in couples that underwent treatment by assisted reproductive technology. *Aging* **2020**, *12*, 8459–8472. [CrossRef] [PubMed]

40. Reinicke, K. "I thought, Oh shit, because I was 19." Discourses and practices on young fatherhood in Denmark. *Fam. Relatsh. Soc.* **2021**, *10*, 463–478. [CrossRef]
41. Xi, Y.P.; Nette, E.G.; King, D.W.; Rosen, M. Age-related changes in normal human basement membrane. *Mech. Ageing Dev.* **1982**, *19*, 315–324. [CrossRef]
42. Jiang, H.; Zhu, W.J.; Li, J.; Chen, Q.J.; Liang, W.B.; Gu, Y.Q. Quantitative histological analysis and ultrastructure of the aging human testis. *Int. Urol. Nephrol.* **2014**, *46*, 879–885. [CrossRef]
43. Dong, S.; Chen, C.; Zhang, J.; Gao, Y.; Zeng, X.; Zhang, X. Testicular aging, male fertility and beyond. *Front. Endocrinol.* **2022**, *13*, 1012119. [CrossRef]
44. Nita, M.; Strzalka-Mrozik, B.; Grzybowski, A.; Mazurek, U.; Romaniuk, W. Age-related macular degeneration and changes in the extracellular matrix. *Med. Sci. Monit.* **2014**, *20*, 1003–1016. [CrossRef]
45. Pohl, E.; Gromoll, J.; Wistuba, J.; Laurentino, S. Healthy ageing and spermatogenesis. *Reproduction* **2021**, *161*, R89–R101. [CrossRef] [PubMed]
46. Johnson, S.L.; Dunleavy, J.; Gemmell, N.J.; Nakagawa, S. Consistent age-dependent declines in human semen quality: A systematic review and meta-analysis. *Ageing Res. Rev.* **2015**, *19*, 22–33. [CrossRef]
47. Oliveira, J.B.A.; Petersen, C.G.; Mauri, A.L.; Vagnini, L.D.; Baruffi, R.L.R.; Franco, J.G., Jr. The effects of age on sperm quality: An evaluation of 1,500 semen samples. *JBRA Assist. Reprod.* **2014**, *18*, 34–41. [CrossRef] [PubMed]
48. Zhu, Q.X.; Meads, C.; Lu, M.L.; Wu, J.Q.; Zhou, W.J.; Gao, E.S. Turning point of age for semen quality: A population-based study in Chinese men. *Fertil. Steril.* **2011**, *96*, 572–576. [CrossRef]
49. Eskenazi, B.; Wyrobek, A.J.; Sloter, E.; Kidd, S.A.; Moore, L.; Young, S.; Moore, D. The association of age and semen quality in healthy men. *Hum. Reprod.* **2003**, *18*, 447–454. [CrossRef]
50. Plas, E.; Berger, P.; Hermann, M.; Pfluger, H. Effects of aging on male fertility? *Exp. Gerontol.* **2000**, *35*, 543–551. [CrossRef]
51. Frattarelli, J.L.; Miller, K.A.; Miller, B.T.; Elkind-Hirsch, K.; Scott, R.T., Jr. Male age negatively impacts embryo development and reproductive outcome in donor oocyte assisted reproductive technology cycles. *Fertil. Steril.* **2008**, *90*, 97–103. [CrossRef]
52. Bellver, J.; Garrido, N.; Remohi, J.; Pellicer, A.; Meseguer, M. Influence of paternal age on assisted reproduction outcome. *Reprod. Biomed. Online* **2008**, *17*, 595–604. [CrossRef] [PubMed]
53. Duran, E.H.; Dowling-Lacey, D.; Bocca, S.; Stadtmauer, L.; Oehninger, S. Impact of male age on the outcome of assisted reproductive technology cycles using donor oocytes. *Reprod. Biomed. Online* **2010**, *20*, 848–856. [CrossRef]
54. Girsh, E.; Katz, N.; Genkin, L.; Girtler, O.; Bocker, J.; Bezdin, S.; Barr, I. Male age influences oocyte-donor program results. *J. Assist. Reprod. Genet.* **2008**, *25*, 137–143. [CrossRef]
55. Begueria, R.; Garcia, D.; Obradors, A.; Poisot, F.; Vassena, R.; Vernaeve, V. Paternal age and assisted reproductive outcomes in ICSI donor oocytes: Is there an effect of older fathers? *Hum. Reprod.* **2014**, *29*, 2114–2122. [CrossRef] [PubMed]
56. Ferreira, R.C.; Braga, D.P.; Bonetti, T.C.; Pasqualotto, F.F.; Iaconelli, A., Jr.; Borges, E., Jr. Negative influence of paternal age on clinical intracytoplasmic sperm injection cycle outcomes in oligozoospermic patients. *Fertil. Steril.* **2010**, *93*, 1870–1874. [CrossRef] [PubMed]
57. Lee, D.M.; Nazroo, J.; O'Connor, D.B.; Blake, M.; Pendleton, N. Sexual Health and Well-being Among Older Men and Women in England: Findings from the English Longitudinal Study of Ageing. *Arch. Sex. Behav.* **2016**, *45*, 133–144. [CrossRef] [PubMed]
58. Kasman, A.M.; Li, S.; Zhao, Q.; Behr, B.; Eisenberg, M.L. Relationship between male age, semen parameters and assisted reproductive technology outcomes. *Andrology* **2021**, *9*, 245–252. [CrossRef] [PubMed]
59. Lai, S.F.; Li, R.H.; Yeung, W.S.; Ng, E.H. Effect of paternal age on semen parameters and live birth rate of in-vitro fertilisation treatment: A retrospective analysis. *Hong Kong Med. J.* **2018**, *24*, 444–450. [CrossRef] [PubMed]
60. Auger, J.; Kunstmann, J.M.; Czyglik, F.; Jouannet, P. Decline in semen quality among fertile men in Paris during the past 20 years. *N. Engl. J. Med.* **1995**, *332*, 281–285. [CrossRef]
61. Veron, G.L.; Tissera, A.D.; Bello, R.; Beltramone, F.; Estofan, G.; Molina, R.I.; Vazquez-Levin, M.H. Impact of age, clinical conditions, and lifestyle on routine semen parameters and sperm kinematics. *Fertil. Steril.* **2018**, *110*, 68–75.e64. [CrossRef]
62. Freour, T.; Jean, M.; Mirallie, S.; Barriere, P. Computer-assisted sperm analysis parameters in young fertile sperm donors and relationship with age. *Syst. Biol. Reprod. Med.* **2012**, *58*, 102–106. [CrossRef]
63. Sloter, E.; Schmid, T.E.; Marchetti, F.; Eskenazi, B.; Nath, J.; Wyrobek, A.J. Quantitative effects of male age on sperm motion. *Hum. Reprod.* **2006**, *21*, 2868–2875. [CrossRef]
64. Baccetti, B.; Renieri, T.; Selmi, M.G.; Soldani, P. Sperm morphogenesis, structure and function in humans over 70 years old. *J. Submicrosc. Cytol.* **1984**, *16*, 585–600.
65. Bastos, P.; Freitas, M.J.; Gomes, A.; Vitorino, R.; Fardilha, M. Unravelling the Power of Omics for the Infertile Aging Male. *Curr. Pharm. Des.* **2017**, *23*, 4451–4469. [CrossRef]
66. Liu, F.J.; Liu, X.; Han, J.L.; Wang, Y.W.; Jin, S.H.; Liu, X.X.; Liu, J.; Wang, W.T.; Wang, W.J. Aged men share the sperm protein PATE1 defect with young asthenozoospermia patients. *Hum. Reprod.* **2015**, *30*, 861–869. [CrossRef]
67. Guo, Y.; Li, J.; Hao, F.; Yang, Y.; Yang, H.; Chang, Q.; Kong, P.; Liu, W.; Jiao, X.; Teng, X. A new perspective on semen quality of aged male: The characteristics of metabolomics and proteomics. *Front. Endocrinol.* **2022**, *13*, 1058250. [CrossRef]
68. Liochev, S.I. Reactive oxygen species and the free radical theory of aging. *Free. Radic. Biol. Med.* **2013**, *60*, 1–4. [CrossRef]
69. Almeida, S.; Rato, L.; Sousa, M.; Alves, M.G.; Oliveira, P.F. Fertility and Sperm Quality in the Aging Male. *Curr. Pharm. Des.* **2017**, *23*, 4429–4437. [CrossRef]

70. Nago, M.; Arichi, A.; Omura, N.; Iwashita, Y.; Kawamura, T.; Yumura, Y. Aging increases oxidative stress in semen. *Investig. Clin. Urol.* **2021**, *62*, 233–238. [CrossRef] [PubMed]
71. Roque, M.; Esteves, S.C. Effect of varicocele repair on sperm DNA fragmentation: A review. *Int. Urol. Nephrol.* **2018**, *50*, 583–603. [CrossRef]
72. Agarwal, A.; Cho, C.L.; Majzoub, A.; Esteves, S.C. The Society for Translational Medicine: Clinical practice guidelines for sperm DNA fragmentation testing in male infertility. *Transl. Androl. Urol.* **2017**, *6*, S720–S733. [CrossRef]
73. Esteves, S.C.; Roque, M.; Bradley, C.K.; Garrido, N. Reproductive outcomes of testicular versus ejaculated sperm for intracytoplasmic sperm injection among men with high levels of DNA fragmentation in semen: Systematic review and meta-analysis. *Fertil. Steril.* **2017**, *108*, 456–467.e451. [CrossRef] [PubMed]
74. Esteves, S.C.; Roque, M.; Garrido, N. Use of testicular sperm for intracytoplasmic sperm injection in men with high sperm DNA fragmentation: A SWOT analysis. *Asian J. Androl.* **2018**, *20*, 1–8. [CrossRef] [PubMed]
75. Nijs, M.; De Jonge, C.; Cox, A.; Janssen, M.; Bosmans, E.; Ombelet, W. Correlation between male age, WHO sperm parameters, DNA fragmentation, chromatin packaging and outcome in assisted reproduction technology. *Andrologia* **2011**, *43*, 174–179. [CrossRef]
76. Garcia-Ferreyra, J.; Luna, D.; Villegas, L.; Romero, R.; Zavala, P.; Hilario, R.; Duenas-Chacon, J. High Aneuploidy Rates Observed in Embryos Derived from Donated Oocytes are Related to Male Aging and High Percentages of Sperm DNA Fragmentation. *Clin. Med. Insights Reprod. Health* **2015**, *9*, 21–27. [CrossRef]
77. Rosiak-Gill, A.; Gill, K.; Jakubik, J.; Fraczek, M.; Patorski, L.; Gaczarzewicz, D.; Kurzawa, R.; Kurpisz, M.; Piasecka, M. Age-related changes in human sperm DNA integrity. *Aging* **2019**, *11*, 5399–5411. [CrossRef]
78. Gonzalez, D.C.; Ory, J.; Blachman-Braun, R.; Nackeeran, S.; Best, J.C.; Ramasamy, R. Advanced Paternal Age and Sperm DNA Fragmentation: A Systematic Review. *World J. Men's Health* **2022**, *40*, 104–115. [CrossRef] [PubMed]
79. Nikitaras, V.; Zander-Fox, D.; McPherson, N.O. Improving Sperm Oxidative Stress and Embryo Quality in Advanced Paternal Age Using Idebenone In Vitro-A Proof-of-Concept Study. *Antioxidants* **2021**, *10*, 1079. [CrossRef]
80. Kaltsas, A. Oxidative Stress and Male Infertility: The Protective Role of Antioxidants. *Medicina* **2023**, *59*, 1769. [CrossRef]
81. Mishra, S.; Kumar, R.; Malhotra, N.; Singh, N.; Dada, R. Mild oxidative stress is beneficial for sperm telomere length maintenance. *World J. Methodol.* **2016**, *6*, 163–170. [CrossRef]
82. McNally, E.J.; Luncsford, P.J.; Armanios, M. Long telomeres and cancer risk: The price of cellular immortality. *J. Clin. Investig.* **2019**, *129*, 3474–3481. [CrossRef] [PubMed]
83. Yang, Q.; Zhao, F.; Dai, S.; Zhang, N.; Zhao, W.; Bai, R.; Sun, Y. Sperm telomere length is positively associated with the quality of early embryonic development. *Hum. Reprod.* **2015**, *30*, 1876–1881. [CrossRef]
84. Eisenberg, D.T.A.; Kuzawa, C.W. The paternal age at conception effect on offspring telomere length: Mechanistic, comparative and adaptive perspectives. *Philos. Trans. R. Soc. B Biol. Sci.* **2018**, *373*, 20160442. [CrossRef]
85. Andreescu, N.I.; Cosma, M.; Farcas, S.S.; Stoian, M.; Amzar, D.G.; Puiu, M. Assessment of chromosomal aneuploidies in sperm of infertile males by using FISH technique. *Rom. J. Morphol. Embryol.* **2016**, *57*, 173–178.
86. Yatsenko, A.N.; Turek, P.J. Reproductive genetics and the aging male. *J. Assist. Reprod. Genet.* **2018**, *35*, 933–941. [CrossRef]
87. Gunes, S.; Hekim, G.N.; Arslan, M.A.; Asci, R. Effects of aging on the male reproductive system. *J. Assist. Reprod. Genet.* **2016**, *33*, 441–454. [CrossRef]
88. Gao, Z.; Moorjani, P.; Sasani, T.A.; Pedersen, B.S.; Quinlan, A.R.; Jorde, L.B.; Amster, G.; Przeworski, M. Overlooked roles of DNA damage and maternal age in generating human germline mutations. *Proc. Natl. Acad. Sci. USA* **2019**, *116*, 9491–9500. [CrossRef]
89. Cai, Y.; Cao, H.; Wang, F.; Zhang, Y.; Kapranov, P. Complex genomic patterns of abasic sites in mammalian DNA revealed by a high-resolution SSiNGLe-AP method. *Nat. Commun.* **2022**, *13*, 5868. [CrossRef]
90. Evenson, D.P.; Djira, G.; Kasperson, K.; Christianson, J. Relationships between the age of 25,445 men attending infertility clinics and sperm chromatin structure assay (SCSA®) defined sperm DNA and chromatin integrity. *Fertil. Steril.* **2020**, *114*, 311–320. [CrossRef]
91. Donatti, L.M.; Martello, C.L.; Andrade, G.M.; Oliveira, N.P.; Frantz, N. Advanced Paternal Age Affects the Sperm DNA Fragmentation Index and May Lead to Lower Good-quality Blastocysts. *Reprod. Sci.* **2023**, *30*, 2489–2494. [CrossRef]
92. Brandt, N.B.; Kristensen, M.L.S.; Catalini, L.; Fedder, J. Effect of paternal health on pregnancy loss-A review of current evidence. *Andrologia* **2022**, *54*, e14259. [CrossRef]
93. Punjabi, U.; Goovaerts, I.; Peeters, K.; Van Mulders, H.; De Neubourg, D. Sperm as a Carrier of Genome Instability in Relation to Paternal Lifestyle and Nutritional Conditions. *Nutrients* **2022**, *14*, 3155. [CrossRef]
94. Horta, F.; Catt, S.; Ramachandran, P.; Vollenhoven, B.; Temple-Smith, P. Female ageing affects the DNA repair capacity of oocytes in IVF using a controlled model of sperm DNA damage in mice. *Hum. Reprod.* **2020**, *35*, 529–544. [CrossRef]
95. Aitken, R.J. Role of sperm DNA damage in creating de-novo mutations in human offspring: The 'post-meiotic oocyte collusion' hypothesis. *Reprod. Biomed. Online* **2022**, *45*, 109–124. [CrossRef] [PubMed]
96. Xavier, M.J.; Nixon, B.; Roman, S.D.; Scott, R.J.; Drevet, J.R.; Aitken, R.J. Paternal impacts on development: Identification of genomic regions vulnerable to oxidative DNA damage in human spermatozoa. *Hum. Reprod.* **2019**, *34*, 1876–1890. [CrossRef] [PubMed]
97. Zweifel, J.E.; Woodward, J.T. The risky business of advanced paternal age: Neurodevelopmental and psychosocial implications for children of older fathers. *Fertil. Steril.* **2022**, *118*, 1013–1021. [CrossRef] [PubMed]

98. Frans, E.M.; Sandin, S.; Reichenberg, A.; Lichtenstein, P.; Langstrom, N.; Hultman, C.M. Advancing paternal age and bipolar disorder. *Arch. Gen. Psychiatry* **2008**, *65*, 1034–1040. [CrossRef]
99. Croen, L.A.; Najjar, D.V.; Fireman, B.; Grether, J.K. Maternal and paternal age and risk of autism spectrum disorders. *Arch. Pediatr. Adolesc. Med.* **2007**, *161*, 334–340. [CrossRef] [PubMed]
100. Malaspina, D.; Corcoran, C.; Fahim, C.; Berman, A.; Harkavy-Friedman, J.; Yale, S.; Goetz, D.; Goetz, R.; Harlap, S.; Gorman, J. Paternal age and sporadic schizophrenia: Evidence for de novo mutations. *Am. J. Med. Genet.* **2002**, *114*, 299–303. [CrossRef]
101. Day, K.; Waite, L.L.; Thalacker-Mercer, A.; West, A.; Bamman, M.M.; Brooks, J.D.; Myers, R.M.; Absher, D. Differential DNA methylation with age displays both common and dynamic features across human tissues that are influenced by CpG landscape. *Genome Biol.* **2013**, *14*, R102. [CrossRef]
102. Milekic, M.H.; Xin, Y.; O'Donnell, A.; Kumar, K.K.; Bradley-Moore, M.; Malaspina, D.; Moore, H.; Brunner, D.; Ge, Y.; Edwards, J.; et al. Age-related sperm DNA methylation changes are transmitted to offspring and associated with abnormal behavior and dysregulated gene expression. *Mol. Psychiatry* **2015**, *20*, 995–1001. [CrossRef] [PubMed]
103. Feinberg, J.I.; Schrott, R.; Ladd-Acosta, C.; Newschaffer, C.J.; Hertz-Picciotto, I.; Croen, L.A.; Daniele Fallin, M.; Feinberg, A.P.; Volk, H.E. Epigenetic changes in sperm are associated with paternal and child quantitative autistic traits in an autism-enriched cohort. *Mol. Psychiatry* **2023**, 1–11. [CrossRef]
104. Menezo, Y.J.; Silvestris, E.; Dale, B.; Elder, K. Oxidative stress and alterations in DNA methylation: Two sides of the same coin in reproduction. *Reprod. Biomed. Online* **2016**, *33*, 668–683. [CrossRef]
105. Liang, K.; Yao, L.; Wang, S.; Zheng, L.; Qian, Z.; Ge, Y.; Chen, L.; Cheng, X.; Ma, R.; Li, C.; et al. miR-125a-5p increases cellular DNA damage of aging males and perturbs stage-specific embryo development via Rbm38-p53 signaling. *Aging Cell* **2021**, *20*, e13508. [CrossRef] [PubMed]
106. Sharma, P.; Ghanghas, P.; Kaushal, N.; Kaur, J.; Kaur, P. Epigenetics and oxidative stress: A twin-edged sword in spermatogenesis. *Andrologia* **2019**, *51*, e13432. [CrossRef] [PubMed]
107. Ashapkin, V.; Suvorov, A.; Pilsner, J.R.; Krawetz, S.A.; Sergeyev, O. Age-associated epigenetic changes in mammalian sperm: Implications for offspring health and development. *Hum. Reprod. Update* **2023**, *29*, 24–44. [CrossRef] [PubMed]
108. Kaarouch, I.; Bouamoud, N.; Madkour, A.; Louanjli, N.; Saadani, B.; Assou, S.; Aboulmaouahib, S.; Amzazi, S.; Copin, H.; Benkhalifa, M.; et al. Paternal age: Negative impact on sperm genome decays and IVF outcomes after 40 years. *Mol. Reprod. Dev.* **2018**, *85*, 271–280. [CrossRef]
109. Ghuman, N.K.; Mair, E.; Pearce, K.; Choudhary, M. Does age of the sperm donor influence live birth outcome in assisted reproduction? *Hum. Reprod.* **2016**, *31*, 582–590. [CrossRef]
110. Robertshaw, I.; Khoury, J.; Abdallah, M.E.; Warikoo, P.; Hofmann, G.E. The effect of paternal age on outcome in assisted reproductive technology using the ovum donation model. *Reprod. Sci.* **2014**, *21*, 590–593. [CrossRef] [PubMed]
111. Campos, I.; Gomez, E.; Fernandez-Valencia, A.L.; Landeras, J.; Gonzalez, R.; Coy, P.; Gadea, J. Effects of men and recipients' age on the reproductive outcome of an oocyte donation program. *J. Assist. Reprod. Genet.* **2008**, *25*, 445–452. [CrossRef] [PubMed]
112. Tiegs, A.W.; Sachdev, N.M.; Grifo, J.A.; McCulloh, D.H.; Licciardi, F. Paternal Age Is Not Associated With Pregnancy Outcomes After Single Thawed Euploid Blastocyst Transfer. *Reprod. Sci.* **2017**, *24*, 1319–1324. [CrossRef]
113. Johnson, S.L.; Zellhuber-McMillan, S.; Gillum, J.; Dunleavy, J.; Evans, J.P.; Nakagawa, S.; Gemmell, N.J. Evidence that fertility trades off with early offspring fitness as males age. *Proc. Biol. Sci.* **2018**, *285*, 20172174. [CrossRef]
114. Hassan, M.A.; Killick, S.R. Effect of male age on fertility: Evidence for the decline in male fertility with increasing age. *Fertil. Steril.* **2003**, *79* (Suppl. S3), 1520–1527. [CrossRef]
115. Wu, Y.; Kang, X.; Zheng, H.; Liu, H.; Liu, J. Effect of Paternal Age on Reproductive Outcomes of In Vitro Fertilization. *PLoS ONE* **2015**, *10*, e0135734. [CrossRef]
116. Reichenberg, A.; Gross, R.; Weiser, M.; Bresnahan, M.; Silverman, J.; Harlap, S.; Rabinowitz, J.; Shulman, C.; Malaspina, D.; Lubin, G.; et al. Advancing paternal age and autism. *Arch. Gen. Psychiatry* **2006**, *63*, 1026–1032. [CrossRef]
117. Crosnoe, L.E.; Kim, E.D. Impact of age on male fertility. *Curr. Opin. Obstet. Gynecol.* **2013**, *25*, 181–185. [CrossRef] [PubMed]
118. Malaspina, D. Paternal factors and schizophrenia risk: De novo mutations and imprinting. *Schizophr. Bull.* **2001**, *27*, 379–393. [CrossRef]
119. Chapuis, A.; Gala, A.; Ferrieres-Hoa, A.; Mullet, T.; Bringer-Deutsch, S.; Vintejoux, E.; Torre, A.; Hamamah, S. Sperm quality and paternal age: Effect on blastocyst formation and pregnancy rates. *Basic Clin. Androl.* **2017**, *27*, 2. [CrossRef] [PubMed]
120. Garcia-Ferreyra, J.; Hilario, R.; Duenas, J. High percentages of embryos with 21, 18 or 13 trisomy are related to advanced paternal age in donor egg cycles. *JBRA Assist. Reprod.* **2018**, *22*, 26–34. [CrossRef]
121. Wu, Y.; Kang, X.; Zheng, H.; Liu, H.; Huang, Q.; Liu, J. Effect of Paternal Age on Reproductive Outcomes of Intracytoplasmic Sperm Injection. *PLoS ONE* **2016**, *11*, e0149867. [CrossRef] [PubMed]
122. Murugesu, S.; Kasaven, L.S.; Petrie, A.; Vaseekaran, A.; Jones, B.P.; Bracewell-Milnes, T.; Barcroft, J.F.; Grewal, K.J.; Getreu, N.; Galazis, N.; et al. Does advanced paternal age affect outcomes following assisted reproductive technology? A systematic review and meta-analysis. *Reprod. Biomed. Online* **2022**, *45*, 283–331. [CrossRef]
123. Wyrobek, A.J.; Eskenazi, B.; Young, S.; Arnheim, N.; Tiemann-Boege, I.; Jabs, E.W.; Glaser, R.L.; Pearson, F.S.; Evenson, D. Advancing age has differential effects on DNA damage, chromatin integrity, gene mutations, and aneuploidies in sperm. *Proc. Natl. Acad. Sci. USA* **2006**, *103*, 9601–9606. [CrossRef]

124. Khandwala, Y.S.; Baker, V.L.; Shaw, G.M.; Stevenson, D.K.; Lu, Y.; Eisenberg, M.L. Association of paternal age with perinatal outcomes between 2007 and 2016 in the United States: Population based cohort study. *BMJ* **2018**, *363*, k4372. [CrossRef]
125. Meijerink, A.M.; Ramos, L.; Fleischer, K.; Veltman, J.A.; Hendriks, J.C.; Braat, D.D. Influence of paternal age on ongoing pregnancy rate at eight weeks' gestation in assisted reproduction. *Reprod. Biomed. Online* **2016**, *32*, 96–103. [CrossRef]
126. Setti, A.S.; Braga, D.; Iaconelli Junior, A.; Borges Junior, E. Increasing paternal age and ejaculatory abstinence length negatively influence the intracytoplasmic sperm injection outcomes from egg-sharing donation cycles. *Andrology* **2020**, *8*, 594–601. [CrossRef]
127. Colaco, S.; Sakkas, D. Paternal factors contributing to embryo quality. *J. Assist. Reprod. Genet.* **2018**, *35*, 1953–1968. [CrossRef]
128. McPherson, N.O.; Zander-Fox, D.; Vincent, A.D.; Lane, M. Combined advanced parental age has an additive negative effect on live birth rates-data from 4057 first IVF/ICSI cycles. *J. Assist. Reprod. Genet.* **2018**, *35*, 279–287. [CrossRef] [PubMed]
129. Klonoff-Cohen, H.S.; Natarajan, L. The effect of advancing paternal age on pregnancy and live birth rates in couples undergoing in vitro fertilization or gamete intrafallopian transfer. *Am. J. Obstet. Gynecol.* **2004**, *191*, 507–514. [CrossRef]
130. Nybo Andersen, A.M.; Hansen, K.D.; Andersen, P.K.; Davey Smith, G. Advanced paternal age and risk of fetal death: A cohort study. *Am. J. Epidemiol.* **2004**, *160*, 1214–1222. [CrossRef] [PubMed]
131. du Fosse, N.A.; van der Hoorn, M.P.; van Lith, J.M.M.; le Cessie, S.; Lashley, E. Advanced paternal age is associated with an increased risk of spontaneous miscarriage: A systematic review and meta-analysis. *Hum. Reprod. Update* **2020**, *26*, 650–669. [CrossRef] [PubMed]
132. Tatsumi, T.; Ishida, E.; Tatsumi, K.; Okada, Y.; Saito, T.; Kubota, T.; Saito, H. Advanced paternal age alone does not adversely affect pregnancy or live-birth rates or sperm parameters following intrauterine insemination. *Reprod. Med. Biol.* **2018**, *17*, 459–465. [CrossRef]
133. Stern, J.E.; Luke, B.; Hornstein, M.D.; Cabral, H.; Gopal, D.; Diop, H.; Kotelchuck, M. The effect of father's age in fertile, subfertile, and assisted reproductive technology pregnancies: A population based cohort study. *J. Assist. Reprod. Genet.* **2014**, *31*, 1437–1444. [CrossRef]
134. Bronet, F.; Martinez, E.; Gaytan, M.; Linan, A.; Cernuda, D.; Ariza, M.; Nogales, M.; Pacheco, A.; San Celestino, M.; Garcia-Velasco, J.A. Sperm DNA fragmentation index does not correlate with the sperm or embryo aneuploidy rate in recurrent miscarriage or implantation failure patients. *Hum. Reprod.* **2012**, *27*, 1922–1929. [CrossRef]
135. Slama, R.; Bouyer, J.; Windham, G.; Fenster, L.; Werwatz, A.; Swan, S.H. Influence of paternal age on the risk of spontaneous abortion. *Am. J. Epidemiol.* **2005**, *161*, 816–823. [CrossRef] [PubMed]
136. Pritts, E.A.; Parker, W.H.; Olive, D.L. Fibroids and infertility: An updated systematic review of the evidence. *Fertil. Steril.* **2009**, *91*, 1215–1223. [CrossRef] [PubMed]
137. Coban, O.; Serdarogullari, M.; Pervaiz, R.; Soykok, A.; Yarkiner, Z.; Bankeroglu, H. Effect of paternal age on assisted reproductive outcomes in ICSI donor cycles. *Andrology* **2023**, *11*, 515–522. [CrossRef] [PubMed]
138. Stabile, L.A.; Mendes, C.M.; Goissis, M.D.; Sousa, R.G.B.; Nichi, M.; Visintin, J.A.; Hamilton, T.; Assumpcao, M. Paternal age impairs in vitro embryo and in vivo fetal development in murine. *Sci. Rep.* **2022**, *12*, 13031. [CrossRef] [PubMed]
139. Setti, A.S.; Braga, D.; Provenza, R.R.; Iaconelli, A., Jr.; Borges, E., Jr. Oocyte ability to repair sperm DNA fragmentation: The impact of maternal age on intracytoplasmic sperm injection outcomes. *Fertil. Steril.* **2021**, *116*, 123–129. [CrossRef] [PubMed]
140. Green, R.F.; Devine, O.; Crider, K.S.; Olney, R.S.; Archer, N.; Olshan, A.F.; Shapira, S.K.; The National Birth Defects Prevention Study. Association of paternal age and risk for major congenital anomalies from the National Birth Defects Prevention Study, 1997 to 2004. *Ann. Epidemiol.* **2010**, *20*, 241–249. [CrossRef] [PubMed]
141. Basso, O.; Wilcox, A.J. Paternal age and delivery before 32 weeks. *Epidemiology* **2006**, *17*, 475–478. [CrossRef] [PubMed]
142. El Rafei, R.; Ghandour, L.; Assaf, G.; Charafeddine, L.; Al Bizri, A.; Alameh, M.; Yunis, K.; National Collaborative Perinatal National Collaborative Perinatal Neonatal Network, American University of Beirut, Lebanon. Children born to mothers in their 20s and fathers in their 40s: Evidence for an increased low birth weight and Cesarean Section deliveries in Lebanon. *Ann. Epidemiol.* **2018**, *28*, 368–371. [CrossRef] [PubMed]
143. Urhoj, S.K.; Andersen, P.K.; Mortensen, L.H.; Davey Smith, G.; Nybo Andersen, A.M. Advanced paternal age and stillbirth rate: A nationwide register-based cohort study of 944,031 pregnancies in Denmark. *Eur. J. Epidemiol.* **2017**, *32*, 227–234. [CrossRef]
144. Mayo, J.A.; Lu, Y.; Stevenson, D.K.; Shaw, G.M.; Eisenberg, M.L. Parental age and stillbirth: A population-based cohort of nearly 10 million California deliveries from 1991 to 2011. *Ann. Epidemiol.* **2019**, *31*, 32–37.e32. [CrossRef]
145. Alio, A.P.; Salihu, H.M.; McIntosh, C.; August, E.M.; Weldeselasse, H.; Sanchez, E.; Mbah, A.K. The effect of paternal age on fetal birth outcomes. *Am. J. Men's Health* **2012**, *6*, 427–435. [CrossRef]
146. Rossen, J.; Klungsoyr, K.; Albrechtsen, S.; Lokkegard, E.; Rasmussen, S.; Bergholt, T.; Skjeldestad, F.E. Can oxytocin augmentation modify the risk of epidural analgesia by maternal age in cesarean sections? *Acta Obstet Gynecol. Scand.* **2018**, *97*, 872–879. [CrossRef] [PubMed]
147. Bernhardt, L.; Dittrich, M.; Prell, A.; Potabattula, R.; Drummer, C.; Behr, R.; Hahn, T.; Schorsch, M.; Muller, T.; Haaf, T. Age-related methylation changes in the human sperm epigenome. *Aging* **2023**, *15*, 1257–1278. [CrossRef]
148. Park, Y.S.; Lee, S.H.; Lim, C.K.; Choi, H.W.; An, J.H.; Park, C.W.; Lee, H.S.; Lee, J.S.; Seo, J.T. Paternal age as an independent factor does not affect embryo quality and pregnancy outcomes of testicular sperm extraction-intracytoplasmic sperm injection in azoospermia. *Andrologia* **2018**, *50*, e12864. [CrossRef]
149. Mathieu, C.; Ecochard, R.; Bied, V.; Lornage, J.; Czyba, J.C. Cumulative conception rate following intrauterine artificial insemination with husband's spermatozoa: Influence of husband's age. *Hum. Reprod.* **1995**, *10*, 1090–1097. [CrossRef]

150. Gu, L.; Zhang, H.; Yin, L.; Bu, Z.; Zhu, G. Effect of male age on the outcome of in vitro fertilization: Oocyte donation as a model. *J. Assist. Reprod. Genet.* **2012**, *29*, 331–334. [CrossRef]
151. Tsai, Y.R.; Lan, K.C.; Kung, F.T.; Lin, P.Y.; Chiang, H.J.; Lin, Y.J.; Huang, F.J. The effect of advanced paternal age on the outcomes of assisted reproductive techniques among patients with azoospermia using cryopreserved testicular spermatozoa. *Taiwan J. Obstet. Gynecol.* **2013**, *52*, 351–355. [CrossRef] [PubMed]
152. Whitcomb, B.W.; Turzanski-Fortner, R.; Richter, K.S.; Kipersztok, S.; Stillman, R.J.; Levy, M.J.; Levens, E.D. Contribution of male age to outcomes in assisted reproductive technologies. *Fertil. Steril.* **2011**, *95*, 147–151. [CrossRef]
153. Tesarik, J.; Greco, E.; Mendoza, C. Late, but not early, paternal effect on human embryo development is related to sperm DNA fragmentation. *Hum. Reprod.* **2004**, *19*, 611–615. [CrossRef]
154. Kim, S.; Kim, M.; Oh, M.Y.; Seo, Y.; Yum, S.K. Impact of increased paternal age on neonatal outcomes in very-low-birth-weight infants. *J. Matern.-Fetal Neonatal Med.* **2023**, *36*, 2257836. [CrossRef]
155. Bu, X.; Ye, W.; Zhou, J. Paternal age, risk of congenital anomalies, and birth outcomes: A population-based cohort study. *Eur. J. Pediatr.* **2023**, *182*, 3519–3526. [CrossRef] [PubMed]
156. Liu, K.; Case, A.; Cheung, A.P.; Sierra, S.; AlAsiri, S.; Carranza-Mamane, B.; Dwyer, C.; Graham, J.; Havelock, J.; Hemmings, R.; et al. RETIRED: Advanced reproductive age and fertility. *J. Obstet. Gynaecol. Can.* **2011**, *33*, 1165–1175. [CrossRef]
157. Toriello, H.V.; Meck, J.M.; Professional Practice and Guidelines Committee. Statement on guidance for genetic counseling in advanced paternal age. *Genet. Med.* **2008**, *10*, 457–460. [CrossRef] [PubMed]
158. Kaltsas, A.; Zikopoulos, A.; Moustakli, E.; Zachariou, A.; Tsirka, G.; Tsiampali, C.; Palapela, N.; Sofikitis, N.; Dimitriadis, F. The Silent Threat to Women's Fertility: Uncovering the Devastating Effects of Oxidative Stress. *Antioxidants* **2023**, *12*, 1490. [CrossRef] [PubMed]
159. Halliwell, B. The antioxidant paradox. *Lancet* **2000**, *355*, 1179–1180. [CrossRef] [PubMed]
160. Symeonidis, E.N.; Evgeni, E.; Palapelas, V.; Koumasi, D.; Pyrgidis, N.; Sokolakis, I.; Hatzichristodoulou, G.; Tsiampali, C.; Mykoniatis, I.; Zachariou, A.; et al. Redox Balance in Male Infertility: Excellence through Moderation—"Muepsilontaurhoomicronnu ἄrhoiotasigmatauomicronnu". *Antioxidants* **2021**, *10*, 1534. [CrossRef]
161. Bertoncelli Tanaka, M.; Agarwal, A.; Esteves, S.C. Paternal age and assisted reproductive technology: Problem solver or trouble maker? *Panminerva Medica* **2019**, *61*, 138–151. [CrossRef] [PubMed]
162. Donnelly, E.T.; Steele, E.K.; McClure, N.; Lewis, S.E. Assessment of DNA integrity and morphology of ejaculated spermatozoa from fertile and infertile men before and after cryopreservation. *Hum. Reprod.* **2001**, *16*, 1191–1199. [CrossRef]
163. Jennings, M.O.; Owen, R.C.; Keefe, D.; Kim, E.D. Management and counseling of the male with advanced paternal age. *Fertil. Steril.* **2017**, *107*, 324–328. [CrossRef]
164. Munne, S.; Sandalinas, M.; Escudero, T.; Velilla, E.; Walmsley, R.; Sadowy, S.; Cohen, J.; Sable, D. Improved implantation after preimplantation genetic diagnosis of aneuploidy. *Reprod. Biomed. Online* **2003**, *7*, 91–97. [CrossRef]
165. Staessen, C.; Verpoest, W.; Donoso, P.; Haentjens, P.; Van der Elst, J.; Liebaers, I.; Devroey, P. Preimplantation genetic screening does not improve delivery rate in women under the age of 36 following single-embryo transfer. *Hum. Reprod.* **2008**, *23*, 2818–2825. [CrossRef] [PubMed]
166. Kaltsas, A.; Dimitriadis, F.; Zachariou, D.; Zikopoulos, A.; Symeonidis, E.N.; Markou, E.; Tien, D.M.B.; Takenaka, A.; Sofikitis, N.; Zachariou, A. From Diagnosis to Treatment: Comprehensive Care by Reproductive Urologists in Assisted Reproductive Technology. *Medicina* **2023**, *59*, 1835. [CrossRef] [PubMed]
167. Marinaro, J.; Goldstein, M. Microsurgical Management of Male Infertility: Compelling Evidence That Collaboration with Qualified Male Reproductive Urologists Enhances Assisted Reproductive Technology (ART) Outcomes. *J. Clin. Med.* **2022**, *11*, 4593. [CrossRef] [PubMed]
168. Stein, L.J.; Rosner, S.; Lo Giudice, A.; Ditzen, B.; Wischmann, T. Analysing medical predictors for the outcome of infertility treatment: A 5-year follow-up survey. *Arch. Gynecol. Obstet.* **2023**, *308*, 1007–1014. [CrossRef] [PubMed]
169. Atsem, S.; Reichenbach, J.; Potabattula, R.; Dittrich, M.; Nava, C.; Depienne, C.; Bohm, L.; Rost, S.; Hahn, T.; Schorsch, M.; et al. Paternal age effects on sperm FOXK1 and KCNA7 methylation and transmission into the next generation. *Hum. Mol. Genet.* **2016**, *25*, 4996–5005. [CrossRef]
170. Yi, H.; Yang, M.; Tang, H.; Lin, M. Risk Factors of Pregnancy Failure in Infertile Patients Undergoing Assisted Reproductive Technology. *Int. J. Gen. Med.* **2022**, *15*, 8807–8817. [CrossRef]

Journal of
Clinical Medicine

MDPI

Review

Culture of Human Embryos at High and Low Oxygen Levels

Ourania Konstantogianni [1,†], Theodoros Panou [1,†], Athanasios Zikopoulos [2], Charikleia Skentou [3], Sofoklis Stavros [4] and Byron Asimakopoulos [1,*]

[1] Laboratory of Reproductive Physiology-IVF, Faculty of Medicine, Democritus University of Thrace, 68100 Alexandroupolis, Greece; theopano2@med.duth.gr (T.P.)
[2] Royal Devon and Exeter Hospital, Barrack Rd, Exeter EX2 5DW, UK; thanzik92@gmail.com
[3] Department of Obstetrics and Gynecology, Medical School of Ioannina, University General Hospital, 45110 Ioannina, Greece
[4] Third Department of Obstetrics and Gynecology, Attikon Hospital, Medical School, National and Kapodistrian University of Athens, 12462 Athens, Greece
* Correspondence: basima@med.duth.gr
† These authors contributed equally to this work.

Abstract: One of the parameters potentially affecting the in vitro growth of preimplantation embryos is the oxygen concentration in the culture environment. An increased oxygen concentration causes the generation of ROS which in turn can cause damage to the cells and seriously disrupt the embryonic development. Previous studies have assessed oxygen concentrations in the fallopian tubes of several mammals of between 5 and 8%, while the oxygen levels in the uterus were found to be even lower; similar measurements have been confirmed in humans. In addition, studies in mammalian embryos showed that low oxygen concentrations improve embryo development. Multiple studies on the effect of the oxygen concentration on human embryos have been conducted so far with diverse methodologies and objectives. Data from these have been included in three meta-analyses. All meta-analyses indicate the potential benefit in favor of a low oxygen concentration, though data are considered to be of a low methodological quality and further studies are considered necessary. However, based on the existing evidence, it is suggested that a low oxygen concentration should be adopted in the routine of the IVF laboratory, especially in the case of blastocyst culture.

Keywords: in vitro embryo culture; oxygen tension; embryo development; ROS; IVF; ICSI

1. Introduction

In the first steps of in vitro fertilization (IVF), Steptoe et al. proposed the adoption of the three gases system (5% CO_2/5% O_2/90% N_2) as suitable for the human blastocyst culture [1,2]. The beneficial effect of a low oxygen concentration on embryo culture has also been confirmed in animal models and particularly in in vitro mouse embryo cultures. The blastocyst development and quality of mice embryos was compared under three different oxygen concentrations (5, 20, and 40%). It was shown that mouse blastocysts cultured under 5% consisted of more blastomeres and numerically exceeded those developed under higher oxygen levels [3].

However, satisfactory results in the embryo culture under 20% O_2 led to the use of N_2 being abandoned in most IVF laboratories due to additional costs [2,3]. In the 1990s, researchers focused on the use of low oxygen in a human embryo culture due to the extension of the culture to the blastocyst stage which aimed to transfer fewer embryos in order to reduce multiple pregnancies [4]. The concept behind the increasing interest in applying lower levels of oxygen lies in the potential dangers associated with atmospheric oxygen concentrations. Several studies confirmed the harmful effect of reactive oxygen species (ROS) derived from the high oxygen levels present in the atmosphere [5,6]. The aim of the current review is to address the benefit of low oxygen levels on mammalian embryo development with particular emphasis on the human embryo development in assisted reproductive technology (ART). It also provides an insight into the physiological shifts induced by the different oxygen levels.

2. Oxygen Concentration in Female Reproductive Tract

There have been repetitive attempts to determine the physiological oxygen levels in the female reproductive tract in several mammals. In a study focusing on oxygen levels in monkeys, hamsters and rabbits, considerable differences were assessed: the oxygen levels varied from 1.5% in the monkey uterus to 8.7% in the rabbit fallopian tube and uterus and hamster uterus [7]. Similar results were presented for the oxygen levels in the rabbit oviduct: the assessed range varied between 40 mmHg (5.3%) and 75 mmHg (9.9%) [8]. A consensus range for the oxygen concentration in the female reproductive tract is 2 to 8% [2,9].

Other experimental studies provided an insight into the effect of different parameters on intrauterine oxygen tension in rats, hamsters and guinea pigs [10–13]. The impact of the menstrual cycle's regulatory hormones (estrogens and progesterones) is of particular importance: the peak of the O_2 levels was found under the effect of low estrogen and high progesterone levels [9,11]. It is noteworthy that oxygen levels are dependent on multiple physiologic (e.g., hormones, uterine cavity anatomy) and pathologic (e.g., cancer, infections) conditions and factors [9,14].

The studies conducted on humans are relatively few. Three major studies assessed the oxygen levels in the human female reproductive tract. The first, by Yedwab et al., compared the oxygen partial pressure among other parameters in women and female rats' uteri throughout the menstrual cycle and observed an increase in oxygen levels by 86–90% in the ovulatory phase in humans (11 mmHg) and by 224% during the late proestrus phase in rats [15]. A more recent study observed a median oxygen pressure of 18.9 mmHg, corresponding to 11.8% oxygen air saturation with a wide range between 4 and 27% assessed. Pregnant women participating in the study exhibited lower levels at 9% oxygen air saturation, whereas non-pregnant women showed oxygen levels of 12.4% [16]. The last study documented uterine oxygen levels in women suffering from three types of gynecological malignancies and healthy controls. The pO_2 levels were 28.5 mmHg for healthy controls and slightly decreased in all individuals suffering from cancer [14]. Overall, the oxygen concentration in the human uterine cavity has been assessed at almost 2%, ranging from 1.4 to 3.8% [14–16]. However, all three studies focused on different objectives and utilized different methods for the measurement of the oxygen levels.

Other studies attempted to assess the use of oxygen by the oocytes and the oxygen levels in the follicular fluid. In a study examining the composition of the human follicular fluid, Shalgi et al. observed the considerable variability of the oxygen levels in the 36 samples assessed. A mean oxygen tension of 54.3 mmHg was reported, corresponding to oxygen levels of almost 7% [17]. The exact way of oxygen utilization by the cumulus–oocyte complex was the objective of a mathematical model: it was concluded that dissolved oxygen is primarily consumed by the cumulus cells and scarcely reaches the oocyte, even under favoring conditions [18]. Contradictory results were the outcome of a different mathematical model undertaken on bovine and murine cumulus–oocyte complexes. It was found that cumulus cells consume only 0.25 to 0.5% of the total oxygen levels available and thus allow the oocyte to absorb most of it [19].

3. The Effect of Oxygen Levels on Early Embryo Metabolism

Throughout the preimplantation period the embryo depends on oxidative phosphorylation. During the cleavage state, the embryo metabolism relies primarily on pyruvate. The same metabolic pattern is evident in the morula stage as well. This substrate utilization analysis was performed in a culture microdroplet using an ultramicrofluorescence assay [20–22]. After compaction (blastomeres become increasingly coherent) and the blastocyst formation, a major metabolic shift occurs. The embryo metabolism becomes increasingly dependent on oxygen. Consequently, the embryo is capable of blastocoele formation and protein synthesis [23,24]. After the blastocoele formation, the blastocyst is comprised of the inner cell mass and the trophectoderm. These cells exhibit different energy requirements, as a mouse study verified. Trophectoderm cells use increasingly specific amino-acids, contain more mitochondria in comparison to the inner cell mass, produce more substrates and energy-containing substances (e.g., ATP) and thus consume greater amounts of oxygen [25].

ROS may result from either cellular metabolic reactions or the surrounding environment of the embryo. The main ROS produced from intracellular procedures include superoxide, hydrogen peroxide and hydroxyl radical [26]. The embryo protects itself from internal and external ROS by the use of specific antioxidant enzymes, including superoxide dismutase, glutathione peroxidase and gamma-glutamylcysteine synthetase [26]. External protective barriers are also present in the follicular and fallopian fluid: hypotaurine, taurine and ascorbic acid [27]. The diverse oxygen levels in the different parts of the female reproductive tract are also strongly associated with the increasing vulnerability due to potential ROS formation. The gradients of oxygen levels throughout the fallopian tubes and the uterus seem to play a stronger protective role for the early-stage embryo than several antioxidant enzymes [24].

The embryos are confronted with excessive amounts of ROS in an ART laboratory setting. The arrest of embryos' development or the presentation of any other developmental disturbance has been accompanied by increased ROS in vitro, but not in vivo [28]. Consequently, ROS from external sources pose an important threat to normal development and pregnancy outcomes. Potential sources of ROS include increased oxygen levels, light or even the sperm cells necessary for fertilization. The potential harmful effect of increased oxygen levels has been confirmed from mouse models. A product of superoxide was targeted using fluorescence. It was demonstrated that mice cultured under lower oxygen levels (under 5% O_2) exhibited the lowest fluorescent emissions compared to higher oxygen levels (20% and 40%) and the effect was dose-dependent [29]. In a similar staining-based study, the peroxide levels were found to be significantly decreased both in the two-cell and four-cell stages of embryo cultures under 5% O_2 [30]. In another study investigating the detrimental impact of light exposure on hamster embryos, it was found that the generation of H_2O_2 during light exposure was significantly greater when the embryos were cultured at 20% O_2 rather than 5% [31].

The direct effect of the ROS on the embryo metabolism of carbohydrates, lipids and amino acids has been studied extensively. Some data are also based on animal models, mostly mice [32,33]. Recent studies have focused on a more comprehensive analysis of the ROS' impact on proteomics and even epigenetics, through the impact of dioxygenases and the paternal protamines on histone modification [34–36]. In a time-of-flight (TOF) spectrometry analysis of five preimplantation mice embryos, 32 proteins were found which could serve as potential biomarkers. Mice cultures under 5% O_2 exhibited a significant resemblance to in vivo developed embryos, whereas the analysis of mice cultures under 20% oxygen showed the decreased expression of 10 proteins [37]. The gene expression patterns are also affected by the oxidative stress. Rinaudo et al. observed that embryos cultured under 5% O_2 showed gene expression patterns that are expected in embryos developed in vivo [38]. The outcome of this study corresponds to the outcome of the study focusing on proteomics. Both of them imply that low oxygen tension creates similar conditions for the embryo's development in vivo. The well-established toxic impact of ROS can be restricted, particularly in the IVF setting. Researchers have proposed potential ways in that direction. Apart from including substances with anti-oxidant actions in the culture medium, restricting light exposure to the culture media and the embryo culture oil and restricting the duration of gamete coincubation in order to avoid ROS production from the sperm metabolism, researchers have particularly emphasized one other method. This method uses lower oxygen tensions in the ART laboratory during insemination, fertilization and other relative procedures [6,39].

4. Culture of Mammalian Embryos under Low Oxygen Levels

The importance of the oxygen levels in embryo cultures is well-established. Since 1978, multiple studies have been conducted on various animal models, demonstrating the need for lowering oxygen levels. The decreased oxygen tension has resulted in better results in all studies carried out so far in various animal species [39].

Most of the animal-model-based studies exploring the benefits of a lower oxygen concentration on embryo cultures were conducted on rodents, including mice, rats and hamsters (Table 1). The first one, by Quinn et al., which took place back in 1978, focused on the oxygen levels' impact on preimplantation embryo culture parameters and subsequent embryo quality. The study examined different oxygen levels: 5% O_2 (classified as low) and 20/40% O_2 (classified as high). It concluded that a culture under 5% O_2 was beneficial for the preimplantation embryos, as this condition allowed more embryos to progress to the blastocyst stage and resulted in better quality embryos with an increased number of blastomeres [3]. The authors also provided an insight into a potential physiological mechanism behind the decreased blastomere number in embryos cultured under high oxygen levels: the blastomeres may perceive the oxygen levels as a marker for their position in the embryo, from the core to the periphery. Under a high oxygen level, they tend to misunderstand their position and thus divide at a slower rate [3]. Another study attempted to clarify the exact stages of embryo development which are affected by different oxygen concentrations. Therefore, they allocated the examined embryos, at first, in two culture groups (under 5% O_2 or 20% O_2) for the first 2 days of culture and afterwards they randomized the embryos for the next 2 days under the two possible oxygen levels, which resulted in four groups. They concluded that the oxygen levels affect the outcome both during the cleavage stage and after the compaction stage. The decrease in the oxygen levels after 48 h was not linked to a substantial improvement of the parameters examined. Likewise, all embryos which were cultured for a certain time interval under high oxygen levels had to withstand damage, which was not reimbursed after the oxygen levels' shift. An additional outcome of the study is the fact that cleavage delay was particularly high in embryos cultured under 20% O_2 [40]. Two other studies with mice primarily examined the genetic status and the way it may be affected by different oxygen levels. In a FISH-based study, BALB/cWT mice, which are susceptible to Y chromosome abnormalities, were examined. Increased mosaicism was observed among embryos cultured under 20% O_2, whereas embryos cultured under 5% oxygen had mosaicism levels comparable to the control branch of the study [41]. Apart from the effect on the gene expression pattern analyzed previously, the microarray study by Rinaudo et al. verified that a culture under 5% oxygen leads to an increased rate of embryo development and an increased cell number [38]. Kishi et al. [42] showed that hamster embryos cultured in hamster embryo culture (HEMC-1) had a higher blastocyst rate under 5% O_2 than under 20% O_2 levels (20.1% vs. 5.5%, respectively). In another study, where multiple parameters were evaluated, it was found that the progression of hamster 2-cell embryos to the blastocyst stage was facilitated under 5% or 10% oxygen levels, whereas 10% O_2 was identified as the optimal oxygen level for hamster embryo cultures [43].

The blastocyst rate and the related parameters were in the epicenter of a rabbit embryo study, carried out under multiple oxygen levels in two groups (5, 10 and 15% O_2 and 1, 5 and 20% O_2). In the first group, cultures under 5, 10 and 15% O_2 resulted in 48, 38 and 21% of the embryos reaching the hatching blastocyst stage, with 258, 226 and 188 cells per embryo, respectively. In the second group, cultures under 1, 5 and 20% O_2 led to a 67, 72 and 29% proportion of hatching embryos, respectively. For the same group, the average cells per embryo were significantly higher under 1% O_2 and 5% O_2 compared to 20% O_2 [44]. The study by Karja et al. examined the effect of different oxygen levels (8–10% and 20%) on the in vitro maturation (IVM) of porcine oocytes, IVF and in vitro embryo production. It was shown that a similar number of oocytes reached the MII phase and were fertilized after IVM. The beneficial character of the low oxygen levels (8–10%) was reflected in the blastocyst formation rates. In addition, DNA fragmentation was found significantly lower under low oxygen levels (8–10%) [45]. Goat two- to four-cell embryos were cultured for a 6-day interval either under 20% O_2 or 7% O_2 in another comparative study. In total, 80% of the embryos reached the expanded or/and hatched blastocyst stage under 7% O_2 in contrast to merely 29% in the other group. Also, the mean embryo cell number was higher under the low oxygen levels' culture (7%) [46]. Leoni et al. examined bovine embryo cultures under 5% and 20% oxygen levels. The blastocyst formation rate, both on the 6th and on the 7th day under 5% O_2, emerged as significantly higher (63.04% vs. 47.36% and 35.10% vs. 26.09%, respectively) [47]. A more recent study focused on the oocyte maturation and embryo culture of the yak species under different oxygen levels (20% O_2, 10% O_2, 5% O_2, 1% O_2) [48]. This study also confirmed that oocyte maturation, blastocyst and hatched blastocyst rates as well as the total blastocyst cell number, the inner cell mass cells and the trophectoderm cells were significantly higher under 5% O_2. The study also addressed the effect of ultra-low oxygen levels: the oocyte maturation, the cleavage, the blastocyst and the hatched blastocyst rates under 1% O_2 were the lowest assessed [48]. In the last two studies mentioned, the cleavage rates were found to be significantly higher under high oxygen levels [47,48] and it was speculated that the detrimental effects of high oxygen levels are mainly manifested on day 3 with blastulation, more than in the earlier development [48]. The latter study also analyzed other molecular parameters, including the apoptosis index of oocytes and blastocyst cells and the expression patterns of genes related to metabolism, antioxidant response, apoptosis, oocyte competence and embryonic developmental markers. All of them were the lowest under 5% O_2 and the highest under 1% O_2 [48]. We could speculate that the lower outcome with 1% O_2 indicates that this extra-low oxygen level is inadequate to support embryo metabolism.

A recent study investigating the effects of oxygen levels on IVM, IVF and the embryo development of common marmosets (*Callithrix jacchus*) gave interesting results which underline the species-specific differences in these processes [49]. IVM and IVF were performed under 8% or 20% O_2 with the latter giving better results, whereas the embryo culture was performed under 5% or 20% O_2, with 5% O_2 resulting in a better embryo morphology and developmental rates [49]. The authors speculated that during IVM and IVF procedures, the cumulus cells surrounding the oocyte act as a barrier which lowers the amount of O_2 available for the oocyte and, at the same time, protects it from excessive oxidation; hence, with 20% O_2, the oocyte has acceptable O_2 tension, whereas with 8% O_2, it is probably in hypoxic conditions. They also suggested that the use of oil covering the microdroplets of the culture medium which hosts the oocytes (during IVM and IVF) and the sperm (during IVF) is also another factor lowering the O_2 tension [49].

It is obvious that the above mentioned animal studies, summarized in Table 1, provide sufficient evidence of the culture in oxygen levels lower than 20% for embryo development. Although the optimal level of oxygen differs by the species, most of the studies found that culture under 5% O_2 is beneficial.

Table 1. Summary of major animal studies KSOM, potassium-supplemented simplex optimized medium; IVM, in vitro maturation; IVF, in vitro fertilization; HECM-1, hamster embryo culture medium-1; Mkrb, modified Krebs–Ringer bicarbonate solution; SOF, synthetic oviduct fluid; TUNEL, terminal deoxynucleotidyl transferase-mediated deoxyuridine triphosphate-nick end labeling; WT, wild type; BSA, bovine serum albumin; FISH, fluorescence in situ hybridization.

Study	Species	Objective	Primary Outcomes	Secondary Outcomes and Additional Remarks	Reproductive Method
Rinaudo et al. (2006) [38]	Mouse	Effect of oxygen levels (5% or 20%) on gene expression patterns	- 5% O_2 levels were correlated to increased rate of embryo development and increased cell number. - The gene expression pattern under 5% O_2 were similar to those present under in vivo development.	- Embryo culture in Whitten's medium or KSOM medium with amino acids under 20% O_2 or 5% O_2. - Results assessed with the use of microarrays.	Not specified
Quinn et al. (1978) [3]	Mouse	Effect of different oxygen levels on preimplantation embryo culture	- More embryos progressed to the blastocyst stage under 5% O_2. - Embryos under 5% O_2 showed an increased number of blastomeres. - Increased time led to fewer blastomeres present.	- Optimal oxygen levels for embryo development were assessed between 2.5% and 5% O_2. - Preimplantation embryo development took place under 5% O_2 and 20/40% O_2.	Not specified
Kishi et al. (1991) [42]	Rat	Effect of HECM-1 medium use on rat 1-cell embryo culture	- Under HECM-1, 57.9%, 32.2%, 17.4% and 9.9% of the pronuclear embryos progressed to the 4-cell, 8-cell, morula and blastocyst stage. - Under mKRB, pronuclear embryos barely reached the 2- and 4-cell stage and never progressed to stages beneath it. - The blastocyst formation rate was assessed at 20.1% under 5% oxygen levels and was significantly higher compared to rate of 5.5% under 20% oxygen levels.	- Embryos were cultured either under hamster embryo culture medium-1 (HECM-1) related to lower oxygen levels or modified Krebs–Ringer bicarbonate solution (mKRB).	Not specified
McKiernan et al. (1990) [43]	Hamster	Effect of different parameters on hamster embryo culture	- Progression of hamster 2-cell embryos to the blastocyst stage was facilitated under reduced oxygen levels. - 10% O_2 among other conditions identified as optimal setting for hamster embryo culture, as 51–57% of the hamster 2-cell embryos progressed to the blastocyst stage.	- Temperature under 37.5 °C emerged as inhibitory for the culture. - Increased CO_2 (7.5% and 10%) supportive for hamster embryo culture. - No significant effect of electrolytes and other chemical substances observed. - Silicone overlay helpful in the culture medium. - Osmolarity above 325 m. Osmols inhibited culture progression.	Not specified
Li et al. (1993) [44]	Rabbit	Effect of different oxygen levels (1–20% O_2) on progression to blastocyst and blastocyst-related parameters	- In the first group, culture under 5, 10 and 15% O_2 resulted in 48, 38 and 21% of the embryos reaching the hatching blastocyst stage with 258, 226 and 188 cells per blastocyst, respectively. - In the second group, culture under 1, 5 and 20% O_2 led to 67, 72 and 29% proportion of hatching embryos, respectively. - In the second group, average cells per embryo were significantly higher under 1% O_2 and 5% O_2 compared to 20% O_2.	- 2 study groups with culture under different oxygen levels (5, 10 and 15% O_2 and 1, 5 and 20% O_2).	Not specified

Table 1. *Cont.*

Study	Species	Objective	Primary Outcomes	Secondary Outcomes and Additional Remarks	Reproductive Method
Karja et al. (2004) [45]	Pig	Effect of different oxygen levels (8–10% or 20%) on oocyte characteristics and embryo quality parameters	- Similar numbers of oocytes reached MII phase and were fertilized. - Progression to blastocyst rates and mean blastocyst cell rates were significantly higher under lower oxygen levels (8–10%). - Significantly lower DNA fragmentation levels in blastocysts under lower oxygen levels (8–10%) were observed.	- Comparison between a standard and a portable incubator. - Comparison between culture under 8–10% O_2 and 20% O_2. - DNA fragmentation assessment in the blastocyst with TUNEL.	IVM/IVF/in vitro culture
Batt et al. (1991) [46]	Goat	Effect of different oxygen levels (7% or 20%) and different protein sources in the culture medium on preimplantation embryo parameters	- Significantly higher number of embryos (80% vs. 29%) reached the expanded or/and hatched blastocyst stage under 7% O_2. - The mean number of cells emerged higher in embryos under 7% O_2.	- 2- to 4-cell goat embryos were examined and cultured in synthetic oviduct fluid (SOF) for a 6day interval under 20% O_2 or 7% O_2. - Miles bovine serum albumin and human serum were the 2 protein sources with the best features in relation to the mean number of embryo cells.	Not specified
Leoni et al. (2007) [47]	Ovine	Effect of oxygen levels (5% or 20%) on ovine embryo culture quality parameters	- Blastocyst formation on the 6th day under 5% O_2 emerged significantly higher (63.04% vs. 47.36%). - Blastocyst formation on the 7th day under 5% O_2 emerged significantly higher (35.10% vs. 26.09%). - Viability rates post vitrification, total cell number and the inner cell mass cells to trophoblastic cells ratio were similar between the cultures under the 2 oxygen levels on 3 consecutive days (6th, 7th and 8th day).	- Fertilization took place either under 5% O_2 or under 20% O_2 and culture under SOF + aa + 0.4% BSA in 5%CO_2 and 5% O_2. - Significantly higher cleavage rate was observed under 20% O_2 (61.2% vs. 50.8%). - No differences in assessed cleavage distribution at 22 h, 26 h and 40 h	IVF
Bean et al. (2002) [41]	Mouse	Effect of oxygen levels (5% or 20%) on genetic status	- Increased mosaicism was observed under 5% CO_2. - Control-level mosaicism was observed under 5% O_2.	- BALB/c WT male mice examined with increased tendency to Y chromosome abnormalities. - FISH was used for the assessment of the sex chromosomes during different cell stages (2-, 4-, 8- and 16-cell stage).	IVF
Wale et al. (2010) [40]	Mouse	Effect of oxygen levels and oxygen level shifts on preimplantation embryo culture	- Cleavage delay was present for embryo culture under 20% O_2 compared to 5% O_2. - The oxygen level shift from 20% O_2 to 5% O_2 after 48 h did not improve culture-related parameters substantially. - All embryo cultures under 20% O_2 for a time period showed significantly lower blastocyst cell numbers. - Oxygen levels affect embryo culture during the cleavage stage and after the compaction stage.	- Mice were cultured under 5% O_2 or 20% O_2 during the first 2 days and then they were randomized in four groups for other 2 days. - Embryo imaging every 15 min took place under time-lapse microscopy.	Not specified

Table 1. *Cont.*

Study	Species	Objective	Primary Outcomes	Secondary Outcomes and Additional Remarks	Reproductive Method
He et al. (2020) [48]	Yak	Effect of different oxygen levels (20% O_2, 10% O_2, 5% O_2 or 1% O_2) on oocyte maturation, embryo preimplantation potential and other parameters	- Oocyte, blastocyst and hatched blastocyst maturation rates emerged as significantly higher under 5% O_2. - Cleavage rate under 10% O_2 and 20% O_2 were significantly higher compared to the 5% O_2 group. - Oocyte, blastocyst and hatched blastocyst maturation rates and the cleavage rate under 1% O_2 were the lowest assessed. - Total blastocyst cell number, the inner cell mass cells and the trophectoderm cells were significantly higher under 5% O_2.	- The apoptosis index of oocytes and blastocyst cells was the lowest under 5% O2 and the highest under 1% O_2. - Expression patterns of genes related to metabolism, antioxidant response, apoptosis, - Oocyte competence and embryonic developmental markers were significantly different under 5% O_2.	IVF
Tkachenko et al. (2017) [49]	Marmoset	Effect of paired oxygen levels (8% O_2–5% O_2, 20% O_2–20% O_2, 20% O_2–5% O_2 and 8% O_2–20% O_2) on in vitro maturation (IVM) and in vitro fertilization (IVF), respectively.	- Oocyte maturation rate emerges as significantly higher under 20% O_2 in comparison to 8% O_2. - Embryo-related morphology parameters and progression rates (from 4-cell embryos to morula stage) showed a comparative benefit for the 5% O_2 group in IVF over the 20% O_2 group.	- No significant difference between cumulus expansion in IVM under 20% O_2 or 8% O_2 was observed. - Progression to the second metaphasis stage was significantly better in the 20–20% group compared to the 8% O_2–5% O_2 and 20% O_2–5% O_2 groups. - Fertilization was impossible for the 8% O_2–20% O_2 group. - The highest normal spindle rate was assessed in the 20–20% group and the difference was statistically significant. - A significantly higher proportion of fertilized oocytes achieved first cleavage in the 20–20% group.	IVM/IVF

5. Culture of Human Embryos under Low Oxygen Levels

Although Steptoe et al. proposed in their monumental study that the human embryo culture should take place under low oxygen levels, the atmospheric oxygen levels dominated for years in the ART laboratories [1]. Some researchers attempted to explain this trend and concluded the following possible explanations: the need for a N_2 supply and new incubators that entail additional costs, the improvement of culture media used in human IVF procedures and the embryo transfer in the four-cell or eight-cell stage on the 2nd or the 3rd day, respectively [4]. However, the culture of human embryos under low (5%) oxygen levels is gaining ground and a lot of studies seem to support the adoption of this method in everyday laboratory setting.

Overall, the results of twelve prospective randomized studies, two randomized studies, four prospective randomized controlled trials, four randomized controlled studies, three comparative studies, one retrospective study, one monocentric retrospective observational study, one cohort study, one retrospective cross-sectional study, one meta-analysis, one review with quantitative synthesis and one systematic review with meta-analysis are presented (Table 2).

All of the studies addressed the impact of low oxygen levels on human embryo cultures and their related parameters. The number of participants in the studies varied significantly, ranging from 100 oocyte donation receivers to 1382 patients. Some studies did not specify the exact number of patients or participants and referred merely to the total number of IVF cycles or the oocyte retrieval cycles undertaken. It is of note that both fertilization methods were used, either IVF, ICSI or a combination of both.

In order to examine whether the human embryo culture under 5% oxygen is indeed advantageous, several parameters have been assessed. The most frequent parameters examined were the fertilization rate, criteria related to blastocyst and embryo quality, developmental rate, implantation and pregnancy rate. One of the first studies published by Dumoulin et al. indicated a significantly increased pregnancy rate under low oxygen levels (24.2% under 5% oxygen in comparison to 19.4% under atmospheric conditions) [50]. In another study by the same researchers, there was a significant improvement to the blastocyst formation rate (25.8% vs. 20.4%) and blastocyst quality under 5% oxygen [51]. The better embryo quality was evaluated as a common finding in many studies, also by de los Santos et al., who referred particularly to the increased blastomere number [52]. In another prospective randomized study simultaneously assessing both fertilization methods, only the embryo score on day 3 significantly improved in cultures under 5% oxygen, without affecting the fertilization rates [53]. Meintjes et al. identified strong proponents of the embryo culture under 5% oxygen, as they found both better preimplantation development (42.9% vs. 30.7%) and an increased living birth rate (57.4% vs. 42.6%) [54].

Sibling oocyte development was a striking feature of another prospective randomized study. The embryos cultured under 5% oxygen exhibited an increased blastocyst formation rate for both fertilization methods (IVF: 73.2% vs. 63.1% and ICSI: 67.4% vs. 54.7%), an increased blastocyst quality (IVF: 31.1% VS. 14.6% and ICSI: 18.9% vs. 11.4%) and a significantly increased optimal blastocyst formation ratio on day 5 (at 2.1 for IVF and 1.7 for ICSI). Although all the previously mentioned outcomes were clearly in favor of the culture under 5% oxygen, the fertilization rates were found to be unaffected with both fertilization methods (IVF: 59% vs. 43.2% and ICSI: 51.2% vs. 28.5%) [55].

Nanassy et al. conducted a retrospective study in order to examine the way in which the oxygen level shifts affected the embryo quality, pregnancy and implantation rate between the 3rd and the 5th day. Until the 3rd day, all embryo cultures took place under 20% O_2. After the 3rd day, 189 and 193 patients were randomized for the group with cultures under 5% O_2 and 20% O_2, respectively. No significant difference could be observed in terms of the embryo quality, implantation rates (44.06% under the 5% O_2 vs. 44.16% under 20% O_2), the pregnancy rate (71.27% under the 5% O_2 vs. 78.72% under 20% O_2) and the clinical pregnancy rate (58.56% under the 5% O_2 vs. 64.36% under 20% O_2). This study confirmed the presumption put forward by another study with mice showing that cultures already damaged un-der high oxygen levels can not improve if the oxygen tension is reduced [40,56]. In another study by Peng et al., higher fertilization and implantation rates were observed primarily for the group of embryos cultured under low oxygen levels. However, this was the first study to indicate that embryos cultured under 20% O_2 showed significantly higher fertilization rates, implantation rates and quality compared to embryos cultured under high oxygen levels for the first 2 days and then cultured under lower oxygen levels. This study speculated that embryos are more sensitive to oxygen level shifts than to oxygen levels per se [57].

The birthweight in embryos developed under low oxygen levels was assessed in the unique cohort study by Van Montfoort et al. The study could not link the oxygen levels to the birthweight. However, a significant increase in embryo quality was reported (45.8% under 5% O_2 and 30.9% under 20% O_2). Although there was no correlation to the live birth rate, embryos of good quality were eligible for cryopreservation [58]. A significant increase in cryopreservation eligibility for embryos cultured under low oxygen levels (30.8% under 5% O_2 and 19.2% under 20% O_2) was also observed by Sepulveda et al., together with better embryo quality (55.4% under 5% O_2 and 41.8% under 20% O_2). All the other parameters assessed did not reach statistical significance, i.e., implantation rates (41.8% under 5% O_2 and 36.8% under 20% O_2) and pregnancy rates (55.3% under 5% O_2 and 54.6% under 20% O_2) [59]. Also, Waldenstrom et al. observed a higher number of eligible blastocysts for cryopreservation (1.7 in the culture under 5% O_2 vs. 1.1 in the culture under 19% O_2) together with a satisfactory blastocyst formation rate (47.8% in the culture under 5% O_2 vs. 42.1% in the culture under 19% O_2) and the mean number of available blastocysts (3.8 in the culture under 5% O_2 vs. 3.3 in the culture under 19% O_2) [60]. In a prospective randomized study, Bahceci et al., found that although the embryo quality in the transfers on day 3 was better in cultures under 5% O_2, the authors concluded that the oxygen levels did not particularly affect the outcome. It is of note that this study did not evaluate the embryos' progression until the blastocyst stage [61]. The better quality of the embryos is a concept shared by another study [62] which reported optimal blastocyst features under 5% O_2. However, the low oxygen levels did not show a significant impact neither on implantation rates (28.8% under 5% O_2 and 25.2% under 20% O_2) nor on ongoing pregnancy rates (31.6% under 5% O_2 and 27.1% under 20% O_2), although they were beneficial for the pregnancy rates in the special subgroup of poor responders (23% under 5% O_2 and 9.8% under 20% O_2) [62]. In contrast to the previous findings, Kasterstein et al. observed a significant increase both in the implantation and pregnancy rates with cultures under 5% O_2 [63]. Only the fertilization rates were found to be relatively similar between the two groups assessed. An increased number of blastomeres and an optimal embryo quality were also parts of the findings, explaining also the significantly higher number of embryos eligible for transfer (31.6% under 5% O_2 vs. 23.1% under 20% O_2). In this study, the live birth rate was significantly higher under the low oxygen levels' culture (34.2% under 5% O_2 vs. 15.8% under 20% O_2) [64]. Like all the previous studies, Ciray et al. emphasized the significantly better embryo and blastocyst quality observed [64].

Paternot et al., in a randomized controlled trial, evaluated the quality of embryos up to day 3 under 5% or 20% O_2 without finding significant differences [65]. This is the only study that actively discourages from the use of low oxygen levels in embryo cultures [65].

Ruiz and her collaborators in IVI performed a prospective randomized controlled trial to evaluate the efficacy of group embryo cultures under 5% O_2 in benchtop incubators, whereas the control group embryos were cultured individually at 20% O_2 in common large incubators. In the statistical analysis, fresh embryo transfers as well as frozen ones were included [66]. With this strategy, the fertilization rate was not different, but there was a higher blastocyst rate, implantation and live birth rate with the fresh embryo transfers [66]. Taking into consideration the frozen embryo transfers, the cumulative implantation rate and cumulative live birth rate were higher as well [66].

Another team from Zagreb performed a prospective randomized trial comparing benchtop incubators with 5% O_2 and conventional incubators with 20% O_2 [67]. The only results in favor of the benchtop incubators with 5% O_2 was the number of blastocysts on day 5 and clinical pregnancy after a single blastocyst transfer; however, there was not any improvement in the clinical pregnancy for all subgroups, nor in the live birth rate, which was the primary outcome of this study [67].

Although almost all the studies compare 5% O_2 to 20% O_2, a Chinese team investigated the effects of continuous embryo culture under ultra-low (2%) O_2 tension vs. 5% O_2 tension [68]. They did not find differences in the embryo development nor in the clinical or ongoing pregnancies between the two groups and, therefore, they concluded that the continuous culture under 2% O_2 does not give any advantage for the in vitro development of human embryos [68]. Similarly, the team of M. Bedaiwy performed a study comparing 3.5% O_2 to 5% O_2. The results were disappointing for the cultures under 3.5% O_2: though the fertilization and cleavage rates were better, the compaction rate, the number of high-quality blastocysts, the implantation rate and the clinical pregnancy rate were in favor of cultures under 5% O_2 [69].

In a meta-analysis, no statistically remarkable difference was assessed between the cultures at 5–6% O_2 or 20% O_2 concerning fertilization, implantation and ongoing pregnancy. The only benefit observed under low oxygen levels referred to embryos transferred on day 5 and day 6. Nevertheless, the authors consider additional studies as advisable [70]. In contrast, a review with quantitative synthesis concluded that low oxygen (5–6%) levels were beneficial as living birth rates, clinical pregnancy rates and ongoing pregnancies were positively affected, leading to an increase in the success rates from 32% to 43%, without any increase in multiple pregnancies, miscarriages and congenital deformities [71]. In the most recent meta-analysis, Nastri et al. found no difference between 5 and 6% O_2 and 20% O_2 regarding fertilization and the cleavage rate, a better morphology at the cleavage stage with 5–6% O_2 and they observed a small improvement in the live birth/ongoing pregnancy and clinical pregnancy rates with the use of 5–6% O_2 [72]. However, they underlined that the available evidence is of very low quality; therefore, more large, well-contacted, randomized clinical trials are needed [72].

Nevertheless, new culture strategies appeared. Several researchers, taking into account the conditions recorded to prevail in the female reproductive system, proposed and tested a shift from 5% O_2 to 2% O_2 after day 2–3, i.e., at the morula and blastocyst stages. It is evident that the strategy of using two phases of low oxygen concentrations (5% in the first 2–3 days of preimplantation development and 2% thereafter) better simulates the physiological conditions to which embryos are exposed within the female reproductive system. However, the reported results are contradictory. In 2016, Yang et al. thawed day-3 embryos that had been cultured at 20% O_2 and further cultured either at 2% O_2, 5% O_2 or 20% O_2 [73]. There were no differences among the three groups in terms of the number of blastocysts and the number of high-quality blastocysts [73]. In the same year, Kaser et al., in a randomized controlled trial, used bipronucleate and tripronucleate embryos allocated either for continuous culture in 5% O_2 or in 5% O_2 from day 1 to day 3 and 2% O_2 from day 3 to day 5 [74]. Although they found that the total yield of blastocysts was higher with the biphasic culture, these blastocysts had fewer cells than the blastocysts derived under 5% O_2 [74]. De Munck et al. used the same biphasic oxygen concentration strategy without finding any improvement in embryo development, quality and the utilization rate of blastocysts [75]. On the contrary, Broillet et al., in an observational retrospective study, reported a significant improvement in the total and usable blastocyst rates as well as a higher cumulative birth rate with the biphasic (5–2%) oxygen concentration strategy [76]. Recently, Li et al. reported that the biphasic strategy (5–2% O_2) resulted in a better blastulation rate for low-quality cleavage embryos, but not for high-quality cleavage embryos [77]. The most recent study is a retrospective cross-sectional one that found only marginal benefits with the biphasic (5–2%) oxygen strategy: they performed both fresh and frozen embryo transfers, finding that there was no difference in the pregnancy and implantation rates although, in fresh embryo transfers, the implantation rate of embryos cultured with the biphasic oxygen strategy was significantly better [78].

Recently, a new embryo culture strategy has been tested. Herbemont et al., based on the results of Wale and Gardner's study in mouse embryos [40], designed and performed a prospective randomized study with multiple arms: culturing preimplantation human embryos initially with either 20% O_2 or 5% O_2 and then (day 5–6) with 20% O_2 and either 5% O_2 or 2% O_2 [79]. The hypothesis for this study was that embryos are particularly susceptible to oxidative stress during the first 2 days of development, whereas after the activation of the embryonic genome, they can develop unhindered even in atmospheric oxygen conditions [79]. The primary study endpoints were the day-2 embryo quality and blastocyst quality. According to the results of this study, on day 2, higher division rates and more high-quality embryos were obtained in the 5% O_2 culture than in the 20% O_2 culture. Culturing blastocysts in either 5% O_2 or 2% O_2 gave better-quality blastocysts than the culture in 20% O_2 [79]. However, there were no statistically significant differences in the clinical outcome of the blastocyst transfer, regardless of whether they were grown under atmospheric oxygen or hypoxic conditions [79]. Therefore, although it has been re-established that embryos are particularly vulnerable to 20% O_2 conditions during the first 2 days of development, the use of low oxygen concentrations (2% or 5%) appears to be advantageous for obtaining good-quality blastocysts [79].

It is obvious that there are considerable differences between the aforementioned studies regarding the settings, the primary outcomes, the size of the study populations and not all of them are randomized clinical trials (Table 2). Therefore, it is not strange that the meta-analysis of Nastri et al. found that the available data are of a low quality [72]. On the other hand, it is clear that all but one of these studies found that cultures of human embryos under 5–6% O_2 give some advantage over the cultures under atmospheric O_2. Hence, we can draw some conclusions with considerable certainty: 1. The fertilization rate, especially with ICSI, seem to not be influenced significantly by the oxygen tension. 2. Embryo development is better under 5% O_2 and this is more obvious in the blastocyst formation rate and quality. 3. In our opinion, an initial culture under 20% O_2 and a shift to 5% O_2 after 2–3 days does not guarantee any advantage. 4. The use of a biphasic oxygen strategy (5% during the first three days, 2% afterwards) is promising as it appears to better reproduce the physiological conditions; however, the existing evidence is not strong enough to support this.

Table 2. Summary of major human studies. IVF, conventional in vitro fertilization; ICSI, intracytoplasmic sperm injection; PNs, pronuclei.

Study	Study Type	Objective	Study Population	Outcome	Reproductive Method
Dumoulin et al. (1995) [50]	Prospective randomized study	Evaluation of oxygen levels (5% CO_2/5% O_2/90% N_2 or 5% CO_2/20% O_2) on fertilization rates, development during transfer day, implantation and pregnancy rates	257 IVF cycles from 186 patients	- Clinically relevant pregnancy rates were assessed at 24.2% under 5% O_2 in comparison to 19.4% under 20% O_2 - No major difference in other parameters between the two groups.	IVF
Dumoulin et al. (1999) [51]	Prospective randomized study	Evaluation of oxygen levels (5% O_2 or 20% O_2) on fertilization rates, implantation rates and development during 2nd or 3rd day	1380 IVF cycles	- No major difference was evaluated in fertilization rate (60% in 5% O_2 vs. 61% in 20% O_2), implantation rates (13.4% vs. 14%) and development during 2nd or 3rd day (26.6% vs. 25.4%). - Statistically significant increased rates in blastocyst formation per cycle were in 5% O_2 group assessed (25.8% vs. 20.4%). - Microscopic blastocyst classification was also higher in O_2 group both for blastocysts fixed at day 5 and day 6 (smaller number of cells in 20% O_2 group). - The authors consider the increase in preimplantation rate as inadequate to produce better pregnancy rates or they speculate that oxygen levels are crucial in the later stages of preimplantation.	IVF
Bahceci et al. (2005) [61]	Prospective randomized study	Comparison of embryo culture under 5% O_2 or 20% O_2 in relation to the ICSI outcome	822 oocyte retrieval cycles, 712 of which led to embryo transfer: - 255 transfers on 2nd day (118 cycles cultured under 5% O_2 and 137 under 20% O_2). - 457 transfers on 3rd day (219 under 5% O_2 and 238 under 20% O_2).	- Quality of embryos and clinical outcomes were similar between the two groups. - Embryos transferred on the 3rd day under 5% O_2 exhibited better features. - ICSI cycles' outcomes were not particularly affected by oxygen levels. - The development of the embryos until the blastocyst formation was not assessed.	ICSI
Kea et al. (2007) [53]	Prospective randomized study	Evaluation of the oxygen levels' effect (5% CO_2/5% O_2/90% N_2 or 5% CO_2) on fertilization rates, embryo development and pregnancy outcomes in IVF patients	1045 oocyte retrievals from 106 patients: - 35 patients underwent IVF, 47 patients underwent ICSI and 2 followed a combined procedure on the 3rd embryo transfer day. - 8 patients underwent IVF, 12 patients underwent ICSI and 2 followed a combined procedure on the 5th embryo transfer day.	- No major differences were concluded in fertilization rates, patients' age and fertilization profile, total number of oocytes and 2PNs and pregnancy rates. - The mean embryo score assessing embryo development was significantly higher on the 3rd day. - 21% of the participants were eligible for blastocyst transfer. - Embryo transfer was performed for 20% under 5% CO_2/5% O_2/90% N2 and 21% under 5% CO_2 on the 5th day.	IVF/ICSI/IVF and ICSI (combination)
Kovacic et al. (2008) [55]	Prospective randomized study	Effect of different oxygen levels (5% O_2 or 20% O_2) on sibling oocyte development until the blastocyst stage and evaluation of fertilization rate and the ratio of optimal embryos and blastocysts	785 cumulus–oocyte complexes (COCs) in the IVF group: - 388 COCs under under 5% O_2. - 397 COCs under 20% O_2. 924 cumulus–oocyte complexes (COCs) in the ICSI group: - 462 COCs under under 5% O_2. - 462 COCs under 20% O_2.	- 5% oxygen levels resulted in increased rate of optimal embryos on the 3rd day (IVF: 59% vs. 43.2% and ICSI: 51.2% vs. 28.5%) without affecting fertilization rates either with IVF or ICSI. - Under 5% O_2, the blastocyst formation rates were increased (IVF: 73.2% vs. 63.1% and ICSI: 67.4% vs. 54.7%) as well as the proportion of the blastocysts with normal inner cell mass (IVF: 31.1% VS. 14.6% and ICSI: 18.9% vs. 11.4%). - The optimal blastocyst formation ratio on the 5th day was assessed at 2.1 for IVF and 1.7 for ICSI, supporting the low (5%) oxygen levels.	IVF/ICSI

Table 2. *Cont.*

Study	Study Type	Objective	Study Population	Outcome	Reproductive Method
Ciray et al. (2009) [64]	Prospective randomized study	Evaluation of the oxygen levels' effect (6% CO_2/5% O_2/89% N_2 or 5% CO_2/20% O_2) on embryo qualities and blastocyst status	75 oocyte retrieval cycles including 2061 oocytes, 74 of which led to embryo transfer: - 869 oocytes for the control group. - 868 oocytes for the study group.	- Statistically significant improvements in embryo quality and in blastocyst status have been observed under 6% CO_2/5% O_2/89% N_2. - It is of note that the shift from the control group (5% CO_2/20% O_2) to other group (6% CO_2/5% O_2/89% N_2) occurred on the 3rd day.	ICSI
Meintjes et al. (2009) [54]	Prospective randomized study	Impact of low oxygen levels (5% O_2) on pregnancy rates	230 patients undergoing IVF or ICSI: 115 control group (20% O_2). 115 group (5% O_2).	- Increased preimplantation rate with 5% O_2 in comparison to 20% O_2 levels (42.9% vs. 30.7%). - Increased living birth rates with 5% O_2 in comparison to 20% O_2 levels (57.4% vs. 42.6%).	IVF/ICSI
Waldenstrom et al. (2009) [60]	Prospective randomized study	Effect of different oxygen levels (5% O_2 vs. 19% O_2) on birth rate	396 patients: 197 patients for culture under 5% O_2. 199 patients for culture under 19% O_2.	- The results showed a statistically significant increase in blastocyst formation (47.8% in the culture under 5% O_2 vs. 42.1% in the culture under 19% O_2), in the average blastocyst number (3.8 in the culture under 5% O_2 vs. 3.3 in the culture under 19% O_2) and in the average number of blastocysts for cryopreservation (1.7 in the culture under 5% O_2 vs. 1.1 in the culture under 19% O_2). - Blastocyst culture under low oxygen levels increased birth rate by 10%.	IVF
Nanassy et al. (2010) [56]	Retrospective study	Impact of oxygen levels' shift (5% O_2 and 20% O_2) on embryo quality, implantation and pregnancy rate between the 3rd and the 5th day	382 patients (until the 3rd day all cultures under 20% O_2): 189 patients for culture under 5% O_2 (after the 3rd day). 193 patients for culture under 20% O_2 (after the 3rd day).	- No statistically significant difference in the embryo quality, the implantation or the pregnancy rate was observed in the 5th day. - Similar implantation rates (44.06% under the 5% O_2 vs. 44.16% under 20% O_2), positive pregnancy tests (71.27% under the 5% O2 vs. 78.72% under 20% O_2) and clinical pregnancies (58.56% under the 5% O2 vs. 64.36% under 20% O_2). - The decrease in the oxygen levels has not proven to be beneficial, presumably due to the damage already caused during the first days of culture under 20% O_2.	IVF
Kovacic et al. (2010) [62]	Prospective randomized study	Impact of embryo culture under different oxygen levels (6% CO_2/5% O_2/89% N_2 or 6% CO_2/20% O_2) on the ICSI outcome	647 patients: 326 patients for culture under 5% O_2. 321 patients for culture under 20% O_2.	- Despite the fact that 5% O_2 levels led to a greater number of better-quality embryos on the 2nd day and optimal blastocysts, implantation rates (28.8% under 5% O_2 and 25.2% under 20% O_2) and rates of ongoing pregnancy (31.6% under 5% O_2 and 27.1% under 20% O_2) were similar in both groups. - The low oxygen levels resulted in higher pregnancy rates in general (38.8% under 5% O_2 and 28.3% under 20% O_2) and in the subgroup of poor responders (23% under 5% O_2 and 9.8% under 20% O_2).	ICSI

Table 2. *Cont.*

Study	Study Type	Objective	Study Population	Outcome	Reproductive Method
Sepulveda et al. (2011) [59]	Prospective randomized study	Comparison between embryo culture under 5% O_2 or 20% O_2	100 oocyte donation receivers randomized for culture under 5% O_2 or 20% O_2	- Fertilization rates were assessed at 72.4% under 5% O_2 and 71.7% under 20% O_2. - There was no significant difference in pregnancy rates (55.3% under 5% O_2 and 54.6% under 20% O_2). An increase in multiple pregnancies was observed (46.2% under 5% O_2 and 29.2% under 20% O_2). - Implantation rates emerged higher under low oxygen levels (41.8% under 5% O_2 and 36.8% under 20% O_2). - Cryopreservation was possible for 30.8% under 5% O_2 and 19.2% under 20% O_2. This difference was statistically significant. - Another statistically significant difference was observed in embryo quality (55.4% under 5% O_2 and 41.8% under 20% O_2).	IVF (not directly mentioned)
Sobrinho et al. (2011) [70]	Meta-analysis	Effect of low oxygen levels on fertilization, implantation and pregnancy rates	7 included studies: Dumoulin et al.(1999) [51], Bahceci et al. (2005) [61], Kea et al. (2007) [53], Kovacic et al. (2008) [55], Ciray et al. (2009) [64], Meintjes et al. (2009) [54] and Kovacic et al. (2010) [62].	- Fertilization rates, implantation rates and ongoing pregnancy rates were not significantly different between the 2 groups (5% O_2 and 20% O_2). - Implantation and ongoing pregnancy rates were similar in studies involving embryo transfer on the 2nd or the 3rd day. - 5% O_2 levels emerged beneficial for embryo transfers on the 5th and 6th day, as confirmed by the statistically significant increase in implantation rates. - More randomized studies are advisable to clarify the effect of low oxygen levels in IVF.	IVF/ICSI
Bontekoe et al. (2012) [71]	Review with quantitative synthesis	Assessment of 5% O_2 levels on IVF- and ICSI-related parameters	1382 patients from 4 included studies: Kovacic et al. (2008) [55], Meintjes et al. (2009) [54], Sepulveda et al. (2011) [59] and Waldestrom et al. (2011) [60].	- Embryo culture under 5% O_2 is beneficial for IVF/ICSI outcomes. - Living birth rates, clinical pregnancy rates and ongoing pregnancies were positively affected. The estimated increase in success levels ranges from 32% to 43%. - An increase in multiple pregnancies, miscarriages and congenital deformities has not been observed.	IVF/ICSI
de los Santos MJ et al. (2013) [52]	Prospective randomized study	Evaluation of oxygen levels (5.5% CO_2/6% O_2/88.5% N_2 or 5.5% CO_2/20% O_2) on ongoing pregnancies from oocyte donation cycles	564 cycles under 6% O_2. 561 cycles under 20% O_2.	- Ongoing pregnancy rates were assessed at 41.3% under 6% O_2 and at 40.8% under 20% O_2. - Blastomere number and optimal embryo quality rate were statistically significantly higher at 6% O_2. - In embryo transfers on the 3rd day, 6% O_2 improved only embryo quality, without improving ongoing pregnancy rates.	IVF/ICSI
Kasterstein et al. (2013) [63]	Prospective randomized study	Evaluation of different oxygen levels (5% O_2 or 20% O_2) on embryo development and clinical outcome (in cycles with more than 8 oocytes collected)	258 patients. 3638 mature oocytes retrieved. 1833 incubated under 5% O_2. 1805 sibling oocytes incubated under 20% O_2.	- Fertilization rates were similar in both groups. - The 5% oxygen levels resulted in statistically significantly increased blastomeres and optimal embryo quality. - More embryos were eligible for transfer in the low-oxygen group (31.6% under 5% O_2 vs. 23.1% under 20% O_2). - A statistically significant increase was observed in implantation and pregnancy rates in the low-oxygen group. - Living birth rates per transfer were also statistically significantly increased (34.2% under 5% O_2 vs. 15.8% under 20% O_2).	ICSI

Table 2. *Cont.*

Study	Study Type	Objective	Study Population	Outcome	Reproductive Method
Paternot et al. (2013) [65]	2 randomized controlled trials	Assessment of embryo incubation in a mini-incubator or a conventional incubator and effect of different oxygen levels (5% O_2 and 20% O_2) on embryo quality	395 embryos in each group	- Embryo cultures in a mini-incubator were similar to the embryo cultures in a conventional incubator on the first 3 days of embryo development. - Low oxygen concentrations did not affect embryo quality substantially.	IVF/ICSI
Peng ZF et al. (2015) [57]	Randomized study	Evaluation of different oxygen levels on fertilization rates, implantation rates, pregnancy rates, multiple pregnancies and miscarriages	3484 IVF and ICSI cycles: 1131 cycles cultured under 5% CO_2 and 20% O_2. 1258 cycles cultured at first under 5% CO_2 and 20% O_2 and after the 2nd day under 5% O_2/5% CO_2/90% N_2 until the 3rd day. 1095 cycles cultured under 5% O_2/5% CO_2/90% N_2.	- Increased fertilization and implantation rates were statistically significant for culture under 5% O_2/5% CO_2/90% N2 in comparison to the other 2 groups. These data concern IVF embryos. - Embryos from IVF cultured under 20% O_2 showed statistically significantly better fertilization rates, implantation rates and quality in comparison to the group with the oxygen levels' shift. - Embryos from ICSI cultured under 20% O_2 showed statistically significantly lower cleavage rates than those from the group with the oxygen levels' shift. - These results lead to the conclusion that embryos are more sensitive to the oxygen levels' shifts than to oxygen levels per se.	IVF/ICSI
Nastri et al. (2016) [72]	Systematic review and meta-analysis	Evaluation of different oxygen levels on embryo cultures	21 included studies	- Low-quality evidence suggested that low (5–6%) oxygen levels were beneficial for living birth and clinical pregnancy rate. - Low quality evidence showed no difference in fertilization and cleavage rate between low (5–6%) and high (20%) oxygen levels. - Low-quality evidence suggested that low (5–6%) oxygen levels resulted in better embryo development at the cleavage stage.	IVF/ICSI
Van Montfoort et al. (2020) [58]	Cohort study	Assessment of different oxygen levels' potential involvement in embryo utilization, IVF success rates and birthweight	871 patients. 195 cycles in the group under 5% O_2 (1627 oocytes). 676 cycles in the group under 20% O_2 (5448 oocytes).	- A statistically significantly increased number of quality embryos has been observed under 5% O_2 (45.8% under 5% O_2 and 30.9% under 20% O_2). - This increased number of quality embryos was not correlated to an increased living birth rate, but allowed embryos of better quality to be cryopreserved. - No correlation between oxygen levels and birthweight could be observed.	IVF or IVF/ICSI
Ruíz et al. (2020) [66]	Prospective randomized controlled trial	Assessment of the embryo culture under low oxygen levels (5% O_2) in benchtop incubator on embryo-related parameters	148 patients: 73 patients in the control group culture under 20% O_2 and in large box-incubators. 75 patients in the study group (culture under 5% O_2 and in benchtop incubators).	- Implantation rate and live birth delivery rate per embryo transfer were significantly higher in the study group compared to the conventional embryo culture group (culture under 20% O_2 and in large box-incubators). - Also, the cumulative implantation rate and the cumulative live birth rate per embryo transfer emerged as significantly higher in the study group compared to the conventional embryo culture group. - Particular benefit was assessed for poor-quality embryos. - Fresh embryo transfers were correlated with higher blastocyst, implantation, live birth, cumulative implantation and cumulative live birth rate in comparison to the frozen embryo transfers assessed.	IVF

Table 2. *Cont.*

Study	Study Type	Objective	Study Population	Outcome	Reproductive Method
Gelo et al. (2019) [67]	Prospective randomized controlled trial	Evaluation of embryo culture under 5% O_2 in a benchtop incubator or 20% O_2 in a classic incubator on embryo-related and clinical parameters	393 patients: 198 patients in the 5% O_2 group. 195 patients in the 20% O_2 group.	- Both for the live birth rates and for the fertilization rates, no statistically significant improvement could be assessed for the 5% O_2 group. However, a statistically beneficial role of the embryo culture under 5% O_2 was confirmed for the blastocyst number on the 5th day and for the fertilization rate. - Clinical pregnancy rates emerged as higher in the 5% O_2 group, but significantly higher only on the 5th day. - Overall, benchtop incubators led to an increase in the number of blastocysts produced and, consequently, to higher pregnancy rates.	IVF/ICSI
Li et al. (2022) [68]	Randomized study	Assessment of ultra-low (2%) oxygen levels on embryo development and clinical parameters	2298 oocytes from 152 patients	- On the 3rd day, no statistically significant difference could be observed in good-quality and available embryos rates between the two groups (culture under 2% O_2 and 5% O_2). - The blastulation rate and the fraction of good-quality blastocysts on the 5th day and the total blastulation rate emerged as similar between the 2 groups. - Clinical and ongoing pregnancy rates were also similar in the first transfer between the 2 groups. - The application of embryo culture under 2% is not recommended based on these results.	IVF
Fawzy et al. (2017) [69]	Comparative study	Evaluation of low oxygen levels (3.5% O_2) on embryo development and clinical parameters	6024 oocytes from 558 patients: 3290 oocytes from 293 patients in the 3.5% O_2 group. 2734 oocytes from 265 patients in the 5% O_2 group.	- Statistically significantly higher fertilization and cleavage emerged in the 3.5% O_2 group compared to the 5% O_2. - However, the compaction rate on the 3rd day and the number of formed, good-quality and cryopreserved blastocysts was assessed as significantly lower in the 3.5% O_2 group. - Significantly lower biochemical pregnancy, clinical pregnancy and implantation rates were assessed for the 3.5% O_2 group.	ICSI
Yang et al. (2016) [73]	Comparative study	Assessment of different oxygen levels (2% O_2, 5% O_2 and 20% O_2) on embryo cultures until the blastocyst stage	155 embryos from 21 couples (120 finally included): 46 embryos in the 2% O_2 group. 44 embryos in the 5% O_2 group. 30 embryos in the 20% O_2 group.	- The blastocyst formation rate was similar in the 3 groups assessed. - The apoptosis rate was significantly lower for blastocyst formation under 5% O_2. - No statistically significant difference in the expression patterns of the genes assessed was found between the 2% O_2 and the 5% O_2 group. - Cryopreserved embryos from the 3rd day until the blastocyst stage will benefit from culture under 5% O_2.	IVF
Kaser et al. (2018) [74]	Randomized controlled trial	Assessment of human preimplantation embryos' culture under 2% O_2 or 5% O_2	203 zygotes: 102 zygotes for culture under 5% O_2 for both periods (days 1 to 3 and days 3 to 5). 101 zygotes for culture under 5% O_2 for days 1 to 3 and under 2% O_2 for days 3 to 5.	- Embryos cultured under 2% O_2 were less likely to arrest in cleavage stage on the 5th day. - A higher blastulation rate was assessed for embryos cultured under 2% O_2. - Statistically significantly fewer cells were found in blastocysts of embryos cultures under 2% O_2. - Metabolic changes, including amino acids' capacity and metabolites' status against oxidative stress, were also found. An overexpression of MUC1 was assessed in the 2% O_2 without clinical significance.	IVF/ICSI

Table 2. *Cont.*

Study	Study Type	Objective	Study Population	Outcome	Reproductive Method
De Munck et al. (2019) [75]	2 prospective randomized controlled trial	Evaluation of the shift in oxygen concentration from 5% to 2% after the 3rd day on blastocyst parameters	1811 embryos (direct exposure). 405 embryos for culture under 2% O_2. 406 embryos for culture under 5% O_2. 1144 embryos (gradual exposure). 572 embryos for culture under 2% O_2. 572 embryos for culture under 5% O_2.	- No statistically significant differences could be assessed in the blastulation rate, the utilization rate and the number of good-quality blastocysts.	IVF/ICSI
Brouillet et al. (2021) [76]	Monocentric retrospective observational study	Evaluation of oxygen levels' shift from 5% to 2% on embryo-related and clinical parameters	120 couples. (1st IVF cycle with embryo culture under 5% O_2 and 2nd IVF cycle with embryo culture under 5% O_2 for the first 3 days and then under 2% O_2 for days 3 to 5/6.)	- Usable blastocyst rate and the cumulative birth rate emerged as statistically significantly increased in the 2nd IVF cycle. - The expression pattern, according to the analysis of 707 RNAs, was significantly different and included genes related to many aspects of embryo development and beyond. - The oxygen levels' shift may improve the effectiveness of IVF.	IVF
Li et al. (2022) [77]	Comparative study	Evaluation of oxygen levels' shift from 5% to 2% in embryo-related and clinical parameters.	510 embryos from 188 patients: 296 embryos from 106 patients for culture under 5% O_2 after the 3rd day until the 5th or the 6th day. 214 embryos from 82 patients for culture under 2% O_2 after the 3rd day until the 5th or the 6th day.	- Blastulation rate and high-quality blastulation rate emerged as similar for high-quality embryos. - For low-quality embryos, culture under 2% O_2 after the 3rd day improved the blastulation rate in a statistically significant way, without any significant improvement in the high-quality blastulation rate. - Prolonged culture until the 7th day led to a statistically significant increase in the blastulation rate for the low-quality embryos, cultured under 2% O_2.	IVF/ICSI
Patel et al. (2023) [78]	Retrospective cross-sectional study	Assessment of low (5% O_2) and ultra-low (2% O_2) oxygen levels on embryo-related and clinical parameters	382 patients; 206 embryos for culture under 2% O_2. 176 embryos for culture under 5% O_2.	- Implantation and pregnancy rates by the oxygen concentration the two groups. - During frozen embryo transfer, the abortion rate was statistically significantly higher in the group of embryos cultured under 5% O_2. - Despite the higher number of good-quality embryos observed in the 5% O_2 group, clinical outcomes did not improve substantially. - Embryos transferred fresh showed a statistically significantly improved implantation rate.	IVF
Herbemont et al. (2021) [79]	Randomized controlled trial	Evaluation of the oxygen levels' importance according to the embryo's developmental stage	773 IVF/ICSI cycles: 265 cycles in culture under 20% O_2 and after the 2nd day, culture of the available good-quality embryos in 88 cycles under 20% O_2. 508 cycles in culture under 5% O_2, after the 2nd day either culture until the 6th day for 195 cycles or shift of the oxygen levels to 20% O_2 until the 6th day for 94 cycles.	- The number of early embryos in the cleavage state and the quality features for embryos on the 2nd day were statistically significantly higher in the group with the 508 cycles performed. A proper model also confirmed the significance of the oxygen levels in that correlation. - The number and the rate of top-quality blastocysts on the 5th day emerged as statistically significantly lower in the group with the 88 cycles performed. The groups with the 195 and 88 cycles performed exhibited similar results. The first outcome was confirmed for the 6th day as well. - After the transfer of the blastocysts, no important differences were observed regarding the clinical parameters. - Overall, the researchers propose the culture of the embryos at an early stage under low oxygen levels, as the oxidative stress acts presumably prior to the genome activation of the embryo.	IVF/ICSI

6. Conclusions

The cultures under low or high oxygen levels have been extensively investigated either in embryos of various mammal species or human embryos. The hasty conclusion from the animal studies is that the culture in low oxygen levels, instead of the culture in atmospheric oxygen levels, offers advantages in embryo development. However, the optimal low oxygen levels vary by species. As for human embryos, most of the studies compared 5% to 20% oxygen levels. Although the quality of the evidence is not good, as the meta-analysis of Nastri et al. [72] indicates, all the relevant studies, with the exception of one [64], showed that the culture under low oxygen levels is, to some extent, beneficial for human embryos. Nevertheless, no study to date could confirm any benefit for embryos, implantation or pregnancy rates related to the use of atmospheric oxygen levels in the human embryo culture in comparison to the culture under 5–6% oxygen levels. The biphasic oxygen concentration strategy (5% in the first three days and 2% afterwards) appears as an interesting and promising method, though additional studies are needed in order to confirm its value.

In conclusion, the currently available evidence does not support the culture of human embryos under atmospheric conditions. The higher cost related to cultures under 5% or 2% O_2 cannot be considered as a reason for not adopting the culture under low oxygen tension.

Author Contributions: Conceptualization, B.A.; writing—original draft preparation, O.K. and T.P.; review and editing, A.Z., C.S. and S.S.; supervision, B.A.; project administration, B.A. All authors have read and agreed to the published version of the manuscript.

Funding: This research received no external funding.

Institutional Review Board Statement: Not applicable.

Informed Consent Statement: Not applicable.

Data Availability Statement: No new data were created.

Conflicts of Interest: The authors declare no conflicts of interest.

References

1. Steptoe, P.C.; Edwards, R.G.; Purdy, J.M. Human Blastocysts grown in Culture. *Nature* **1971**, *229*, 132–133. [CrossRef] [PubMed]
2. Sciorio, R.; Smith, G.D. Embryo culture at a reduced oxygen concentration of 5%: A mini review. *Zygote* **2019**, *27*, 355–361. [CrossRef] [PubMed]
3. Quinn, P.; Harlow, G.M. The effect of oxygen on the development of preimplantation mouse embryos in vitro. *J. Exp. Zool.* **1978**, *206*, 73–80. [CrossRef] [PubMed]
4. Higdon, H.L., 3rd; Blackhurst, D.W.; Boone, W.R. Incubator management in an assisted reproductive technology laboratory. *Fertil. Steril.* **2008**, *89*, 703–710. [CrossRef] [PubMed]
5. Bedaiwy, M.A.; Falcone, T.; Mohamed, M.S.; Aleem, A.A.N.; Sharma, R.K.; Worley, S.E.; Thornton, J.; Agarwal, A. Differential growth of human embryos in vitro: Role of reactive oxygen species. *Fertil. Steril.* **2004**, *82*, 593–600. [CrossRef] [PubMed]
6. Catt, J.W.; Henman, M. Toxic effects of oxygen on human embryo development. *Hum. Reprod.* **2000**, *15* (Suppl. S2), 199–206. [CrossRef] [PubMed]
7. Fischer, B.; Bavister, B.D. Oxygen tension in the oviduct and uterus of rhesus monkeys, hamsters and rabbits. *J. Reprod. Fertil.* **1993**, *99*, 673–679. [CrossRef] [PubMed]
8. Mastroianni, L., Jr.; Jones, R. Oxygen Tension Within the rabbit fallopian tube. *Reproduction* **1965**, *9*, 99–102. [CrossRef] [PubMed]
9. Ng, K.Y.B.; Mingels, R.; Morgan, H.; Macklon, N.; Cheong, Y. In vivo oxygen, temperature and pH dynamics in the female reproductive tract and their importance in human conception: A systematic review. *Hum. Reprod. Updat.* **2017**, *24*, 15–34. [CrossRef] [PubMed]
10. Mitchell, J.A.; Yochim, J.M. Measurement of Intrauterine Oxygen Tension in the Rat and Its Regulation by Ovarian Steroid Hormones. *Endocrinology* **1968**, *83*, 691–700. [CrossRef]
11. Kaufman, D.L.; Mitchell, J.A. Intrauterine oxygen tension during the oestrous cycle in the hamster: Patterns of change. *Comp. Biochem. Physiol. Part A Physiol.* **1994**, *107*, 673–678. [CrossRef] [PubMed]
12. Garris, D.R.; Mitchell, J.A. Intrauterine Oxygen Tension during the Estrous Cycle in the Guinea Pig: Its Relation to Uterine Blood Volume and Plasma Estrogen and Progesterone Levels. *Biol. Reprod.* **1979**, *21*, 149–159. [CrossRef] [PubMed]

13. Mitchell, J.A.; Van Kainen, B.R. Effects of Alcohol on Intrauterine Oxygen Tension in the Rat. *Alcohol. Clin. Exp. Res.* **1992**, *16*, 308–310. [CrossRef] [PubMed]
14. Kigawa, J. Studies on the levels of pO2 and pCO2 in the uterine cavity and uterine tissue (author's transl). *Nihon Sanka Fujinka Gakkai Zasshi* **1981**, *33*, 1646–1654. [PubMed]
15. Yedwab, G.A.; Paz, G.; Homonnai, T.Z.; David, M.P.; Kraicer, P.F. The Temperature, pH, and Partial Pressure of Oxygen in the Cervix and Uterus of Women and Uterus of Rats During the Cycle. *Fertil. Steril.* **1976**, *27*, 304–309. [CrossRef] [PubMed]
16. Ottosen, L.D.; Hindkjær, J.; Husth, M.; Petersen, D.E.; Kirk, J.; Ingerslev, H.J. Observations on intrauterine oxygen tension measured by fibre-optic microsensors. *Reprod. Biomed. Online* **2006**, *13*, 380–385. [CrossRef] [PubMed]
17. Shalgi, R.; Kraicer, P.F.; Soferman, N. Gases and electrolytes of human follicular fluid. *Reproduction* **1972**, *28*, 335–340. [CrossRef] [PubMed]
18. Gosden, R.; Byatt-Smith, J. Oxygen concentration gradient across the ovarian follicular epithelium: Model, predictions and implications. *Hum. Reprod.* **1986**, *1*, 65–68. [CrossRef] [PubMed]
19. Clark, A.R.; Stokes, Y.M.; Lane, M.; Thompson, J.G. Mathematical modelling of oxygen concentration in bovine and murine cumulus–oocyte complexes. *Reproduction* **2006**, *131*, 999–1006. [CrossRef] [PubMed]
20. Hardy, K.; Hooper, M.; Handyside, A.; Rutherford, A.; Winston, R.; Leese, H. Non-invasive measurement of glucose and pyruvate uptake by individual human oocytes and preimplantation embryos. *Hum. Reprod.* **1989**, *4*, 188–191. [CrossRef] [PubMed]
21. Gott, A.; Hardy, K.; Winston, R.; Leese, H. Non-invasive measurement of pyruvate and glucose uptake and lactate production by sigle human preimplantation embryos. *Hum. Reprod.* **1990**, *5*, 104–108. [CrossRef] [PubMed]
22. Leese, H.J. Metabolic control during preimplantation mammalian development. *Hum. Reprod. Updat.* **1995**, *1*, 63–72. [CrossRef] [PubMed]
23. Leese, H.J.; Conaghan, J.; Martin, K.L.; Hardy, K. Early human embryo metabolism. *BioEssays* **1993**, *15*, 259–264. [CrossRef] [PubMed]
24. Leese, H.J. Metabolism of the preimplantation embryo: 40 years on. *Reproduction* **2012**, *143*, 417–427. [CrossRef] [PubMed]
25. Houghton, F.D. Energy metabolism of the inner cell mass and trophectoderm of the mouse blastocyst. *Differentiation* **2006**, *74*, 11–18. [CrossRef] [PubMed]
26. Guérin, P.; El Mouatassim, S.; Ménézo, Y. Oxidative stress and protection against reactive oxygen species in the pre-implantation embryo and its surroundings. *Hum. Reprod. Update* **2001**, *7*, 175–189. [CrossRef] [PubMed]
27. Guérin, P.; Ménézo, Y. Hypotaurine and taurine in gamete and embryo environments: De novo synthesis via the cysteine sulfinic acid pathway in oviduct cells. *Zygote* **1995**, *3*, 333–343. [CrossRef] [PubMed]
28. Johnson, M.H.; Nasresfahani, M.H. Radical solutions and cultural problems: Could free oxygen radicals be responsible for the impaired development of preimplantation mammalian embryos in vitro? *BioEssays* **1994**, *16*, 31–38. [CrossRef] [PubMed]
29. Goto, Y.; Noda, Y.; Mori, T.; Nakano, M. Increased generation of reactive oxygen species in embryos cultured in vitro. *Free Radic. Biol. Med.* **1993**, *15*, 69–75. [CrossRef] [PubMed]
30. Kwon, H.-C.; Yang, H.-W.; Hwang, K.-J.; Yoo, J.-H.; Kim, M.-S.; Lee, C.-H.; Ryu, H.S.; Oh, K.S. Effects of Low Oxygen Condition on the Generation of Reactive Oxygen Species and the Development in Mouse Embryos Cultured in vitro. *J. Obstet. Gynaecol. Res.* **1999**, *25*, 359–366. [CrossRef] [PubMed]
31. Nakayama, T.; Noda, Y.; Goto, Y.; Mori, T. Effects of visible light and other environmental factors on the production of oxygen radicals by hamster embryos. *Theriogenology* **1994**, *41*, 499–510. [CrossRef] [PubMed]
32. Martín-Romero, F.J.; Miguel-Lasobras, E.M.; Domínguez-Arroyo, J.A.; González-Carrera, E.; Álvarez, I.S. Contribution of culture media to oxidative stress and its effect on human oocytes. *Reprod. Biomed. Online* **2008**, *17*, 652–661. [CrossRef] [PubMed]
33. Wale, P.L.; Gardner, D.K. Oxygen Regulates Amino Acid Turnover and Carbohydrate Uptake During the Preimplantation Period of Mouse Embryo Development1. *Biol. Reprod.* **2012**, *87*, 1–8. [CrossRef] [PubMed]
34. Gu, T.-P.; Guo, F.; Yang, H.; Wu, H.-P.; Xu, G.-F.; Liu, W.; Xie, Z.-G.; Shi, L.; He, X.; Jin, S.-G.; et al. The role of Tet3 DNA dioxygenase in epigenetic reprogramming by oocytes. *Nature* **2011**, *477*, 606–610. [CrossRef] [PubMed]
35. Morgan, H.D.; Santos, F.; Green, K.; Dean, W.; Reik, W. Epigenetic reprogramming in mammals. *Hum. Mol. Genet.* **2005**, *14*, R47–R58. [CrossRef] [PubMed]
36. Marcho, C.; Cui, W.; Mager, J. Epigenetic dynamics during preimplantation development. *Reproduction* **2015**, *150*, R109–R120. [CrossRef] [PubMed]
37. Katz-Jaffe, M.G.; Linck, D.W.; Schoolcraft, W.B.; Gardner, D.K. A proteomic analysis of mammalian preimplantation embryonic development. *Reproduction* **2005**, *130*, 899–905. [CrossRef] [PubMed]
38. Rinaudo, P.F.; Giritharan, G.; Talbi, S.; Dobson, A.T.; Schultz, R.M. Effects of oxygen tension on gene expression in preimplantation mouse embryos. *Fertil. Steril.* **2006**, *86*, 1265.e1–1265.e36. [CrossRef] [PubMed]
39. Otsuki, J.; Nagai, Y.; Chiba, K. Peroxidation of mineral oil used in droplet culture is detrimental to fertilization and embryo development. *Fertil. Steril.* **2007**, *88*, 741–743. [CrossRef] [PubMed]
40. Wale, P.; Gardner, D. Time-lapse analysis of mouse embryo development in oxygen gradients. *Reprod. Biomed. Online* **2010**, *21*, 402–410. [CrossRef] [PubMed]
41. Bean, C.J.; Hassold, T.J.; Judis, L.; Hunt, P.A. Fertilization in vitro increases non-disjunction during early cleavage divisions in a mouse model system. *Hum. Reprod.* **2002**, *17*, 2362–2367. [CrossRef] [PubMed]

42. Kishi, J.; Noda, Y.; Narimoto, K.; Umaoka, Y.; Mori, T. Block to development in cultured rat 1-cell embryos is overcome using medium HECM-1. *Hum. Reprod.* **1991**, *6*, 1445–1448. [CrossRef] [PubMed]
43. McKiernan, S.H.; Bavister, B.D. Environmental Variables Influencing in Vitro Development of Hamster 2-Cell Embryos to the Blastocyst Stage1. *Biol. Reprod.* **1990**, *43*, 404–413. [CrossRef] [PubMed]
44. Li, J.; Foote, R.H. Culture of rabbit zygotes into blastocysts in protein-free medium with one to twenty per cent oxygen. *Reproduction* **1993**, *98*, 163–167. [CrossRef] [PubMed]
45. Karja, N.W.K.; Wongsrikeao, P.; Murakami, M.; Agung, B.; Fahrudin, M.; Nagai, T.; Otoi, T. Effects of oxygen tension on the development and quality of porcine in vitro fertilized embryos. *Theriogenology* **2004**, *62*, 1585–1595. [CrossRef] [PubMed]
46. Batt, P.; Gardner, D.; Cameron, A. Oxygen concentration and protein source affect the development of preimplantation goat embryos in vitro. *Reprod. Fertil. Dev.* **1991**, *3*, 601–607. [CrossRef] [PubMed]
47. Leoni, G.; Rosati, I.; Succu, S.; Bogliolo, L.; Bebbere, D.; Berlinguer, F.; Ledda, S.; Naitana, S. A Low Oxygen Atmosphere during IVF Accelerates the Kinetic of Formation of In Vitro Produced Ovine Blastocysts. *Reprod. Domest. Anim.* **2007**, *42*, 299–304. [CrossRef] [PubMed]
48. He, H.; Zhang, H.; Li, Q.; Fan, J.; Pan, Y.; Zhang, T.; Robert, N.; Zhao, L.; Hu, X.; Han, X.; et al. Low oxygen concentrations improve yak oocyte maturation and enhance the developmental competence of preimplantation embryos. *Theriogenology* **2020**, *156*, 46–58. [CrossRef] [PubMed]
49. Tkachenko, O.Y.; Delimitreva, S.; Wedi, E.; Scheerer-Bernhard, J.U.; Valle, R.R.; Nayudu, P.L. Effects of oxygen concentration in IVM/IVF on marmoset monkey oocyte maturation and embryo development. *Anim. Reprod.* **2017**, *14*, 1170–1178. [CrossRef]
50. Dumoulin, J.C.; Vanvuchelen, R.C.; Land, J.A.; Pieters, M.H.; Geraedts, J.P.; Evers, J.L. Effect of oxygen concentration on in vitro fertilization and embryo culture in the human and the mouse. *Fertil. Steril.* **1995**, *63*, 115–119. [CrossRef] [PubMed]
51. Dumoulin, J.C.; Meijers, C.J.; Bras, M.; Coonen, E.; Geraedts, J.P.; Evers, J.L. Effect of oxygen concentration on human in-vitro fertilization and embryo culture. *Hum. Reprod.* **1999**, *14*, 465–469. [CrossRef] [PubMed]
52. De los Santos, M.J.d.L.; Gámiz, P.; Albert, C.; Galán, A.; Viloria, T.; Pérez, S.; Romero, J.L.; Remohï, J. Reduced oxygen tension improves embryo quality but not clinical pregnancy rates: A randomized clinical study into ovum donation cycles. *Fertil. Steril.* **2013**, *100*, 402–407. [CrossRef] [PubMed]
53. Kea, B.; Gebhardt, J.; Watt, J.; Westphal, L.M.; Lathi, R.B.; Milki, A.A.; Behr, B. Effect of reduced oxygen concentrations on the outcome of in vitro fertilization. *Fertil. Steril.* **2007**, *87*, 213–216. [CrossRef] [PubMed]
54. Meintjes, M.; Chantilis, S.J.; Douglas, J.D.; Rodriguez, A.J.; Guerami, A.R.; Bookout, D.M.; Barnett, B.D.; Madden, J.D. A controlled randomized trial evaluating the effect of lowered incubator oxygen tension on live births in a predominantly blastocyst transfer program. *Hum. Reprod.* **2008**, *24*, 300–307. [CrossRef] [PubMed]
55. Kovačič, B.; Vlaisavljević, V. Influence of atmospheric versus reduced oxygen concentration on development of human blastocysts in vitro: A prospective study on sibling oocytes. *Reprod. Biomed. Online* **2008**, *17*, 229–236. [CrossRef] [PubMed]
56. Nanassy, L.; Wilcox, A.L.; Peterson, C.M.; Hammoud, A.; Carrell, D.T. Comparison of 5% and ambient oxygen during days 3–5 of in vitro culture of human embryos. *Fertil. Steril.* **2010**, *93*, 579–585. [CrossRef] [PubMed]
57. Peng, Z.F.; Shi, S.L.; Jin, H.X.; Yao, G.D.; Wang, E.Y.; Yang, H.Y.; Song, W.; Sun, Y. Impact of oxygen concentrations on fertilization; cleavage; implantation; and pregnancy rates of in vitro generated human embryos. *Int. J. Clin. Exp. Med.* **2015**, *8*, 6179–6185. [PubMed]
58. Van Montfoort, A.P.A.; Arts, E.; Wijnandts, L.; Sluijmer, A.; Pelinck, M.J.; Land, J.A.; Van Echten-Arends, J. Reduced oxygen concentration during human IVF culture improves embryo utilization and cumulative pregnancy rates per cycle. *Hum. Reprod. Open* **2020**, *2020*, hoz036. [CrossRef] [PubMed]
59. Sepulveda, S.; Steurer, I.; Gazzo, E.; Escudero, E.; Noriega, L. Effect of oxygen conditions on the results of an oocyte donation program: A prospective randomized trial [Efeito das condicoes de oxigenio no resultado de um programa de ovo–doacao: Estudo prospectivo e randomizado]. *J. Bras. De Reprod. Assist.* **2011**, *15*, 32–33.
60. Waldenström, U.; Engström, A.-B.; Hellberg, D.; Nilsson, S. Low-oxygen compared with high-oxygen atmosphere in blastocyst culture, a prospective randomized study. *Fertil. Steril.* **2009**, *91*, 2461–2465. [CrossRef] [PubMed]
61. Bahçeci, M.; Çray, H.N.; Karagenc, L.; Ulug, U.; Bener, F. Effect of oxygen concentration during the incubation of embryos of women undergoing ICSI and embryo transfer: A prospective randomized study. *Reprod. Biomed. Online* **2005**, *11*, 438–443. [CrossRef] [PubMed]
62. Kovačič, B.; Sajko, M.; Vlaisavljević, V. A prospective, randomized trial on the effect of atmospheric versus reduced oxygen concentration on the outcome of intracytoplasmic sperm injection cycles. *Fertil. Steril.* **2010**, *94*, 511–519. [CrossRef] [PubMed]
63. Kasterstein, E.; Strassburger, D.; Komarovsky, D.; Bern, O.; Komsky, A.; Raziel, A.; Friedler, S.; Ron-El, R. The effect of two distinct levels of oxygen concentration on embryo development in a sibling oocyte study. *J. Assist. Reprod. Genet.* **2013**, *30*, 1073–1079. [CrossRef] [PubMed]
64. Ciray, H.N.; Aksoy, T.; Yaramanci, K.; Karayaka, I.; Bahceci, M. In vitro culture under physiologic oxygen concentration improves blastocyst yield and quality: A prospective randomized survey on sibling oocytes. *Fertil. Steril.* **2009**, *91*, 1459–1461. [CrossRef] [PubMed]
65. Paternot, G.; Debrock, S.; D'Hooghe, T.; Spiessens, C. Can embryo quality be improved by in vitro exposure to low oxygen concentration or by using a mini-incubator? two randomized controlled trials. *Fertil. Steril.* **2013**, *100*, S247–S248. [CrossRef]

66. Ruíz, M.; Santamaría-López, E.; Blasco, V.; Hernáez, M.J.; Caligara, C.; Pellicer, A.; Fernández-Sánchez, M.; Prados, N. Effect of Group Embryo Culture under Low Oxygen Tension in Benchtop Incubators on Human Embryo Culture: Prospective, Randomized, Controlled Trial. *Reprod. Sci.* **2020**, *27*, 1522–1533. [CrossRef] [PubMed]
67. Gelo, N.; Kirinec, G.; Baldani, D.P.; Vrčić, H.; Ježek, D.; Milošević, M.; Stanić, P. Influence of human embryo cultivation in a classic CO_2 incubator with 20% oxygen versus benchtop incubator with 5% oxygen on live births: The randomized prospective trial. *Zygote* **2019**, *27*, 131–136. [CrossRef] [PubMed]
68. Li, M.; Wang, M.; Xue, X. Effect of ultra-low O_2 (2%) tension on human in-vitro embryo development. *Pak. J. Pharm. Sci.* **2022**, *35*, 135–139.
69. Fawzy, M.; Emad, M.; AbdelRahman, M.Y.; Abdelghafar, H.; Hafez, F.F.A.; Bedaiwy, M.A. Impact of 3.5% O_2 culture on embryo development and clinical outcomes: A comparative study. *Fertil. Steril.* **2017**, *108*, 635–641. [CrossRef] [PubMed]
70. Sobrinho, D.B.G.; Oliveira, J.B.A.; Petersen, C.G.; Mauri, A.L.; Silva, L.F.; Massaro, F.C.; Baruffi, R.L.; Cavagna, M.; Franco, J.G. IVF/ICSI outcomes after culture of human embryos at low oxygen tension: A meta-analysis. *Reprod. Biol. Endocrinol.* **2011**, *9*, 143. [CrossRef]
71. Bontekoe, S.; Mantikou, E.; van Wely, M.; Seshadri, S.; Repping, S.; Mastenbroek, S. Low oxygen concentrations for embryo culture in assisted reproductive technologies. *Cochrane Database Syst. Rev.* **2012**. [CrossRef] [PubMed]
72. Nastri, C.O.; Nóbrega, B.N.; Teixeira, D.M.; Amorim, J.; Diniz, L.M.; Barbosa, M.W.; Giorgi, V.S.; Pileggi, V.N.; Martins, W.P. Low versus atmospheric oxygen tension for embryo culture in assisted reproduction: A systematic review and meta-analysis. *Fertil. Steril.* **2016**, *106*, 95–104.e17. [CrossRef]
73. Yang, Y.; Xu, Y.; Ding, C.; Khoudja, R.Y.; Lin, M.; Awonuga, A.O.; Dai, J.; Puscheck, E.E.; Rappolee, D.A.; Zhou, C. Comparison of 2, 5, and 20% O_2 on the development of post-thaw human embryos. *J. Assist. Reprod. Genet.* **2016**, *33*, 919–927. [CrossRef] [PubMed]
74. Kaser, D.J.; Bogale, B.; Sarda, V.; Farland, L.V.; Williams, P.L.; Racowsky, C. Randomized controlled trial of low (5%) versus ultralow (2%) oxygen for extended culture using bipronucleate and tripronucleate human preimplantation embryos. *Fertil. Steril.* **2018**, *109*, 1030–1037.e2. [CrossRef] [PubMed]
75. De Munck, N.; Janssens, R.; Segers, I.; Tournaye, H.; Van de Velde, H.; Verheyen, G. Influence of ultra-low oxygen (2%) tension on in-vitro human embryo development. *Hum. Reprod.* **2018**, *34*, 228–234. [CrossRef] [PubMed]
76. Brouillet, S.; Baron, C.; Barry, F.; Andreeva, A.; Haouzi, D.; Gala, A.; Ferrières-Hoa, A.; Loup, V.; Anahory, T.; Ranisavljevic, N.; et al. Biphasic (5–2%) oxygen concentration strategy significantly improves the usable blastocyst and cumulative live birth rates in in vitro fertilization. *Sci. Rep.* **2021**, *11*, 7580. [CrossRef] [PubMed]
77. Li, M.; Xue, X.; Shi, J. Ultralow Oxygen Tension (2%) Is Beneficial for Blastocyst Formation of In Vitro Human Low-Quality Embryo Culture. *BioMed Res. Int.* **2022**, *2022*, 9603185. [CrossRef] [PubMed]
78. Patel, D.; Patel, R.G.; Patel, T.; Patel, N.; Maheshwari, N. Limited Effects of Ultra-low Oxygen Concentration during Extended Embryo Culture on In vitro Fertilisation Outcomes in Indian Women: A Retrospective Cross-sectional Study. *J. Hum. Reprod. Sci.* **2023**, *16*, 324–332. [CrossRef] [PubMed]
79. Herbemont, C.; Labrosse, J.; Bennani-Smires, B.; Cedrin-Durnerin, I.; Peigne, M.; Sermondade, N.; Sarandi, S.; Vivot, A.; Vicaut, E.; Talib, Z.; et al. Impact of oxygen tension according to embryo stage of development: A prospective randomized study. *Sci. Rep.* **2021**, *11*, 22313. [CrossRef] [PubMed]

Journal of
Clinical Medicine

MDPI

Review

Evolution of Minimally Invasive and Non-Invasive Preimplantation Genetic Testing: An Overview

Efthalia Moustakli [1], Athanasios Zikopoulos [2], Charikleia Skentou [3], Ioanna Bouba [1], Konstantinos Dafopoulos [4] and Ioannis Georgiou [1,*]

1 Laboratory of Medical Genetics, Faculty of Medicine, School of Health Sciences, University of Ioannina, 45110 Ioannina, Greece; thaleia.moustakli@gmail.com (E.M.); ioannabouba@gmail.com (I.B.)
2 Obstetrics and Gynecology, Royal Devon and Exeter Hospital Barrack Rd, Exeter EX2 5DW, UK; thanzik92@gmail.com
3 Department of Obstetrics and Gynecology, Medical School of Ioannina, University General Hospital, 45110 Ioannina, Greece; haraskentou@gmail.com
4 IVF Unit, Department of Obstetrics and Gynecology, Faculty of Medicine, School of Health Sciences University of Thessaly, 41500 Larissa, Greece; kdafop@yahoo.gr
* Correspondence: igeorgio@uoi.gr

Abstract: Preimplantation genetic testing (PGT) has become a common supplementary diagnostic/testing tool for in vitro fertilization (IVF) cycles due to a significant increase in cases of PGT for monogenic conditions (PGT-M) and de novo aneuploidies (PGT-A) over the last ten years. This tendency is mostly attributable to the advancement and application of novel cytogenetic and molecular techniques in clinical practice that are capable of providing an efficient evaluation of the embryonic chromosomal complement and leading to better IVF/ICSI results. Although PGT is widely used, it requires invasive biopsy of the blastocyst, which may harm the embryo. Non-invasive approaches, like cell-free DNA (cfDNA) testing, have lower risks but have drawbacks in consistency and sensitivity. This review discusses new developments and opportunities in the field of preimplantation genetic testing, enhancing the overall effectiveness and accessibility of preimplantation testing in the framework of developments in genomic sequencing, bioinformatics, and the integration of artificial intelligence in the interpretation of genetic data.

Keywords: blastocoel fluid; blastocentesis; spent culture media; embryo biopsy; mosaicism; next-generation sequencing

1. Introduction

Preimplantation testing of embryos is an idea that was historically put forward and experimentally tested a few decades before the clinical application of preimplantation genetic testing (PGT) [1]. Although medically assisted reproduction and molecular methods had not evolved up to the standards needed for their clinical application at the time, biopsies were feasible in embryos from experimental animals [2]. The floor was set by the emergence of leading technologies such as FISH and PCR at almost the same time as IVF and, later, intracytoplasmic sperm injection (ICSI) [3]. The ability of both fluorescent in situ hybridization (FISH) and polymerase chain reaction (PCR) to highlight the genetic contents of single or several cells by hybridization and amplification, respectively, met the concept and the criteria for the revolutionary application of PGT.

Later technological advancements in chromosome arrays and deep sequencing shifted the appropriate timeline for embryo biopsy from polar bodies and day-3 blastomeres to the blastocyst stage [4]. Blastocysts became popular at the beginning of the millennium, and it was only a matter of time until blastocyst biopsy took the upper hand in biopsies, shortly after the year 2010 (according to ESHRE data). Several reasons supported the shift towards blastocyst biopsy [5]. The first was the emergence of sequential media, supporting efficient blastocyst culture with no need to replenish or recondition the medium throughout the culture period [6]. The second was the better selection of compatible embryos for biopsy and the number of trophectoderm cells excised for better and deeper analysis [7]. The third was the advent of multiple parallel sequencing and its potential to extend future applications in chromosome sequences, aneuploidies, and structural variations using the same robust technology for all genetic abnormalities [8]. Consequently, in theory, irrespective of the initial indication for PGT—either monogenic disorders (PGT-M) or structural rearrangements (PGT-SR)—next-generation sequencing (NGS) would result in a diagnostic yield that also covered partial- or whole-chromosome aneuploidies (PGT-A), and vice versa (Figure 1) [9].

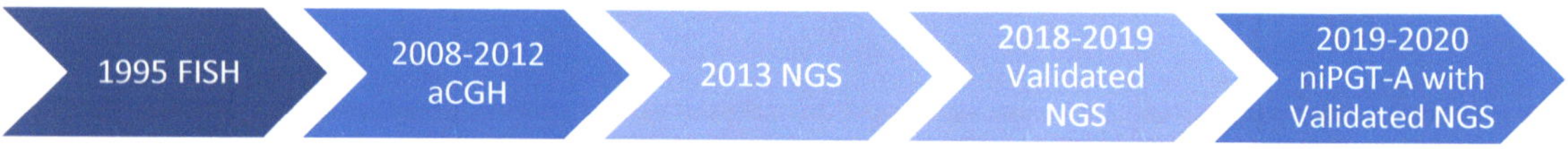
1995 FISH
2008-2012 aCGH
2013 NGS
2018-2019 Validated NGS
2019-2020 niPGT-A with Validated NGS

Figure 1. The schematic progression of PGT-A toward non-invasive and minimally invasive methods is depicted in the diagram below.

2. Schematic Evolution of PGT-A towards the Minimally Invasive and Non-Invasive Approaches

The ultimate goal of PGT-A, in particular, was to increase the implantation rate and the live birth rate, reduce the time of pregnancy, decrease pregnancy losses, and precisely diagnose harmful mosaicisms [10]. Although randomized controlled trials (RCTs) and other studies have been conducted to validate the high expectations related to PGT-A, the results were either inconclusive, weak, or negative (Table 1) [11].

Table 1. The invasive and non-invasive methods that have been and/or are currently being utilized to assess PGT.

Invasive PGT		
FISH	**aCGH**	**NGS**
• By measuring the copy number of the particular loci, target-specific DNA probes tagged with various fluorochromes or haptens can be used to identify chromosome imbalances linked to meiotic segregation of chromosome rearrangements. • Sporadic chromosomal aneuploidy screening in an effort to increase assisted reproduction's effectiveness. • In most cases, predictive value remains low, and routine clinical use in not advised.	• Comprehensive examination of an individual's genome to detect any genetic material gains or losses. • Determine whether certain tiny chromosomal regions are duplicated or absent. • Green: DNA problem Red: DNA control • A DNA "chip" that has a collection of DNA molecules covering the entire human genome is hybridized with a mixture of two fluorescent markers. • A scanner examines the hybridization result. Normal DNA content → yellow Green: chromosomal region in excess Red: chromosomal region in defect	• Parallel genome sequencing. • Facilitates the detection and screening of embryos with chromosomal mosaicism, euploidy, and aneuploidy. • NGS-based PGT enhances the success of IVF pregnancy outcomes. • Involvement of cleavage-stage biopsies, the transfer of new embryos, and the rate of implantation for recurrent implantation failure (RIF). • NGS provide a useful addition to the existing methods for screening for aneuploidy.

Table 1. *Cont.*

Minimally invasive PGT	Non-invasive PGT
Blastocoel fluid (BF)	**Spent Culture Media (SCM)**
• Blastocentesis → a minimally invasive procedure. • A puncture of the blastocoelic cavity with an ICSI needle is required to aspirate the fluid during this technique. • The fluid includes embryonic cells and cfDNA. NGS or PCR genetic study of fluid to detect any chromosomal abnormalities. • Compared to embryos with chromosomal defects, euploid embryos have a higher chance of implantation and a lower risk of miscarriage, which is why genetic analysis indicates that euploid embryos are chosen for embryo transfer.	• Embryos cultivated in a particular medium that offers the environment and nutrients required for development. Molecules such as cfDNA, RNA, and metabolites are released into the culture media as the cells grow. • Following around five to six days of embryo cultivation, a small sample is taken from every embryo. • The cfDNA and RNA contained in the medium can be examined by NGS, PCR, or microarray analysis. • During IVF cycles, embryos that are euploid and have appropriate metabolic profiles are chosen for transfer to the uterus. • The validity of the results may be questioned due to bias in the ploidy comparison and determination process.

3. Standard Sources of Preimplantation Embryo Genetic Information

Polar body (PB) biopsy was introduced as an approach to preimplantation testing with minimal risk of embryo damage, as its most prominent positive feature [12]. In addition, PB biopsy is applicable in countries with strict legislation against day-three biopsy or biopsy after syngamy. Nevertheless, the major drawback of this type of biopsy is the need for primary and secondary PBs; it is also relatively labor-intensive, only maternal chromosomes are examined, and it is not applicable in cases of abnormal paternal genetic contribution [13].

There are advantages and disadvantages to day-three preimplantation embryo biopsy as well [14]. The most positive aspects are that genetic information from both parents and the embryo is present, it can be performed with 6–10 cells, and blastomeres at this stage are assumed to be totipotent, representing the whole embryo, before differentiating to trophectoderm and inner cell mass [15]. This type of biopsy was the prevalent biopsy method for almost two decades (1990–2010), in conjunction with FISH for aneuploidies and structural variations, and with PCR for monogenic disorders. Initially, two cells were biopsied, and later only one cell was biopsied, due to the observed and reported reduction in pregnancy rates, along with the measurable impact on the embryo [16].

The blastocyst biopsy of the trophectoderm was introduced in 2011 and has remained the method of choice since then [17]. The more cells available (5–10 cells), the lesser the impact on the embryo's inner cell mass, rendering this type of biopsy safe, reliable, and effective, with no effect on the reproductive potential [18–20]. Nevertheless, in recent years, considerations have emerged, as the cells originate from the trophectoderm only, meaning that the mosaic inner cell mass remains undiagnosed [21]. Furthermore, mosaicism in the trophectoderm generates uncertainty over the safety of mosaic embryo transfers [22]. Blastocyst culture conditions per se produce fewer embryos to test, and biopsy conditions and operators create variability between labs concerning the percentages of normal embryos. Other drawbacks in blastocyst biopsy are the additional costs to standard IVF-ICSI, the need for extensive training, and the discarding of potentially viable embryos [23].

4. Origin of Embryonic DNA

Finding the source of the DNA is crucial for evaluating the blastocoel fluid (BF) and spent culture medium (SCM) DNA and how closely they reflect the growing embryo [24]. Extraembryonic DNA is thought to be released in small amounts as a result of the embryo's cell death mechanisms. DNA fragmentation is linked to certain processes, such as necrosis and apoptosis. Apoptosis may play a part in controlling the number of cells in the body or eliminating the presence of cells that are genetically aberrant or potentially detrimental to development [25]. It consequently manifests in human blastocysts that are in good condition. Neighboring cells can phagocytose apoptotic cells or shed them into the peritoneal space or blastocoel cavity [26]. Extraembryonic DNA may yield more significant information about the lineage that will ultimately produce the fetus than traditional trophectoderm (TE) biopsies if apoptosis is mainly restricted to the inner cell mass (ICM). Bolton and colleagues (2016) used individual cell tracking in a chimeric preimplantation mouse model of mosaicism to find that aneuploid cells in the murine TE continue to proliferate abnormally, while those in the ICM undergo apoptosis to eliminate them [27].

According to Fabian et al. (2005), apoptotic cells can be ejected into the blastocoel cavity or perivitelline space, or they can be phagocytosed by nearby cells. When exposed and accessible internucleosomal linker DNA is cleaved by endonuclease, apoptosis occurs [28]. This results in oligomers and multiples that are approximately 180 bp in size [29]. According to Zhang et al. (2016), NGS analysis of pooled BF samples ($n = 3$) indicated two native populations of DNA fragments: the first spanning 160–220 bp in length, and the second spanning 300–400 bp [30]. These findings are consistent with the theory that extraembryonic DNA originates from apoptotic cells [31]. Many mammals have been reported to experience waves of apoptosis in their ICMs; however, levels of both ICM and TE lineages in human IVF embryos seem to be comparable (7–8% of cells) [32,33].

Comprehending the release of DNA from the BF and SCM as a result of normal or pathological events is crucial. Which embryos—those with poor viability and morphology, which may have higher rates of cell death—have more DNA available in the BF/SCM? Those with good morphology have numerous cells. Regarding the relationship between successful extraembryonic DNA retrieval and embryo quality, research to date has produced contradictory findings [34].

Although Zhang and colleagues found no correlation between the amount of BF-DNA and embryo quality, other teams have found that blastocyst morphology and whole-genome amplification (WGA) efficiency are positively correlated, and that fully expanded day-5 blastocysts are more likely than less-developed embryos to yield detectable extraembryonic DNA [24,35]. Apoptosis marker caspase-3 activity and BF-DNA content were found to be positively correlated with each other, as well as with embryo quality, according to Rule and colleagues [36]. On the other hand, a cohort of embryos with an aneuploid trophectoderm biopsy diagnosis (81% of 185 samples) had WGA rates (SurePlex, Illumina) that were significantly higher than those with a euploid diagnosis (45% of 71 samples) [35].

Furthermore, the group with unsuccessful BF amplification had higher clinical pregnancy rates (77% vs. 37%) when 53 paired embryos were used for IVF [37]. The authors conjectured that, in light of these findings, failed BF amplification could function as an extra selection factor to help prioritize embryos for transfer during in vitro fertilization. Moreover, it is possible that the embryo was harmed by the sampling processes, resulting in at least some of the DNA found in the blastocoel. When cells accidentally lyse during blastocentesis, their nuclear contents may leak into the BF and be aspirated [38]. This could happen if the TE layer is penetrated. Furthermore, it is not known whether extraembryonic DNA is always found outside of cells, or if it is occasionally found inside membrane-enclosed cells that are not part of the embryo [31].

Owing to the diameter of the ICSI pipette that is usually used to collect BF, it is not completely possible to avoid sampling of whole cells floating in the BF. According to studies conducted in 2015 and 2019 by Poli and by Battaglia and colleagues, respectively, the identification of proteins, extracellular vesicles, and micro-RNAs (miRNAs) in human BF suggests that the blastocoel may actively contribute to intercellular communication during embryo development and implantation [39,40]. Such extracellular vesicles might also include a fraction of extraembryonic DNA [41].

5. Alternative Sources of Preimplantation Embryo Genetic Materialla

The sources of genetic material competent for clinical preimplantation testing, apart from the TE, are mainly two extraembryonic sources: the BF, alternatively termed blastocoel cavity fluid (BCF), and the spent embryo culture medium (SCM), which both contain embryonic DNA and other nucleic acids with value for prognostic embryo testing [42]. BCF fills the blastocoelic cavity synchronously to the formation of the blastocyst and is therefore valuable to aspirate and use as a cell-free sample. BCF aspiration is a minimally invasive approach targeting a volume of almost 4 nL, without any kind of cell extraction or cell damage [36]. The aspiration of the BCF has been suggested and implemented as a preparative step for blastocyst freezing, with validated clinical results, and is therefore appropriate for the preservation of blastocysts following the aspiration step [43]. SCM testing is the epitome of the non-invasive approach, as it simply requires the collection of the remaining medium when the blastocyst is removed to a new culture medium droplet [44]. Nevertheless, the collection of the SCM requires a change of culture medium, even if it is not required by the process implemented when using one-step culture media. This may also require an additional culture day for the collection of a richer nucleic acid medium [45].

6. Recommendation of Trophectoderm Biopsy Replacement

What can now be tested by the invasive PGT on the biopsied trophectoderm (TE) cells is a broad spectrum of genetic information residing in the blastocyst, such as numeric (including ploidy) and structural chromosome constitution, mosaicism, copy number variations (CNVs), single-nucleotide variants (SNVs), methylation, DNA fingerprinting, contamination, and mRNAs and microRNAs (including piRNA, snoRNA, etc.) (ESHRE data, Dagan Wells JUNO Genetics).

The contemporary gold standard, with TE biopsy and 24-chromosome testing, has proven to be efficient and safe in several RCTs, to reduce chromosomally abnormal pregnancies, and also to reduce the time to pregnancy and the overall treatment costs, with no impact on the so-called cumulative live birth rate (CLBR). In addition, TE biopsy has proven high reliability when applying strict criteria for mosaicism stratification [46–51].

Nevertheless, TE biopsy has some characteristic features that the community acknowledges as limitations to the broad and uncompromised use of PGT [17]. First, the training in biopsy is time-consuming, and the practice itself is delicate and time-consuming, requiring dedicated and expensive equipment to perform. There is also a risk of embryo damage and stress, as well as high variability in the results between operators and laboratories [52]. As TE biopsy broadly depends on the chance to extract cells from the unaffected part of the embryo in case of mosaicism, the probability of wrongly diagnosing an embryo is high, and the risk of discarding a healthy embryo is also high due to the opposite chances [53].

7. Non-Invasive Methods for Embryo Assessment

In the fields of in vitro fertilization (IVF) and assisted reproductive technology (ART), non-invasive techniques for evaluating embryos are becoming more and more significant. These techniques aspire to offer important insights on the health and development potential of embryos by employing non-invasive techniques like embryo biopsy [54]. First of all, time-lapse imaging requires taking ongoing pictures of the growing embryos at consistent intervals, without interfering with the environment of their culture. Embryologists can employ this technique to evaluate the regularity and timing of cell divisions, as well as to observe important developmental milestones. Embryos with the best development patterns can be identified owing to this continuous monitoring [55].

Metabolomic profiling is an additional non-invasive technique for evaluating embryos. Specifically, this approach examines the metabolic waste products generated by developing embryos [56]. Researchers can learn more about an embryo's metabolic activities by examining the chemical composition of the culture media used to cultivate it. Variations in metabolite levels may provide information about the health and viability of embryos. Furthermore, morphokinetic analysis falls under the same category as this approach, which assesses the morphological traits and the kinetics of embryonic development [57].

8. Automated Assessment

Automated techniques can assess features like cell symmetry, blastomere size, and timing of cell divisions by analyzing images or footage of growing embryos. Embryo quality may be indicated by deviations from typical developmental patterns [58].

Time-lapse systems provide digital images of embryos at frequent intervals, allowing embryologists to assess their quality without removing them from their culture environment [59]. Embryos can be transferred to the uterus at the cleavage or blastocyst stages. The blastocyst stage may increase the likelihood of selectively transferring viable embryos [60]. Correct identification of cell numbers is significant in determining the timing parameters for embryo quality evaluation [61].

Though advances in cell detection and tracking have been made, topological alterations and image noise continue to pose significant challenges to computer vision research. In medical imaging applications, variables in pertinent data influence decision-making [58]. Artificial intelligence has not received much attention as a tool for assessing human embryo development quality. A crucial method for upcoming human support technology is deep learning. Convolutional neural networks (CNNs) have enormous promise for use in medical diagnostics, imaging, and overall healthcare [62]. Time-lapse photos have been used to analyze embryos objectively and automatically through the development of a technique called STORK [63]. An extremely encouraging outcome was that the method could predict blastocyst quality with an area under the curve (AUC) [63]. According to a recent study, individual time-lapse imaging for mouse and human embryos up to the four-cell stage can be classified using a framework based on Inception-V3 CNNs [64].

For the assessment of embryos, oxygen consumption and culture conditions are two additional non-invasive methods. Information regarding the metabolic activity of growing embryos can be obtained by tracking their rate of oxygen consumption. Understanding of the energy needs and general health of embryos can be gained by using this non-invasive technique [65]. Regarding embryo culture conditions, optimizing the culture environment in which embryos develop is a critical aspect of non-invasive assessment. Factors such as temperature, pH, and nutrient concentrations can impact embryo quality [66]. Maintaining optimal culture conditions is essential for supporting healthy embryo development. It is important to note that time-lapse imaging and carefully regulated culture conditions are combined in a technique known as an EmbryoScope [67].

9. Benefits of Minimally Invasive and Non-Invasive PGT

Despite TE biopsy being the gold standard, its safety and reliability have been called into question by the emergence of PGT in embryo assessment [9]. Still, as long as they adhere to the established protocols, non-invasive and minimally invasive techniques are seen as unique innovations because they are less costly and easier to perform [68]. One of the main advantages is that less invasive biopsy stress is applied to the embryos due to less embryo manipulation [69]. Minimal intervention may be advantageous for the fetus's growth and well-being. The TE biopsy procedure requires appropriate handling as well as appropriate training [52].

This approach is expensive for both the couple undergoing IVF and the facility [70]. Deviating TE biopsy with alternative approaches may also result in higher rates of pregnancy, a broader range of patients receiving treatment, and lower costs. However, the use of embryo biopsy for genetic testing raises many moral and ethical questions, and this is something that needs to be acknowledged. Their beliefs and ideals support avoiding this process [4]. Clinical misdiagnosis and confusion surrounding PGT-A will persist even in the presence of the most precise genetic analysis. This is because there is proof that the present biopsy procedures may be hazardous, and because of the discrepancy between TE and inner cell mass (ICM) [71]. Nevertheless, to apply new technology, attempts have been made to make it less intrusive and to create complex algorithms. Promising methods include measuring DNA in spent embryonic culture medium and blastocoel fluid, measuring mitochondrial DNA, metabolomics, measuring nutritional glucose intake, proteomics, and life-span microscopy [72].

When developing algorithms for the appropriate selection of embryos for transfer to humans in in vitro fertilization (IVF), for instance, the quick screening of glucose metabolism in the human embryo on day 4 and day 5 (morulae stage) may turn out to be beneficial [73]. The notion that male and female human embryos have different physiologies as a result of having two active X chromosomes and having a modified proteome for a limited period during preimplantation is further supported by the detected sex-related metabolic differences [74]. Hence, according to Gardner and colleagues, glucose consumption may be used as a marker to help identify competent embryos capable of supporting implantation, development, and live birth [73].

10. Blastocoel Fluid Aspiration

A typical human embryo develops into a fully developed blastocyst from 120 to 144 h after fertilization. The embryo typically has a fully formed blastocoel at this point, which is a cavity filled with fluid and enclosed in a layer of trophectoderm (TE) cells. The inner cell mass (ICM), a collection of cells connected to the inner side of the TE layer and expanding into the cavity, is in contact with the blastocoelic fluid, which we will refer to as blastosol in this instance [39].

The cavity known as a blastocoel, which has an average capacity of 4–6 nL, begins to form on day 4 and fully develops between days 5 and 6. The genetic material is amplified to a great degree of variety, as suggested by the variations in amplification rates [39]. Significant differences in the outcomes between PGT-A and blastocoel are also observed. A related concern that emerges and can be addressed is related to the variations in the genetic coherence between trophectoderm and blastocoel cells [11].

Embryonic proteins are discharged into the blastocoel, where they may accumulate. According to the study conducted by Watson and colleagues, there is strict regulation over the movement of molecules into and out of the enclosed blastocoel fluid [75]. The surrounding monolayer of TE cells forms a solid barrier separating the blastocoel from the external environment through tight connections. Due to the absence of impurities from the culture medium, the blastocoel can offer an extremely pure sample of embryo secretions. To acquire blastosol samples from viable embryos, a micromanipulation technique known as blastocentesis was developed. Embryonic DNA was collected using this methodology for preimplantation genetic screening before invasive biopsy techniques were developed (Figure 2) [76–78].

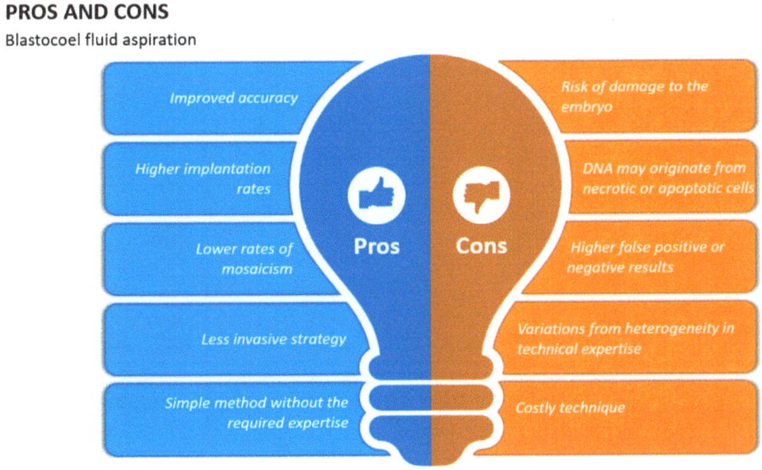

Figure 2. The benefits and drawbacks of blastocoel fluid aspiration.

11. Spent Embryo Culture Medium (SCM)

Research has concentrated on metabolites, proteins, interleukins, and microRNAs, and it has been investigated whether measuring specific chemicals produced could be useful in predicting the reproductive competence of embryos [79]. The wide range of substances that embryos leak into the medium—known as the secretome—have been the subject of multiple studies over the last ten years. Assessing the spent culture medium (SCM) of the embryo presents a viable substitute for the non-invasive genetic evaluation of preimplantation embryos.

Examining genetic information, it appears that SCM may occasionally contain more DNA than the blastocoel fluid (BF). In contrast to blastocentesis, which still involves some degree of embryo manipulation, this implies that SCM could provide a source of material for a completely non-invasive genetic testing technique [38]. There have been reports of the discovery of mitochondrial DNA (mtDNA) and genomic DNA (gDNA) in SCM as early as days 2–3 of development [80]. The amount of DNA has been seen to rise during embryo culture, indicating that a significant portion of the genetic material found in SCM has an embryonic origin, even though various media formulations may contain DNA contaminants, which is a reason for concern when thinking about genetic testing [81].

Nucleic acids are expected to be able to move from the preimplantation embryo into the medium with little resistance because, despite the zona pellucida protective glycoprotein barrier surrounding it, it has a high degree of flexibility, even the relatively large macromolecules [82]. Nevertheless, it is still unknown what processes lead to the release of embryonic DNA. The gDNA in the SCM is most likely extremely low in quantity, degraded, and/or the product of cell death processes, similar to the blastocoel, according to a comparison of the observed PCR amplification rates from SCM with those from cellular biopsies [69].

Even though apoptosis and the resulting DNA release seem to be typical aspects of blastocyst development, other mechanisms might be required to account for the embryonic DNA found in SCM at earlier stages. According to studies, cell death that occurs before compaction is related to fragmentation and embryo arrest, and healthy, normally developing human embryos do not exhibit any signs of apoptosis before the blastocyst stage [83,84]. Consequently, Stigliani and colleagues set out to examine the role of gDNA and mtDNA in day-3 SCM as a biomarker of embryo quality. It is interesting to note that, when comparing SCM samples from poor-to-average morphological grades to samples from high-quality embryos, the amounts of total double-stranded DNA (dsDNA) were higher. Furthermore, the dsDNA was primarily of mitochondrial origin, according to further qPCR for single-copy nuclear and mitochondrial genes. The number of copies of mtDNA in the medium was also significantly correlated with increasing maternal age and the degree of embryonic fragmentation [85].

Based on these findings, it was believed that nuclear–cytoplasmic fragments, not apoptotic bodies, were the primary source of DNA in the SCM. Since a single-copy nuclear gene was employed for normalization, which is not ideal for quantifying mtDNA in samples with very low DNA concentrations (especially if the DNA is degraded), care must be taken when interpreting this data. In the study conducted by Hammond and colleagues, it was noted that cleavage-stage embryos with low or no fragmentation in the SCM included mtDNA and gDNA, after using single- and multi-copy gene quantitative PCR (qPCR) markers [86].

In addition, Stigliani's group subsequently demonstrated that implantation results, trophectoderm quality, and subsequent blastulation rates were all favorably correlated with the mtDNA-to-gDNA ratio in day-3 SCM [85]. There is yet no confirmation of the degree to which the relative ratio of gDNA or mtDNA, or their total levels in the SCM, signal embryo viability. Certain results are in line with those of blastocoel. Initially, a significant fluctuation in the nucleic acid DNA content amplification rate is noted. Furthermore, there are differences in consistency between PGT-A and SCM. Overall, compared to blastocentesis, the outcomes of SCM were generally more in line with those of invasive biopsies [11].

Before being used in clinical practice, SCM presents with extra difficulties. Such obstacles include significant variances in analytical techniques, as well as sample contamination. The outcomes, however, are encouraging when certain changes are made to the existing techniques for embryo culture [87]. First, a modification should be made the day after the culture medium; that is, on day 4, when sequential media are utilized and appropriate for the SCM procedure to be applied, rather than on day 3 [88]. Additionally, it is advised to reduce the volume of the embryo culture medium, with a value range of 5 to 30 milliliters, since smaller volumes may be handled and processed more easily and do not require further procedures. Furthermore, blastocysts that are fully grown by day 5 can be obtained by prolonging the culture period to day 6 or even 7 [89]. Finally, the advent of single-stage media that can maintain embryo development throughout the blastocyst stage may mean that numerous changes to the culture media are not required (Figure 3) [23].

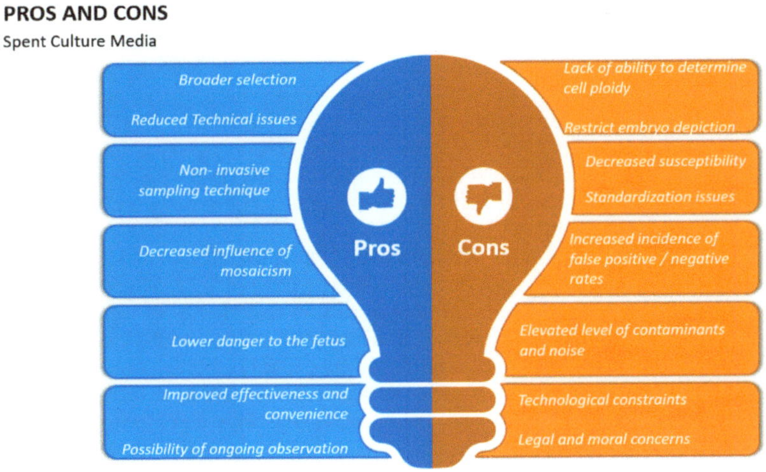

Figure 3. Advantages and disadvantages of spent culture media (SCM) concerning non-invasive PGT.

12. Diagnostic Performance of Blastocyst Culture Media in Non-Invasive PGT

Employing trophectoderm (TE) biopsy in conjunction with preimplantation genetic testing (PGT) has proven beneficial for millions of couples in conceiving healthy offspring by identifying embryos that have chromosomal and/or genetic abnormalities [90]. Nonetheless, numerous issues persist concerning the precision of diagnosis and the security of this method. A five-to-ten TE cell biopsy still cannot be considered a perfect reflection of the inner cell mass (ICM)'s true chromosomal state. Furthermore, chromosomal mosaicism in blastocyst-stage embryos may impair the diagnostic precision of a single TE biopsy [91,92]. A single sample containing two or more cell lines with distinct genotypes is known as chromosomal mosaicism [93].

In human preimplantation embryos, this has been widely detected, in contrast to later placental samples. Currently, several studies have shown that the rising number of chromosomal mosaicism reports may be associated with the greater sensitivity of the TE biopsy itself [50,93,94], as well as with the NGS platform [94,95]. A healthy live birth could nonetheless occur from the transfer of embryos identified as "abnormal" by TE biopsy in PGT for aneuploidy (PGT-A), indicating the limitations of TE biopsy's diagnostic accuracy [46]. Furthermore, there is always a chance that the viability of embryos will be compromised by invasive biopsy procedures [5,96]. In this case, investigations are being carried out to confirm whether utilizing cell-free DNA (cfDNA) for non-invasive preimplantation genetic testing for aneuploidy (niPGT-A) could be promoted as a viable method for aneuploidy screening.

A new era of possibilities for niPGT-A was opened by Palini and colleagues, who successfully amplified cell-free DNA samples in blastocoel fluid (BF) to identify embryos with X-linked illness [97]. It was subsequently discovered that the extracellular cfDNA in discarded culture media included a greater amount of genetic material related to medicine than that in BF [98]. Even though the use of cfDNA in niPGT has been encouraged, its initial source and makeup remain unknown; it may have been contaminated with a combination of maternal cells and embryonic DNA [99]. Furthermore, there is ongoing debate regarding the consistency of ICM and cfDNA from BF or spent culture media [69,100–102].

Previous studies were conducted to compare the diagnostic efficacy of niPGT-A and TE biopsy, or to assess the concordance between niPGT-A and TE biopsy PGT-A, using the remaining portion of the embryo or the entire embryo as the standard reference [46,100,103–105]. Nonetheless, a growing body of research has shown that mosaicism may cause the TE biopsy results and the remainder of the embryo mixed with ICM and TE to inaccurately represent the genetic state of the blastocyst-stage embryo [46,106–108].

Comparing BCM with many embryonic biopsy sites, especially the ICM samples, would be a more cautious and advisable method to confirm the diagnostic efficacy of niPGT-A [109]. The diagnostic effectiveness of niPGT-A has never been thoroughly assessed before, as far as we are aware. It compares the concordance of ICM, BCM, and TE (i.e., initial TE and TE re-biopsy) samples. Chen et al.'s study revealed that three partially "mosaic" embryos identified by initial TE biopsies were euploid upon analyzing TE re-biopsies, BCM, and ICM samples. This implies that TE biopsy might not be a trustworthy marker of ICM's true chromosomal condition.

The self-correcting process in mosaic embryos [110], which allows mosaic cells in the cleavage-stage embryo to be incorporated into TE cells but not ICM cells, may help to explain this. The actual manipulation of the biopsy could be another reason. According to reports, laser biopsy manipulation can cause mosaicism, cell injury, and the loss of cellular DNA [93]. This can therefore cause bias in the development of libraries. Furthermore, higher-resolution NGS-based PGT-A shows improved sensitivity to detect lower-level mosaicism [111,112], in contrast to earlier technologies like array comparative genomic hybridization (aCGH) [113].

An additional issue in diagnosing lower-level mosaicism arises from the fact that euploid/aneuploid mosaic embryos are regarded as abnormal in between euploid and abnormal embryos. Carefully determining the threshold for mosaicism is necessary to classify the embryos as euploid, aneuploid, or mosaic. According to the Preimplantation Genetic Diagnosis International Society [93], the mosaic spectrum runs from 20% (much-reduced risk) to 80% (greater risk), and this information should be taken into account and reported. Various laboratories may have different cutoff values for reporting mosaic levels because of varying degrees of ability to detect mosaicism. This could potentially impact the precision of TE biopsies and wasted BCM.

Based on NGS results, Maxwell and colleagues found that 31.6% of the embryos that were miscarried but had previously been identified as euploid were found to be mosaic using the 20% to 80% mosaic criterion [111]. A different study showed that similar pregnancy outcomes to euploid embryos were associated with mosaic embryos that had fewer defective cells (<50%) [114]. In their PGT laboratory, the lower cutoff value for mosaic was 40%, while the upper value was 70%, to reduce the false positive rate (FPR) and false negative rate (FNR). Three "mosaic" embryos in Chen and colleagues' investigation had mosaicism values of 40% (monosomy 5), 30% (monosomy X, trisomy 18 and 21), and 50% (monosomy X). However, the uniform cupidity of the samples from the TE re-biopsies, ICM, and BCM shown by the test findings suggested that the mosaics in the first TE biopsies were related to false positives rather than the incorrect threshold for mosaicism.

It should be highlighted that embryos with the first TE biopsy diagnosed with chromosomal mosaicism are often discarded. Nonetheless, it has been demonstrated that PGT-A embryos transferred with TE biopsy diagnoses of "aneuploidy" might nevertheless produce live, healthy children, demonstrating the limitations of TE biopsy's diagnostic precision [106,113,115,116]. Alternatively, BCM sampling, being a non-invasive procedure, may reduce the bias previously described, making it more dependable for predicting the ICM karyotypes, and potentially preventing the loss of normal embryos [106,113,115].

Furthermore, niPGT-A with a BCM sample may attain diagnostic efficacy comparable to that of TE biopsy, and in the three aforementioned partial "mosaic" cases it proved to be congruent with the ICM findings. Additionally, niPGT-A with BCM in conjunction with an initial TE biopsy could result in a more promising diagnostic accuracy. For instance, the highest priority for transfer is given to embryos that show the same euploid results from both the TE biopsy and niPGT-A [90]. Similarly, the lowest priority for transfer is given to embryos that show euploid results from niPGT-A and mosaic results from the first TE biopsy, rather than them being disposed of directly. More research is required on the combination of TE biopsy and niPGT-A, and in clinical applications the test costs should be taken into account.

The clinical applicability of niPGT-A is contingent upon its efficacy in amplifying sufficient cfDNA, in addition to its diagnostic capabilities. Both TE and ICM may theoretically leak cfDNA into the culture material, but TE comes into direct contact with the medium, while ICM does not [109]. Through artificial blastocyst collapse by laser, cfDNA was released from BF into the spent BCM, increasing the concentration of cfDNA with the least amount of damage. The 26 donated embryos used in this investigation all produced effective DNA amplification, which was higher than the efficiency shown in other studies [69,97,117]. Furthermore, it is reasonable to assume that this manipulation, when used in sample collection in niPGT, may not cause much damage to the embryos, since it artificially collapses the blastocoel cavity in enlarged blastocysts, which may enhance the vitrification result [69,97,117,118].

13. Diagnostic Performance of BF and SCM as PGT DNA Sources in Clinical Settings

The genotypes of the embryos produced during PGT-M cycles were compared among the various specimens in the first section of this investigation. The spent culture medium collected from the blastocyst-stage (SBM) samples yielded a considerably higher diagnosis rate than the BF samples, albeit inferior to that of the TE samples. Even though SBM can be diagnosed, 10.1% of the loci studied had a high detection of artifacts or allele drop-in (ADI). The inclusion of foreign DNA in the culture media is one of the possible causes of this noteworthy rate of detectable nonembryonic DNA material [24]. Indeed, many brands of new, unused media have been observed to contain trace levels of DNA [86,99]. The most likely way that these contaminants are added to the media is by adding non-pure DNA-binding proteins, including albumin. PCR is a useful tool for detecting this kind of DNA contamination in culture media samples, even though it is rare and potentially innocuous during traditional IVF procedures.

Interestingly, in both the BF and SBM groups, the allele dropout (ADO) rates for paternal alleles were statistically considerably greater than those for maternal ones. This initial finding indicated that mother DNA was more represented in DNA than paternal DNA [24]. Accordingly, it is likely that genetic material from the polar bodies or cumulus complex is still present in the culture system and is retrieved using embryonic DNA for analysis. Further support for this notion came from the discovery of the mutant allele of maternal origin in the SBM samples, even if the corresponding TE was homozygous for the wild-type gene. These findings offered strong proof of the significant amount of maternal DNA present in SBM samples (Table 2) [24].

While some recent research has recommended the clinical use of SBM for aneuploidy testing [105,119] or PGT-M [120], these findings show that more research is necessary before this diagnostic strategy can be taken into consideration in clinical settings. To increase the proportion of embryonic DNA and stop nonembryonic DNA carryover, different approaches could be used. We suggest pretreatment DNA depletion in culture media, total oocyte elimination, and temporal standardization (with regard to blastocyst growth) for BF and SBM collection, among other things. A modified variation of Chan et al.'s second-generation non-invasive fetal DNA analysis could be used to amplify embryo-specific DNA [30]. A different, efficient method of obtaining embryonic DNA for genetic testing selectively could be the isolation and focused examination of exosomes released by the blastocyst in the culture medium [121].

Table 2. An overview of the main findings concerning the systematic reviews of non-invasive PGT-A.

Cell-Free DNA SCM	Cell-Free DNA BF
The ploidy of the embryo was unaffected by cfDNA.	Cells separate into TE and ICM on the 4th day of blastocyst development. Blastocoel forms withing the blastocyst during cavitation.
An estimated 86–94% of instances involve contamination with maternal genetic material.	Through blastocentesis → BF aspirated. About 0.01 μL of BF can be isolated.
The seed embryo's embryonic DNA content ranged from 0% to 100%. Not every embryo's embryonic genome may be evenly represented in the seed embryo.	Only 34.8% of BF samples were able to produce a signal suitable for embryo karyotyping. This outcome might have been caused by the fact that fresh blastocysts were used for the blastocentesis.

According to the PGT-A data from the study by Capalbo and colleagues, only 34.8% of the BF samples were able to produce a signal suitable for embryo karyotyping [24]. Before the embryos were cryopreserved or had a biopsy (under experimental circumstances), BFs were obtained in sizable investigations of the usage of BF for PGT. On the other hand, their study replicated a real PGT cycle therapy (under clinical circumstances) by collecting blastocoel samples from fresh, untreated blastocysts [24]. When compared to the results that we obtained under clinical conditions, the amplification rates under experimental conditions were higher (62%, 82%, and 96%) [35,102]. Perhaps increased DNA availability in the cavity as a result of cell lysis induced by cryopreservation or micromanipulation led to the higher DNA amplification rates seen in these investigations [122].

According to published data from Tobler's and Werner's groups, only a small percentage (37.5%) of the amplified samples in our dataset produced results consistent with those obtained from TE biopsies (53% and 72% of amplified samples matched the initial embryo diagnosis, respectively) [102,123]. Only a small percentage of the incongruous instances identified can be associated with the application of various methods for aneuploidy evaluation, as qPCR and VeriSeq PGT-A techniques generated concordant results for uniform aneuploidies when examined on cell line specimens. It is extremely difficult to identify the biological basis of such discordances, because functional research on the biological mechanisms of embryonic DNA release in the extracellular environment is inadequate [24]. Membrane-encapsulated DNA may come from DNA-containing pieces from apoptotic cells, from selective degeneration of aberrant cells in mosaic diploid/aneuploid embryos, or from improper (or corrected) chromosome segregation mechanisms during cell division [102].

The analytical sample may be seriously contaminated by this kind of non-representative DNA, seriously endangering the diagnostic sample's accuracy [124]. However, at this time, there is not enough evidence to confirm that human preimplantation embryos have aneuploidy correction mechanisms. Enigmatically, fluidic samples may prove to be even more accurate in forecasting the genetic makeup of the blastocyst than TE biopsies if all embryonic cells release their DNA uniformly [38].

Through the comparison of vitrified and/or warmed embryos and culture media ploidy results, Xu and colleagues stated that a detailed examination of non-invasive chromosomal screening (NICS) revealed that the test was confirmed under experimental settings [105]. Of the 42 pairings of samples, 38 showed diagnostic consistency at the embryo stage, while only 62% of the samples had full karyotype concordance. Additionally, by withholding genotyping data, the investigators were unable to determine whether nonembryonic DNA contamination was present in the samples, or where they originated. Moreover, given the absence of a control group in the research, the six live births that seven couples who underwent NICS-based embryo selection were able to achieve did not constitute sufficient proof to back up the therapeutic efficacy of the NICS intervention [105].

14. Mosaicism

The existence of multiple genotypically different cell populations within a single zygote is known as mosaicism. It is believed that, during post-zygotic cell division, mosaic cellular populations result from post-zygotic mitotic mistakes [125]. Mosaicism in PGT-A is characterized by a 20% to 80% mixture of euploid and aneuploid DNA; euploid DNA is found in less than 20% of the sample, while aneuploid DNA is found in more than 80% of the sample. Although 5% is the stated incidence of mosaic embryos, some researchers have used PGT-A to find rates as high as 20% to 30%. Embryos in the cleavage stage (30–70%) are more likely to exhibit mosaicism than those in the blastocyst stage (5–15%) [72].

Depending on the timing of mitotic mistakes in the blastocyst stage, and on the cell lineage, there are four types of mosaicism: A "total mosaic" embryo has both euploid and aneuploid cells in both the TE and the inner cell mass (ICM). The embryo is classified as "ICM mosaic" if the mosaic population is solely ICM, and as "TE mosaic" if it is purely TE. Finally, an embryo is considered to be "ICM/TE mosaic" if every cell in the ICM is euploid and every cell in the TE is aneuploid, or vice versa [126].

Euploidization in mosaic embryos may cause DNA to be liberated from aneuploid cells, increasing the likelihood of a false positive aneuploidy diagnosis. As euploid cells remain in the ICM, the DNA expelled into the BF would be aneuploid. According to several studies, it is known that certain mosaic embryos can implant and produce euploid offspring, indicating the possibility of mechanisms for the removal of defective cells [113,116,127].

Aneuploidy and chromosomal mosaicism are known to result from aberrant cell division in embryos. A study based on the theory that euploid and aneuploid cells would not contribute equally to the DNA contained in the culture media revealed that such embryos could occasionally deliver healthy blastocysts [128]. Despite the euploid nature of the biopsies taken from these developing embryos, it was shown that the excluded cells in these chromosomally normal blastocysts were aneuploid, and that compaction often resulted in the exclusion of some cells. If apoptosis or other mechanisms of cell death or exclusion can be used to repair mosaic embryos, more studies on human embryos are required to validate this conclusion. Based on published research with limited data on extraembryonic DNA, BF and SCM samples may have more aneuploid events than paired TE biopsies [35,129]. If confirmed, this would cast doubt on the idea underlying the PGT-A study of extraembryonic DNA or shed light on the fraction of aneuploidies undiagnosed by PGT-A.

Mosaic human embryos refer to embryos that have a mixture of normal and abnormal cells, often due to genetic mutations or chromosomal abnormalities. These embryos can result from errors in cell division during early embryonic development. The concept of mosaic embryos has significant implications in the field of reproductive medicine and assisted reproductive technology, particularly in the context of in vitro fertilization (IVF) and preimplantation genetic testing (PGT) (Figure 4) [130].

In preimplantation diagnostic research, the detection of mosaicism carries significant implications for genetic counseling. During oogenesis, as opposed to spermatogenesis, nondisjunction is more frequent. In cases where the offspring has a non-mosaic trisomy for a particular chromosome, gonadal mosaicism should be considered, as the recurring risk of mosaicism is unclear. The presence of germline mosaicism provides a basic explanation for the recurrence of uncommon mutations within a single family, and it may aid in the familial aggregation of affected people. Genetic counseling is dependent on the type of mosaicism, as each chromosome that is afflicted presents with unique clinical signs [125].

In monosomies, mosaicism has an impact on survival rates. While monosomies in humans are lethal, mosaic monosomies, which occur when more than 70% of cells are normal and the remaining monosomes persist, may not result in death after delivery.

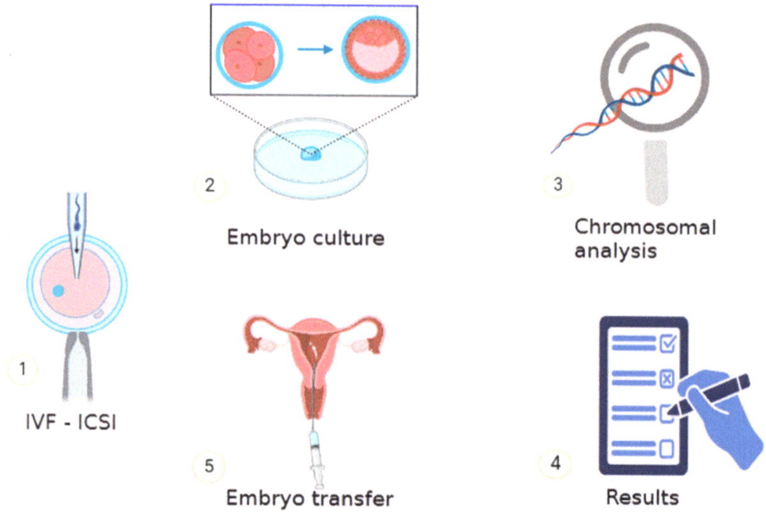

Figure 4. The chromosomal composition of the embryo can be ascertained without an embryo biopsy through non-invasive preimplantation genetic testing, or niPGT-A.

Malignant conditions are caused by mosaicism. As people age, there is a noticeable, gradual loss of certain human genes, which causes tissue to become mosaic. Malignant tissue (such as neurofibromatosis) may also develop from the mosaic tissue.

15. Conclusions

In clinical practice, niPGT may lower expenditures per couple and increase the number of couples seeking PGT if it is validated and successfully applied. Furthermore, it might result in important developments for IVF/ICSI procedures in the future. In the first instance, it will enable and facilitate genetic analysis in embryos that, according to existing standards, are not appropriate for biopsy. Furthermore, because of technological advancements, this procedure can be used without running the risk of harming the fetus. In terms of where the genetic material derives from, it seems that blastocoel fluid aspiration (blastocentesis) is not as efficient a source of cfDNA as SCM (spent culture medium). Undoubtedly, investigations that significantly deviate from mainstream embryological procedures seem to obtain the best niPGT results.

Author Contributions: Conceptualization, I.G. and E.M.; methodology, E.M.; validation, I.G. and I.B.; resources, A.Z., K.D. and C.S.; data curation, E.M.; writing—original draft preparation, E.M.; writing—review and editing, I.B.; visualization, I.G.; supervision, I.G. All authors have read and agreed to the published version of the manuscript.

Funding: This research received no external funding.

Institutional Review Board Statement: Not applicable.

Informed Consent Statement: Not applicable.

Data Availability Statement: Data are unavailable due to privacy or ethical restrictions.

Conflicts of Interest: The authors declare no conflicts of interest.

References

1. Edwards, R.G.; Gardner, R.L. Sexing of Live Rabbit Blastocysts. *Nature* **1967**, *214*, 576–577. [CrossRef]
2. Chen, H.; Zhang, L.; Meng, L.; Liang, L.; Zhang, C. Advantages of vitrification preservation in assisted reproduction and potential influences on imprinted genes. *Clin. Epigenet.* **2022**, *14*, 141. [CrossRef]
3. Wang, J.; Sauer, M.V. In vitro fertilization (IVF): A review of 3 decades of clinical innovation and technological advancement. *Ther. Clin. Risk Manag.* **2006**, *2*, 355–364. [CrossRef]
4. Takeuchi, K. Pre-implantation genetic testing: Past, present, future. *Reprod. Med. Biol.* **2021**, *20*, 27–40. [CrossRef]
5. Bar-El, L.; Kalma, Y.; Malcov, M.; Schwartz, T.; Raviv, S.; Cohen, T.; Amir, H.; Cohen, Y.; Reches, A.; Amit, A.; et al. Blastomere biopsy for PGD delays embryo compaction and blastulation: A time-lapse microscopic analysis. *J. Assist. Reprod. Genet.* **2016**, *33*, 1449–1457. [CrossRef]
6. Chronopoulou, E.; Harper, J.C. IVF culture media: Past, present and future. *Hum. Reprod. Update* **2015**, *21*, 39–55. [CrossRef]
7. Lal, A.; Roudebush, W.E.; Chosed, R.J. Embryo Biopsy Can Offer More Information Than Just Ploidy Status. *Front. Cell Dev. Biol.* **2020**, *8*, 78. [CrossRef]
8. Koboldt, D.C.; Steinberg, K.M.; Larson, D.E.; Wilson, R.K.; Mardis, E.R. The Next-Generation Sequencing Revolution and Its Impact on Genomics. *Cell* **2013**, *155*, 27–38. [CrossRef]
9. De Rycke, M.; Berckmoes, V. Preimplantation Genetic Testing for Monogenic Disorders. *Genes* **2020**, *11*, 871. [CrossRef] [PubMed]
10. Murtinger, M.; Schuff, M.; Wirleitner, B.; Miglar, S.; Spitzer, D. Comment on the recent PGDIS Position Statement on the Transfer of Mosaic Embryos 2021. *J. Assist. Reprod. Genet.* **2022**, *39*, 2563–2570. [CrossRef] [PubMed]
11. Viotti, M. Preimplantation Genetic Testing for Chromosomal Abnormalities: Aneuploidy, Mosaicism, and Structural Rearrangements. *Genes* **2020**, *11*, 602. [CrossRef] [PubMed]
12. Montag, M.; Van Der Ven, K.; Rösing, B.; Van Der Ven, H. Polar body biopsy: A viable alternative to preimplantation genetic diagnosis and screening. *Reprod. Biomed. Online* **2009**, *18*, 6–11. [CrossRef]
13. Schenk, M.; Groselj-Strele, A.; Eberhard, K.; Feldmeier, E.; Kastelic, D.; Cerk, S.; Weiss, G. Impact of polar body biopsy on embryo morphokinetics—Back to the roots in preimplantation genetic testing? *J. Assist. Reprod. Genet.* **2018**, *35*, 1521–1528. [CrossRef] [PubMed]
14. Wang, A.Y.; Sullivan, E.A.; Li, Z.; Farquhar, C. Day 5 versus day 3 embryo biopsy for preimplantation genetic testing for monogenic/single gene defects. *Cochrane Database Syst. Rev.* **2018**, *2018*, CD013233. [CrossRef]
15. Toyooka, Y. Trophoblast lineage specification in the mammalian preimplantation embryo. *Reprod. Med. Biol.* **2020**, *19*, 209–221. [CrossRef] [PubMed]
16. Burks, C.; Van Heertum, K.; Weinerman, R. The Technological Advances in Embryo Selection and Genetic Testing: A Look Back at the Evolution of Aneuploidy Screening and the Prospects of Non-Invasive PGT. *Reprod. Med.* **2021**, *2*, 26–34. [CrossRef]
17. Aoyama, N.; Kato, K. Trophectoderm biopsy for preimplantation genetic test and technical tips: A review. *Reprod. Med. Biol.* **2020**, *19*, 222–231. [CrossRef]
18. Scott, R.T.; Upham, K.M.; Forman, E.J.; Zhao, T.; Treff, N.R. Cleavage-stage biopsy significantly impairs human embryonic implantation potential while blastocyst biopsy does not: A randomized and paired clinical trial. *Fertil. Steril.* **2013**, *100*, 624–630. [CrossRef]
19. Forman, E.J.; Hong, K.H.; Ferry, K.M.; Tao, X.; Taylor, D.; Levy, B.; Treff, N.R.; Scott, R.T. In vitro fertilization with single euploid blastocyst transfer: A randomized controlled trial. *Fertil. Steril.* **2013**, *100*, 100–107.e1. [CrossRef]
20. Sunkara, S.K.; LaMarca, A.; Polyzos, N.P.; Seed, P.T.; Khalaf, Y. Live birth and perinatal outcomes following stimulated and unstimulated IVF: Analysis of over two decades of a nationwide data. *Hum. Reprod.* **2016**, *31*, 2261–2267. [CrossRef]
21. Capalbo, A.; Rienzi, L. Mosaicism between trophectoderm and inner cell mass. *Fertil. Steril.* **2017**, *107*, 1098–1106. [CrossRef]
22. Lee, C.I.; Cheng, E.H.; Lee, M.S.; Lin, P.Y.; Chen, Y.C.; Chen, C.H.; Huang, L.-S.; Huang, C.-C.; Lee, T.-H. Healthy live births from transfer of low-mosaicism embryos after preimplantation genetic testing for aneuploidy. *J. Assist. Reprod. Genet.* **2020**, *37*, 2305–2313. [CrossRef]
23. Deng, J.; Zhao, Q.; Cinnioglu, C.; Kayali, R.; Lathi, R.B.; Behr, B. The impact of culture conditions on blastocyst formation and aneuploidy rates: A comparison between single-step and sequential media in a large academic practice. *J. Assist. Reprod. Genet.* **2020**, *37*, 161–169. [CrossRef]
24. Capalbo, A.; Romanelli, V.; Patassini, C.; Poli, M.; Girardi, L.; Giancani, A.; Stoppa, M.; Cimadomo, D.; Ubaldi, F.M.; Rienzi, L. Diagnostic efficacy of blastocoel fluid and spent media as sources of DNA for preimplantation genetic testing in standard clinical conditions. *Fertil. Steril.* **2018**, *110*, 870–879.e5. [CrossRef]
25. Fulda, S.; Gorman, A.M.; Hori, O.; Samali, A. Cellular Stress Responses: Cell Survival and Cell Death. *Int. J. Cell Biol.* **2010**, *2010*, 214074. [CrossRef]
26. Pisko, J.; Špirková, A.; Čikoš, Š.; Olexiková, L.; Kovaříková, V.; Šefčíková, Z.; Fabian, D. Apoptotic cells in mouse blastocysts are eliminated by neighbouring blastomeres. *Sci. Rep.* **2021**, *11*, 9228. [CrossRef]
27. Bolton, H.; Graham, S.J.L.; Van Der Aa, N.; Kumar, P.; Theunis, K.; Fernandez Gallardo, E.; Voet, T.; Zernicka-Goetz, M. Mouse model of chromosome mosaicism reveals lineage-specific depletion of aneuploid cells and normal developmental potential. *Nat. Commun.* **2016**, *7*, 11165. [CrossRef]

28. Fabian, M.A.; Biggs, W.H.; Treiber, D.K.; Atteridge, C.E.; Azimioara, M.D.; Benedetti, M.G.; Carter, T.A.; Ciceri, P.; Edeen, P.T.; Floyd, M.; et al. A small molecule–kinase interaction map for clinical kinase inhibitors. *Nat. Biotechnol.* **2005**, *23*, 329–336. [CrossRef]
29. Matassov, D.; Kagan, T.; Leblanc, J.; Sikorska, M.; Zakeri, Z. Measurement of Apoptosis by DNA Fragmentation. In *Apoptosis Methods and Protocols*; Humana Press: Totowa, NJ, USA, 2004; pp. 1–18. Available online: http://link.springer.com/10.1385/1-59259-812-9:001 (accessed on 15 January 2024).
30. Zhang, Y.; Li, N.; Wang, L.; Sun, H.; Ma, M.; Wang, H.; Xu, X.; Zhang, W.; Liu, Y.; Cram, D.S.; et al. Molecular analysis of DNA in blastocoele fluid using next-generation sequencing. *J. Assist. Reprod. Genet.* **2016**, *33*, 637–645. [CrossRef] [PubMed]
31. Thowfeequ, S.; Srinivas, S. Embryonic and extraembryonic tissues during mammalian development: Shifting boundaries in time and space. *Philos. Trans. R. Soc. B Biol. Sci.* **2022**, *377*, 20210255. [CrossRef] [PubMed]
32. Hardy, K.; Handyside, A.H.; Winston, R.M.L. The human blastocyst: Cell number, death and allocation during late preimplantation development in vitro. *Development* **1989**, *107*, 597–604. [CrossRef]
33. Brison, D.R. Apoptosis in mammalian preimplantation embryos: Regulation by survival factors. *Hum. Fertil.* **2000**, *3*, 36–47. [CrossRef]
34. Kakourou, G.; Mamas, T.; Vrettou, C.; Traeger-Synodinos, J. An Update on Non-invasive Approaches for Genetic Testing of the Preimplantation Embryo. *Curr. Genom.* **2022**, *23*, 337–352. [CrossRef]
35. Magli, M.C.; Pomante, A.; Cafueri, G.; Valerio, M.; Crippa, A.; Ferraretti, A.P.; Gianaroli, L. Preimplantation genetic testing: Polar bodies, blastomeres, trophectoderm cells, or blastocoelic fluid? *Fertil. Steril.* **2016**, *105*, 676–683.e5. [CrossRef]
36. Rule, K.; Chosed, R.J.; Arthur Chang, T.; David Wininger, J.; Roudebush, W.E. Relationship between blastocoel cell-free DNA and day-5 blastocyst morphology. *J. Assist. Reprod. Genet.* **2018**, *35*, 1497–1501. [CrossRef]
37. Magli, M.C.; Albanese, C.; Crippa, A.; Tabanelli, C.; Ferraretti, A.P.; Gianaroli, L. Deoxyribonucleic acid detection in blastocoelic fluid: A new predictor of embryo ploidy and viable pregnancy. *Fertil. Steril.* **2019**, *111*, 77–85. [CrossRef]
38. Shi, W.; Zhao, Z.; Xue, X.; Li, Q.; Yao, Y.; Wang, D.; Wang, J.; Lu, S.; Shi, J. Ploidy Testing of Blastocoel Fluid for Screening May Be Technically Challenging and More Invasive Than That of Spent Cell Culture Media. *Front. Physiol.* **2022**, *13*, 794210. [CrossRef]
39. Poli, M.; Ori, A.; Child, T.; Jaroudi, S.; Spath, K.; Beck, M.; Wells, D. Characterization and quantification of proteins secreted by single human embryos prior to implantation. *EMBO Mol. Med.* **2015**, *7*, 1465–1479. [CrossRef]
40. Battaglia, R.; Palini, S.; Vento, M.E.; La Ferlita, A.; Lo Faro, M.J.; Caroppo, E.; Borzì, P.; Falzone, L.; Barbagallo, D.; Ragusa, M.; et al. Identification of extracellular vesicles and characterization of miRNA expression profiles in human blastocoel fluid. *Sci. Rep.* **2019**, *9*, 84. [CrossRef] [PubMed]
41. Simon, B.; Bolumar, D.; Amadoz, A.; Jimenez-Almazán, J.; Valbuena, D.; Vilella, F.; Moreno, I. Identification and Characterization of Extracellular Vesicles and Its DNA Cargo Secreted During Murine Embryo Development. *Genes* **2020**, *11*, 203. [CrossRef] [PubMed]
42. Tomic, M.; Vrtacnik Bokal, E.; Stimpfel, M. Non-Invasive Preimplantation Genetic Testing for Aneuploidy and the Mystery of Genetic Material: A Review Article. *Int. J. Mol. Sci.* **2022**, *23*, 3568. [CrossRef] [PubMed]
43. Michailov, Y.; Friedler, S.; Saar-Ryss, B. Methods to improve frozen-thawed blastocyst transfer outcomes- the IVF laboratory perspective. *J. IVF-Worldw.* **2023**, *1*, 1–15. [CrossRef]
44. Sialakouma, A.; Karakasiliotis, I.; Ntala, V.; Nikolettos, N.; Asimakopoulos, B. Embryonic Cell-free DNA in Spent Culture Medium: A Non-invasive Tool for Aneuploidy Screening of the Corresponding Embryos. *In Vivo* **2021**, *35*, 3449–3457. [CrossRef] [PubMed]
45. Brouillet, S.; Martinez, G.; Coutton, C.; Hamamah, S. Is cell-free DNA in spent embryo culture medium an alternative to embryo biopsy for preimplantation genetic testing? A systematic review. *Reprod. Biomed. Online* **2020**, *40*, 779–796. [CrossRef] [PubMed]
46. Popovic, M.; Dheedene, A.; Christodoulou, C.; Taelman, J.; Dhaenens, L.; Van Nieuwerburgh, F.; Deforce, D.; Van den Abbeel, E.; De Sutter, P.; Menten, B.; et al. Chromosomal mosaicism in human blastocysts: The ultimate challenge of preimplantation genetic testing? *Hum. Reprod.* **2018**, *33*, 1342–1354. [CrossRef] [PubMed]
47. Victor, A.R.; Griffin, D.K.; Brake, A.J.; Tyndall, J.C.; Murphy, A.E.; Lepkowsky, L.T.; Lal, A.; Zouves, C.G.; Barnes, F.L.; McCoy, R.C.; et al. Assessment of aneuploidy concordance between clinical trophectoderm biopsy and blastocyst. *Hum. Reprod.* **2019**, *34*, 181–192. [CrossRef] [PubMed]
48. Lawrenz, B.; El Khatib, I.; Liñán, A.; Bayram, A.; Arnanz, A.; Chopra, R.; De Munck, N.; Fatemi, H.M. The clinicians' dilemma with mosaicism—An insight from inner cell mass biopsies. *Hum. Reprod.* **2019**, *34*, 998–1010. [CrossRef] [PubMed]
49. Chuang, T.H.; Hsieh, J.Y.; Lee, M.J.; Lai, H.H.; Hsieh, C.L.; Wang, H.L.; Chang, Y.-J.; Chen, S.-U. Concordance between different trophectoderm biopsy sites and the inner cell mass of chromosomal composition measured with a next-generation sequencing platform. *MHR Basic Sci. Reprod. Med.* **2018**, *24*, 593–601. [CrossRef] [PubMed]
50. Popovic, M.; Dhaenens, L.; Taelman, J.; Dheedene, A.; Bialecka, M.; De Sutter, P.; Lopes, S.M.C.d.S.; Menten, B.; Heindryckx, B. Extended in vitro culture of human embryos demonstrates the complex nature of diagnosing chromosomal mosaicism from a single trophectoderm biopsy. *Hum. Reprod.* **2019**, *34*, 758–769. [CrossRef]
51. Girardi, L.; Figliuzzi, M.; Poli, M.; Serdarogullari, M.; Patassini, C.; Caroselli, S.; Pergher, I.; Cogo, F.; Coban, O.; Boynukalin, F.K.; et al. The use of copy number loads to designate mosaicism in blastocyst stage PGT-A cycles: Fewer is better. *Hum. Reprod.* **2023**, *38*, 982–991. [CrossRef]

52. Cimadomo, D.; Capalbo, A.; Ubaldi, F.M.; Scarica, C.; Palagiano, A.; Canipari, R.; Rienzi, L. The Impact of Biopsy on Human Embryo Developmental Potential during Preimplantation Genetic Diagnosis. *BioMed Res. Int.* **2016**, *2016*, 7193075. [CrossRef] [PubMed]
53. Capalbo, A.; Ubaldi, F.M.; Rienzi, L.; Scott, R.; Treff, N. Detecting mosaicism in trophectoderm biopsies: Current challenges and future possibilities. *Hum. Reprod.* **2017**, *32*, 492–498. [CrossRef] [PubMed]
54. Pandit, S.; Sharma, R. Non invasive assessment of human oocytes and embryos in assisted reproduction: Review on present practices and future trends. *Med. J. Armed. Forces India* **2022**, *78*, 7–16. [CrossRef]
55. Armstrong, S.; Bhide, P.; Jordan, V.; Pacey, A.; Farquhar, C. Time-lapse systems for embryo incubation and assessment in assisted reproduction. *Cochrane Database Syst. Rev.* **2018**, *2018*, CD011320. [CrossRef] [PubMed]
56. Zheng, W.; Zhang, S.; Gu, Y.; Gong, F.; Kong, L.; Lu, G.; Lin, G.; Liang, B.; Hu, L. Non-invasive Metabolomic Profiling of Embryo Culture Medium Using Raman Spectroscopy With Deep Learning Model Predicts the Blastocyst Development Potential of Embryos. *Front. Physiol.* **2021**, *12*, 777259. [CrossRef] [PubMed]
57. Pinto, S.; Guerra-Carvalho, B.; Crisóstomo, L.; Rocha, A.; Barros, A.; Alves, M.G.; Oliveira, P.F. Metabolomics Integration in Assisted Reproductive Technologies for Enhanced Embryo Selection beyond Morphokinetic Analysis. *Int. J. Mol. Sci.* **2023**, *25*, 491. [CrossRef] [PubMed]
58. Raudonis, V.; Paulauskaite-Taraseviciene, A.; Sutiene, K.; Jonaitis, D. Towards the automation of early-stage human embryo development detection. *Biomed. Eng. OnLine* **2019**, *18*, 120. [CrossRef] [PubMed]
59. Paulson, R.J.; Reichman, D.E.; Zaninovic, N.; Goodman, L.R.; Racowsky, C. Time-lapse imaging: Clearly useful to both laboratory personnel and patient outcomes versus just because we can doesn't mean we should. *Fertil. Steril.* **2018**, *109*, 584–591. [CrossRef] [PubMed]
60. Wang, S.S.; Sun, H.X. Blastocyst transfer ameliorates live birth rate compared with cleavage-stage embryos transfer in fresh in vitro fertilization or intracytoplasmic sperm injection cycles: Reviews and meta-analysis. *Yonsei Med. J.* **2014**, *55*, 815–825. [CrossRef]
61. Wong, C.C.; Loewke, K.E.; Bossert, N.L.; Behr, B.; De Jonge, C.J.; Baer, T.M.; Reijo Pera, R.A. Non-invasive imaging of human embryos before embryonic genome activation predicts development to the blastocyst stage. *Nat. Biotechnol.* **2010**, *28*, 1115–1121. [CrossRef]
62. Lundervold, A.S.; Lundervold, A. An overview of deep learning in medical imaging focusing on MRI. *Z. Med. Phys.* **2019**, *29*, 102–127. [CrossRef]
63. Khosravi, P.; Kazemi, E.; Zhan, Q.; Malmsten, J.E.; Toschi, M.; Zisimopoulos, P.; Sigaras, A.; Lavery, S.; Cooper, L.A.D.; Hickman, C.; et al. Deep learning enables robust assessment and selection of human blastocysts after in vitro fertilization. *NPJ Digit. Med.* **2019**, *2*, 21. [CrossRef]
64. Malmsten, J.; Zaninovic, N.; Zhan, Q.; Toschi, M.; Rosenwaks, Z.; Shan, J. Automatic prediction of embryo cell stages using artificial intelligence convolutional neural network. *Fertil. Steril.* **2018**, *110*, e360. [CrossRef]
65. Motiei, M.; Vaculikova, K.; Cela, A.; Tvrdonova, K.; Khalili, R.; Rumpik, D.; Rumpikova, T.; Glatz, Z.; Saha, T. Non-Invasive Human Embryo Metabolic Assessment as a Developmental Criterion. *J. Clin. Med.* **2020**, *9*, 4094. [CrossRef]
66. Bartolacci, A.; Tondo, F.; Alteri, A.; Solano Narduche, L.; De Girolamo, S.; D'Alessandro, G.; Rabellotti, E.; Papaleo, E.; Pagliardini, L. The Task Matters: A Comprehensive Review and Proposed Literature Score of the Effects of Chemical and Physical Parameters on Embryo Developmental Competence. *Life* **2023**, *13*, 2161. [CrossRef]
67. Lundin, K.; Park, H. Time-lapse technology for embryo culture and selection. *Upsala J. Med. Sci.* **2020**, *125*, 77–84. [CrossRef]
68. Villena Gonzales, W.; Mobashsher, A.; Abbosh, A. The Progress of Glucose Monitoring—A Review of Invasive to Minimally and Non-Invasive Techniques, Devices and Sensors. *Sensors* **2019**, *19*, 800. [CrossRef]
69. Li, P.; Song, Z.; Yao, Y.; Huang, T.; Mao, R.; Huang, J.; Ma, Y.; Dong, X.; Huang, W.; Huang, J.; et al. Preimplantation Genetic Screening with Spent Culture Medium/Blastocoel Fluid for in Vitro Fertilization. *Sci. Rep.* **2018**, *8*, 9275. [CrossRef]
70. Wu, A.K.; Elliott, P.; Katz, P.P.; Smith, J.F. Time costs of fertility care: The hidden hardship of building a family. *Fertil. Steril.* **2013**, *99*, 2025–2030. [CrossRef]
71. Wilton, L.; Thornhill, A.; Traeger-Synodinos, J.; Sermon, K.D.; Harper, J.C. The causes of misdiagnosis and adverse outcomes in PGD. *Hum. Reprod.* **2009**, *24*, 1221–1228. [CrossRef]
72. Bouba, I.; Hatzi, E.; Ladias, P.; Sakaloglou, P.; Kostoulas, C.; Georgiou, I. Biological and Clinical Significance of Mosaicism in Human Preimplantation Embryos. *J. Dev. Biol.* **2021**, *9*, 18. [CrossRef]
73. Gardner, D.K.; Wale, P.L.; Collins, R.; Lane, M. Glucose consumption of single post-compaction human embryos is predictive of embryo sex and live birth outcome. *Hum. Reprod.* **2011**, *26*, 1981–1986. [CrossRef] [PubMed]
74. Gardner, D.K.; Larman, M.G.; Thouas, G.A. Sex-related physiology of the preimplantation embryo. *Mol. Hum. Reprod.* **2010**, *16*, 539–547. [CrossRef] [PubMed]
75. Watson, A.J.; Natale, D.R.; Barcroft, L.C. Molecular regulation of blastocyst formation. *Anim. Reprod. Sci.* **2004**, *82–83*, 583–592. [CrossRef]
76. Perloe, M.; Welch, C.; Morton, P.; Venier, W.; Wells, D.; Palini, S. Validation of blastocoele fluid aspiration for preimplantation genetic screening using array comparative genomic hybridization (aCGH). *Fertil. Steril.* **2013**, *100*, S208. [CrossRef]
77. Gianaroli, L.; Magli, M.C.; Pomante, A.; Crivello, A.M.; Cafueri, G.; Valerio, M.; Ferraretti, A.P. Blastocentesis: A source of DNA for preimplantation genetic testing. Results from a pilot study. *Fertil. Steril.* **2014**, *102*, 1692–1699.e6. [CrossRef] [PubMed]

78. Poli, M.; Jaroudi, S.; Sarasa, J.; Spath, K.; Child, T.; Wells, D. The blastocoel fluid as a source of DNA for preimplantation genetic diagnosis and screening. *Fertil. Steril.* **2013**, *100*, S37. [CrossRef]
79. Fang, F.; Li, Z.; Yu, J.; Long, Y.; Zhao, Q.; Ding, X.; Wu, L.; Shao, S.; Zhang, L.; Xiang, W. MicroRNAs secreted by human embryos could be potential biomarkers for clinical outcomes of assisted reproductive technology. *J. Adv. Res.* **2021**, *31*, 25–34. [CrossRef] [PubMed]
80. Stigliani, S.; Anserini, P.; Venturini, P.L.; Scaruffi, P. Mitochondrial DNA content in embryo culture medium is significantly associated with human embryo fragmentation. *Hum. Reprod.* **2013**, *28*, 2652–2660. [CrossRef]
81. Lledo, B.; Morales, R.; Antonio Ortiz, J.; Bernabeu, A.; Bernabeu, R. Noninvasive preimplantation genetic testing using the embryo spent culture medium: An update. *Curr. Opin. Obstet. Gynecol.* **2023**, *35*, 294–299. [CrossRef]
82. Ma, Y.; Gu, M.; Chen, L.; Shen, H.; Pan, Y.; Pang, Y.; Miao, S.; Tong, R.; Huang, H.; Zhu, Y.; et al. Recent advances in critical nodes of embryo engineering technology. *Theranostics* **2021**, *11*, 7391–7424. [CrossRef] [PubMed]
83. Hardy, K.; Spanos, S.; Becker, D.; Iannelli, P.; Winston, R.M.; Stark, J. From cell death to embryo arrest: Mathematical models of human preimplantation embryo development. *Proc. Natl. Acad. Sci. USA* **2001**, *98*, 1655–1660. [CrossRef] [PubMed]
84. Cecchele, A.; Cermisoni, G.C.; Giacomini, E.; Pinna, M.; Vigano, P. Cellular and Molecular Nature of Fragmentation of Human Embryos. *Int. J. Mol. Sci.* **2022**, *23*, 1349. [CrossRef] [PubMed]
85. Stigliani, S.; Persico, L.; Lagazio, C.; Anserini, P.; Venturini, P.L.; Scaruffi, P. Mitochondrial DNA in Day 3 embryo culture medium is a novel, non-invasive biomarker of blastocyst potential and implantation outcome. *MHR Basic Sci. Reprod. Med.* **2014**, *20*, 1238–1246. [CrossRef] [PubMed]
86. Hammond, E.R.; McGillivray, B.C.; Wicker, S.M.; Peek, J.C.; Shelling, A.N.; Stone, P.; Chamley, L.W.; Cree, L.M. Characterizing nuclear and mitochondrial DNA in spent embryo culture media: Genetic contamination identified. *Fertil. Steril.* **2017**, *107*, 220–228.e5. [CrossRef] [PubMed]
87. Sousa, L.N.; Monteiro, P.B. Non-invasive preimplantation genetic testing: A literature review. *JBRA Assist. Reprod.* **2022**, *26*, 554–558.
88. Sepúlveda, S.; Garcia, J.; Arriaga, E.; Diaz, J.; Noriega-Portella, L.; Noriega-Hoces, L. In vitro development and pregnancy outcomes for human embryos cultured in either a single medium or in a sequential media system. *Fertil. Steril.* **2009**, *91*, 1765–1770. [CrossRef] [PubMed]
89. Minasi, M.G.; Fabozzi, G.; Casciani, V.; Lobascio, A.M.; Colasante, A.; Scarselli, F.; Greco, E. Improved blastocyst formation with reduced culture volume: Comparison of three different culture conditions on 1128 sibling human zygotes. *J. Assist. Reprod. Genet.* **2015**, *32*, 215–220. [CrossRef] [PubMed]
90. Chen, J.; Jia, L.; Li, T.; Guo, Y.; He, S.; Zhang, Z.; Su, W.; Zhang, S.; Fang, C. Diagnostic efficiency of blastocyst culture medium in noninvasive preimplantation genetic testing. *F&S Rep.* **2021**, *2*, 88–94.
91. Popovic, M.; Dhaenens, L.; Boel, A.; Menten, B.; Heindryckx, B. Chromosomal mosaicism in human blastocysts: The ultimate diagnostic dilemma. *Hum. Reprod. Update* **2020**, *26*, 313–334. [CrossRef]
92. Esfandiari, N.; Bunnell, M.E.; Casper, R.F. Human embryo mosaicism: Did we drop the ball on chromosomal testing? *J. Assist. Reprod. Genet.* **2016**, *33*, 1439–1444. [CrossRef] [PubMed]
93. Cram, D.S.; Leigh, D.; Handyside, A.; Rechitsky, L.; Xu, K.; Harton, G.; Grifo, J.; Rubio, C.; Fragouli, E.; Kahraman, S.; et al. PGDIS Position Statement on the Transfer of Mosaic Embryos 2019. *Reprod. Biomed. Online* **2019**, *39*, e1–e4. [CrossRef] [PubMed]
94. Munné, S.; Wells, D. Detection of mosaicism at blastocyst stage with the use of high-resolution next-generation sequencing. *Fertil. Steril.* **2017**, *107*, 1085–1091. [CrossRef]
95. Gajecka, M. Unrevealed mosaicism in the next-generation sequencing era. *Mol. Genet. Genom.* **2016**, *291*, 513–530. [CrossRef]
96. Neal, S.A.; Franasiak, J.M.; Forman, E.J.; Werner, M.D.; Morin, S.J.; Tao, X.; Treff, N.R.; Scott, R.T. High relative deoxyribonucleic acid content of trophectoderm biopsy adversely affects pregnancy outcomes. *Fertil. Steril.* **2017**, *107*, 731–736.e1. [CrossRef] [PubMed]
97. Palini, S.; Galluzzi, L.; De Stefani, S.; Bianchi, M.; Wells, D.; Magnani, M.; Bulletti, C. Genomic DNA in human blastocoele fluid. *Reprod. Biomed. Online* **2013**, *26*, 603–610. [CrossRef]
98. Galluzzi, L.; Palini, S.; Stefani, S.D.; Andreoni, F.; Primiterra, M.; Diotallevi, A.; Bulletti, C.; Magnani, M. Extracellular embryo genomic DNA and its potential for genotyping applications. *Future Sci. OA* **2015**, *1*, fso.15.62. [CrossRef] [PubMed]
99. Vera-Rodriguez, M.; Diez-Juan, A.; Jimenez-Almazan, J.; Martinez, S.; Navarro, R.; Peinado, V.; Mercader, A.; Meseguer, M.; Blesa, D.; Moreno, I.; et al. Origin and composition of cell-free DNA in spent medium from human embryo culture during preimplantation development. *Hum. Reprod.* **2018**, *33*, 745–756. [CrossRef] [PubMed]
100. Rubio, C.; Rienzi, L.; Navarro-Sánchez, L.; Cimadomo, D.; García-Pascual, C.M.; Albricci, L.; Soscia, D.; Valbuena, D.; Capalbo, A.; Ubaldi, F.; et al. Embryonic cell-free DNA versus trophectoderm biopsy for aneuploidy testing: Concordance rate and clinical implications. *Fertil. Steril.* **2019**, *112*, 510–519. [CrossRef]
101. Huang, L.; Bogale, B.; Tang, Y.; Lu, S.; Xie, X.S.; Racowsky, C. Noninvasive preimplantation genetic testing for aneuploidy in spent medium may be more reliable than trophectoderm biopsy. *Proc. Natl. Acad. Sci. USA* **2019**, *116*, 14105–14112. [CrossRef]
102. Tobler, K.J.; Zhao, Y.; Ross, R.; Benner, A.T.; Xu, X.; Du, L.; Broman, K.; Thrift, K.; Brezina, P.R.; Kearns, W.G. Blastocoel fluid from differentiated blastocysts harbors embryonic genomic material capable of a whole-genome deoxyribonucleic acid amplification and comprehensive chromosome microarray analysis. *Fertil. Steril.* **2015**, *104*, 418–425. [CrossRef] [PubMed]

103. Jiao, J.; Shi, B.; Sagnelli, M.; Yang, D.; Yao, Y.; Li, W.; Shao, L.; Lu, S.; Li, D.; Wang, X. Minimally invasive preimplantation genetic testing using blastocyst culture medium. *Hum. Reprod.* **2019**, *34*, 1369–1379. [CrossRef] [PubMed]
104. Yeung, Q.S.Y.; Zhang, Y.X.; Chung, J.P.W.; Lui, W.T.; Kwok, Y.K.Y.; Gui, B.; Kong, G.W.S.; Cao, Y.; Li, T.C.; Choy, K.W. A prospective study of non-invasive preimplantation genetic testing for aneuploidies (NiPGT-A) using next-generation sequencing (NGS) on spent culture media (SCM). *J. Assist. Reprod. Genet.* **2019**, *36*, 1609–1621. [CrossRef] [PubMed]
105. Xu, J.; Fang, R.; Chen, L.; Chen, D.; Xiao, J.P.; Yang, W.; Wang, H.; Song, X.; Ma, T.; Bo, S.; et al. Noninvasive chromosome screening of human embryos by genome sequencing of embryo culture medium for in vitro fertilization. *Proc. Natl. Acad. Sci. USA* **2016**, *113*, 11907–11912. [CrossRef] [PubMed]
106. Patrizio, P.; Shoham, G.; Shoham, Z.; Leong, M.; Barad, D.H.; Gleicher, N. Worldwide live births following the transfer of chromosomally "Abnormal" embryos after PGT/A: Results of a worldwide web-based survey. *J. Assist. Reprod. Genet.* **2019**, *36*, 1599–1607. [CrossRef] [PubMed]
107. Vera-Rodriguez, M.; Rubio, C. Assessing the true incidence of mosaicism in preimplantation embryos. *Fertil. Steril.* **2017**, *107*, 1107–1112. [CrossRef] [PubMed]
108. Ou, Z.; Chen, Z.; Yin, M.; Deng, Y.; Liang, Y.; Wang, W.; Yao, Y.; Sun, L. Re-analysis of whole blastocysts after trophectoderm biopsy indicated chromosome aneuploidy. *Hum. Genom.* **2020**, *14*, 3. [CrossRef] [PubMed]
109. Leaver, M.; Wells, D. Non-invasive preimplantation genetic testing (niPGT): The next revolution in reproductive genetics? *Hum. Reprod. Update* **2020**, *26*, 16–42. [CrossRef] [PubMed]
110. Sachdev, N.M.; Maxwell, S.M.; Besser, A.G.; Grifo, J.A. Diagnosis and clinical management of embryonic mosaicism. *Fertil. Steril.* **2017**, *107*, 6–11. [CrossRef]
111. Maxwell, S.M.; Colls, P.; Hodes-Wertz, B.; McCulloh, D.H.; McCaffrey, C.; Wells, D.; Munné, S.; Grifo, J.A. Why do euploid embryos miscarry? A case-control study comparing the rate of aneuploidy within presumed euploid embryos that resulted in miscarriage or live birth using next-generation sequencing. *Fertil. Steril.* **2016**, *106*, 1414–1419.e5. [CrossRef]
112. Wells, D.; Kaur, K.; Grifo, J.; Glassner, M.; Taylor, J.C.; Fragouli, E.; Munne, S. Clinical utilisation of a rapid low-pass whole genome sequencing technique for the diagnosis of aneuploidy in human embryos prior to implantation. *J. Med. Genet.* **2014**, *51*, 553–562. [CrossRef] [PubMed]
113. Greco, E.; Minasi, M.G.; Fiorentino, F. Healthy Babies after Intrauterine Transfer of Mosaic Aneuploid Blastocysts. *N. Engl. J. Med.* **2015**, *373*, 2089–2090. [CrossRef] [PubMed]
114. Spinella, F.; Fiorentino, F.; Biricik, A.; Bono, S.; Ruberti, A.; Cotroneo, E.; Baldi, M.; Cursio, E.; Minasi, M.G.; Greco, E. Extent of chromosomal mosaicism influences the clinical outcome of in vitro fertilization treatments. *Fertil. Steril.* **2018**, *109*, 77–83. [CrossRef] [PubMed]
115. Zore, T.; Kroener, L.L.; Wang, C.; Liu, L.; Buyalos, R.; Hubert, G.; Shamonki, M. Transfer of embryos with segmental mosaicism is associated with a significant reduction in live-birth rate. *Fertil. Steril.* **2019**, *111*, 69–76. [CrossRef] [PubMed]
116. Fragouli, E.; Alfarawati, S.; Spath, K.; Babariya, D.; Tarozzi, N.; Borini, A.; Wells, D. Analysis of implantation and ongoing pregnancy rates following the transfer of mosaic diploid–aneuploid blastocysts. *Hum. Genet.* **2017**, *136*, 805–819. [CrossRef] [PubMed]
117. Ho, J.R.; Arrach, N.; Rhodes-Long, K.; Ahmady, A.; Ingles, S.; Chung, K.; Bendikson, K.A.; Paulson, R.J.; McGinnis, L.K. Pushing the limits of detection: Investigation of cell-free DNA for aneuploidy screening in embryos. *Fertil. Steril.* **2018**, *110*, 467–475.e2. [CrossRef] [PubMed]
118. Darwish, E.; Magdi, Y. Artificial shrinkage of blastocoel using a laser pulse prior to vitrification improves clinical outcome. *J. Assist. Reprod. Genet.* **2016**, *33*, 467–471. [CrossRef] [PubMed]
119. Shamonki, M.I.; Jin, H.; Haimowitz, Z.; Liu, L. Proof of concept: Preimplantation genetic screening without embryo biopsy through analysis of cell-free DNA in spent embryo culture media. *Fertil. Steril.* **2016**, *106*, 1312–1318. [CrossRef]
120. Wu, H.; Ding, C.; Shen, X.; Wang, J.; Li, R.; Cai, B.; Xu, Y.; Zhong, Y.; Zhou, C. Medium-Based Noninvasive Preimplantation Genetic Diagnosis for Human α-Thalassemias-SEA. *Medicine* **2015**, *94*, e669. [CrossRef]
121. Giacomini, E.; Vago, R.; Sanchez, A.M.; Podini, P.; Zarovni, N.; Murdica, V.; Rizzo, R.; Bortolotti, D.; Candiani, M.; Viganò, P. Secretome of in vitro cultured human embryos contains extracellular vesicles that are uptaken by the maternal side. *Sci. Rep.* **2017**, *7*, 5210. [CrossRef]
122. Bankoglu, E.E.; Stipp, F.; Gerber, J.; Seyfried, F.; Heidland, A.; Bahner, U.; Stopper, H. Effect of cryopreservation on DNA damage and DNA repair activity in human blood samples in the comet assay. *Arch. Toxicol.* **2021**, *95*, 1831–1841. [CrossRef] [PubMed]
123. Werner, M.D.; Scott, K.; Bohrer, C.; Gabriele, D.; Tao, X.; Hong, K.H.; Taylor, D.; Treff, N.; Scott, R. The accuracy of blastocoel fluid comprehensive chromosomal screening (CCS) is dependent on amplification yield and sequencing depth when using nextgen sequencing. *Fertil. Steril.* **2014**, *102*, e308–e309. [CrossRef]
124. Anvari, M.; Gharib, A.; Abolhasani, M.; Azari-Yaam, A.; Gharalari, F.; Safavi, M.; Zare-Mirzaie, A.; Vasei, M. Pre-analytical Practices in the Molecular Diagnostic Tests, A Concise Review. *Iran. J. Pathol.* **2021**, *16*, 1–19. [CrossRef] [PubMed]
125. Thorpe, J.; Osei-Owusu, I.A.; Avigdor, B.E.; Tupler, R.; Pevsner, J. Mosaicism in Human Health and Disease. *Annu. Rev. Genet.* **2020**, *54*, 487–510. [CrossRef] [PubMed]
126. Mourad, A.; Antaki, R.; Bissonnette, F.; Al Baini, O.; Saadeh, B.; Jamal, W. Evidence-based clinical prioritization of embryos with mosaic results: A systematic review and meta-analysis. *J. Assist. Reprod. Genet.* **2021**, *38*, 2849–2860. [CrossRef] [PubMed]

127. Lledó, B.; Morales, R.; Ortiz, J.A.; Blanca, H.; Ten, J.; Llácer, J.; Bernabeu, R. Implantation potential of mosaic embryos. *Syst. Biol. Reprod. Med.* **2017**, *63*, 206–208. [CrossRef] [PubMed]
128. Tšuiko, O.; Zhigalina, D.I.; Jatsenko, T.; Skryabin, N.A.; Kanbekova, O.R.; Artyukhova, V.G.; Svetlakov, A.V.; Teearu, K.; Trošin, A.; Salumets, A.; et al. Karyotype of the blastocoel fluid demonstrates low concordance with both trophectoderm and inner cell mass. *Fertil. Steril.* **2018**, *109*, 1127–1134.e1. [CrossRef] [PubMed]
129. McCoy, R.C. Mosaicism in Preimplantation Human Embryos: When Chromosomal Abnormalities Are the Norm. *Trends Genet.* **2017**, *33*, 448–463. [CrossRef]
130. Li, X.; Hao, Y.; Elshewy, N.; Zhu, X.; Zhang, Z.; Zhou, P. The mechanisms and clinical application of mosaicism in preimplantation embryos. *J. Assist. Reprod. Genet.* **2020**, *37*, 497–508. [CrossRef]

Journal of
Clinical Medicine

MDPI

Review

The Contribution of Proteomics in Understanding Endometrial Protein Expression in Women with Recurrent Implantation Failure

Anastasios Potiris [1,*,†], Eleni Alyfanti [1,†], Eirini Drakaki [2], Despoina Mavrogianni [2], Theodoros Karampitsakos [1], Pavlos Machairoudias [1], Spyridon Topis [1], Athanasios Zikopoulos [3], Chara Skentou [4], Periklis Panagopoulos [1], Peter Drakakis [1] and Sofoklis Stavros [1]

1 Third Department of Obstetrics and Gynecology, Medical School, University General Hospital "ATTIKON", National and Kapodistrian University of Athens, 12462 Athens, Greece; elenalyfanti@med.uoa.gr (E.A.); theokarampi@med.uoa.gr (T.K.); pavlosmach@med.uoa.gr (P.M.); spyrostopis@med.uoa.gr (S.T.); perpanag@med.uoa.gr (P.P.); pdrakakis@med.uoa.gr (P.D.); sfstavrou@med.uoa.gr (S.S.)
2 First Department of Obstetrics and Gynecology, Medical School, Alexandra Hospital, National and Kapodistrian University of Athens, 11528 Athens, Greece; eirinidrak@med.uoa.gr (E.D.); dmavrogianni@med.uoa.gr (D.M.)
3 Department of Obstetrics and Gynecology, Royal Cornwall Hospital, Treliske, Truro TR1 3LQ, UK; thanzik92@gmail.com
4 Department of Obstetrics and Gynecology, Medical School of the University of Ioannina, 45110 Ioannina, Greece; haraskentou@uoi.gr
* Correspondence: apotiris@med.uoa.gr; Tel.: +30-(210)-5832237
† These authors contributed equally to this work.

Abstract: Recurrent implantation failure (RIF) poses a significant challenge in assisted reproductive technology (ART) outcomes. The endometrium plays a crucial role in embryo implantation, and its protein expression profile is integral in determining receptivity. Proteomics has emerged as a valuable tool in unraveling the molecular intricacies underlying endometrial receptivity and RIF. The aim of the present review is to analyze the contribution of proteomics to the understanding of endometrial protein expression in women with RIF, based on the results of significant proteomic studies. Medline/Pubmed databases were searched using keywords pertaining to proteomics combined with terms related to RIF. 15 studies were included in the present review. Several proteins have been found to exhibit differential expression in endometrial biopsies and fluid samples between fertile women and women with RIF during the receptive endometrial phase. The profile of endometrial proteins varied significantly among the studies. Nevertheless, similar changes in the expression levels of annexin-6, progesterone receptor, MMP-2, and MMP-9 in the endometrium of women with RIF, were found in more than one study indicating that certain proteins could potentially be effective biomarkers of endometrial receptivity. Proteomics contributes significantly to the understanding of protein expression in the endometrium of women with RIF and the analysis of proteins in endometrial fluid are promising for improving the clinical management of RIF.

Keywords: proteomics; recurrent implantation failure (RIF); endometrial protein expression; biomarkers; endometrial receptivity

1. Introduction

Recurrent implantation failure (RIF) is a highly demanding and complex clinical phenomenon that, despite advancements in assisted reproductive technology, remains a major issue affecting approximately 15% of women undergoing in vitro fertilization [1]. Despite the extensive relevant literature, there is still no widely accepted definition. The definition that until recently had the broadest acceptance for RIF is that of Coughlan et al., who define RIF as the failure to achieve clinical pregnancy after the transfer of at least four high-quality embryos following at least three fresh or frozen IVF cycles, in women under the age of 40 [2]. The European Society of Human Reproduction and Embryology (ESHRE) has recently defined RIF as the scenario in which the transfer of embryos considered to be viable has failed to result in a positive pregnancy test sufficiently often in a specific patient to warrant consideration of further investigations and/or interventions [3].

The implantation of the embryo is of utmost importance for the success of IVF and although it is well known that is a very complex process, it is a fact that the precise mechanisms have not yet been fully elucidated. Recurrent implantation failure can be caused by maternal, paternal, and fetal factors, as well as a combination of different factors. Maternal factors include disorders of endometrial receptivity, the immune system, thrombophilia, chronic endometritis and inflammation, endocrine disorders, uterine polyps, and uterine anatomical abnormalities [4,5]; additionally, thin endometrium and additional factors such as maternal age, BMI, smoking, alcohol consumption, and stress. Embryonic factors include various types of chromosomal abnormalities in the embryo, translocations, inversions, deletions, and mosaicism [6,7]. It is important to note that disorders related to endometrial receptivity and biochemical alterations of the dialogue between the endometrium and the blastocyst account for approximately two-thirds of cases of recurrent implantation failure [8,9]. Despite the extensive research and suggestions that have been made for the correct diagnosis, prognosis and various treatment options for RIF, there are still knowledge gaps that need further investigation.

Proteomics, a high-throughput approach enabling the comprehensive analysis of protein expression, post-translational modifications, and protein–protein interactions, has emerged as a powerful tool in reproductive medicine providing exceptionally high-precision qualitative and quantitative results. There are numerous techniques applied in proteomic analysis and can be divided into four categories. These include conventional techniques, used for protein purification and based on chromatography, advanced techniques, quantitative techniques, and high-performance techniques [10]. The use of proteomics offers the ability to reveal the mechanisms of complex biological processes and conditions, including fertilization, embryo implantation, embryo development, and pregnancy [11]. Proteomic analysis has been widely applied in modern research, which aims to gain a deeper understanding of the pathology of recurrent implantation failure and to find reliable biomarkers of endometrial receptivity.

This review aims to summarize the current state of knowledge, regarding the contribution of several proteomic studies carried out in the last two decades, in deciphering endometrial protein expression patterns in women with RIF, with a focus on its potential implications for improving ART outcomes.

2. Materials and Methods

To provide a comprehensive review of the literature published up to November 2023, Medline/PubMed databases were searched using keywords pertaining to proteomics, including "proteomic analysis", "proteome", "protein expression profiles", combined with terms related to recurrent implantation failure (RIF) such as "implantation failure", "endometrial receptivity", "embryo implantation", and "endometrial receptivity biomarkers". These terms were either used separately or in combination with the help of the Boolean administration (OR, AND). All articles published after 2003 and with an English title and abstract were initially accepted. Reviews, systematic reviews, and studies that examined the endometrium of women who, apart from RIF, were diagnosed with other pathological conditions were not included.

In the screening process, the title and abstract of 20 studies were screened independently by two reviewers (A.P. and E.A.). Subsequently, a full-text assessment was performed. If a study was selected only by one reviewer, the decision was taken by a third reviewer (D.M.). 17 studies were selected for full-text assessment and after careful evaluation 15 articles were included in the present review. Data extraction was performed by a single reviewer (E.A.) and validated by a second reviewer (A.P.).

3. Results

3.1. Comparison of Protein Expression in Endometrial Tissue Samples between Fertile Women and Women with Recurrent Implantation Failure

The study by Brosens et al., published in 2010, demonstrated that changes in the expression, modification, or regulation of apolipoprotein-A1 (apoA-I) by paracrine embryonic signals play a significant role, as they can lead to implantation failure. apoA-I is the major protein component of high-density lipoprotein (HDL) particles and is a key part in lipid metabolism. The research team employed a series of proteomic techniques, such as surface-enhanced laser desorption/ionization time-of-flight mass spectrometry (SELDI-TOF-MS), immunohistochemistry, Western blot analysis, and enzyme-linked immunosorbent assay (ELISA). A comparison was made between endometrial samples during the mid-secretory phase from women with recurrent implantation failure and fertile women. The analysis using SELDI-TOF-MS showed higher levels of apoA-I expression in women with RIF (p-value = 0.0002); however, verification via Western blotting did not reveal a significant increase in apoA-I levels in samples from women with RIF compared to fertile controls. To investigate the response of apolipoprotein-A1, which is a potent anti-inflammatory molecule, to embryonic hormonal stimuli, human chorionic gonadotropin (hCG) was injected into the histological samples. The administration of hCG resulted in a strong inhibition of apoA-I expression in differentiated endometrial tissue cultures from the comparison groups [12].

The team of Mariee et al., in 2012 applied the method of immunohistochemistry to compare the levels of interleukin-15 (IL-15) and leukemia inhibitory factor (LIF) in the endometrium of women with recurrent implantation failure (RIF) and in the endometrium of women with normal fertility. Furthermore, they examined the relationship between the levels of IL-15 and LIF with the number of uterine natural killer cells (uNK cells). IL-15 is a pleiotropic cytokine that belongs to the four α-helix bundle family of cytokines and plays an important role in both innate and adaptive immunity. One of its basic functions is the stimulation of Natural Killer (NK) cells. LIF belongs to the interleukin-6 (IL-6) cytokine family and participates in various biological processes, particularly in the regulation of stem cell pluripotency, inflammation, and the immune response, while it has been proven that LIF produced by the endometrial tissue is involved in the crosstalk between the embryo and the uterus during implantation. The results of this study showed that the quantity of LIF in the epithelial tissue of the endometrial glands in women with recurrent implantation failure (RIF) was lower compared to fertile women (p-value = 0.01). In contrast, the level of IL-15 in stromal cells of women with RIF was higher than that of the control group (p-value = 0.009). Finally, a significant correlation was observed between the number of uNK cells and the expression of IL-15 in the stromal cells (r = 0.427, p-value = 0.001), while there was no correlation between the expression of LIF and the number of uNK cells [13].

In 2014, the team of Garrido-Gómez et al. conducted a comparison between endometrial biopsy samples from women undergoing hormone replacement therapy, which had been characterized as receptive and non-receptive based on evaluation with the ERA (Endometrial Receptivity Analysis) test. These samples were taken following administration of progesterone for 5 consecutive days. Protein isolation was performed, followed by differential gel electrophoresis (DIGE) and MALDI-MS analysis, which identified 24 proteins with differential expression between receptive and non-receptive endometrial samples. Subsequently, through in silico analysis, a network was created with these 24 proteins along with various introduced nodes, aiming to determine if any pathway or group of proteins was involved in the differential receptivity status of the endometrium between the two comparison groups. Two statistically significant pathways were identified in comparison between samples from receptive (ERA-R) and non-receptive endometria (ERA-NR): the "carbohydrate biosynthesis pathway" and the "nuclear mRNA splicing through spliceosome pathway". This network highlighted phosphoglucomutase 1 (PGM1), alpha-enolase (ENO1), and sialic acid synthase (SIAS) as dysregulated proteins associated with carbohydrate metabolism pathways, which may be involved in altering the metabolic state of the endometrium and thereby increasing its receptivity. The results of the DIGE analysis were validated using Western blotting and immunohistochemistry for two proteins: annexin-6 (ANXA6) and progesterone receptor membrane component 1 (PGRMC1). ANXA6 belongs to the annexin family of calcium-dependent phospholipid-binding proteins and is involved in membrane binding, endocytosis, intracellular trafficking, and signaling pathways, including apoptosis signaling pathway. PGRMC1 is a versatile protein involved in steroid hormone signaling, cellular signaling pathways, gene expression regulation, and membrane organization. The results obtained by Western blot and immunohistochemistry confirmed the increased expression of ANXA6 and PGRMC1 in ERA-NR endometrial samples compared to ERA-R samples. Based on these results, the research team proposed ANXA6 and PGRMC1 proteins as new molecular targets and the "carbohydrate biosynthesis pathway" and "nuclear mRNA splicing through the spliceosome" as significant pathways associated with the creation of receptive endometrium [14].

The scientific team of Long et al. investigated in 2016 the relationship between telomerase and the expression of steroid hormone receptors in recurrent implantation failure (RIF). Telomerase is a ribonucleoprotein which adds guanine-rich repetitive sequences to the 3′ end of telomeres, to maintain the length of DNA telomeres. Estrogen receptor alpha (ER alpha) and progesterone receptor (PR) are two nuclear receptors, that are activated by estrogens and progesterone, respectively, influence gene expression and they play an essential role during the implantation window. Endometrial biopsies were collected from patients with RIF and from fertile women. Using the real-time PCR technique, changes were detected at the transcriptional level of the expression of telomerase reverse transcriptase (Tert), estrogen receptor alpha (ER alpha) and progesterone receptor (PR). Subsequently, Western blotting and immunohistochemistry techniques were applied to analyze the expression of TERT and ER alpha at the protein level. The protein expression of TERT was increased in patients with RIF (p-value < 0.0001) and was localized in the endometrial epithelium and stromal cells. However, the signal from the ER alpha in the stromal cells of women with RIF was weaker compared to the control samples (p-value = 0.0056). In conclusion, this study demonstrated that induction of TERT is significantly correlated with reduced production of ER alpha, which in turn directly affects the protein environment of the endometrium and contributes to embryo implantation failure [15].

The research study by Dhaenes et al. in 2018 investigated the protein profile of in vitro cultured endometrial stromal cells obtained from women with recurrent implantation failure (RIF), recurrent pregnancy loss (RPL) and from fertile women. The study compared the protein profile on the first day (non-decidualized samples) of culture with that on the fifth day (decidualized samples). Proteins were isolated and analyzed using high-resolution mass spectrometry. The results showed an increase in ANXA6 (annexin 6), PSMC5 (26S proteasome regulatory subunit 8), and FSCN1 (fascin) in the RIF group, while PBXIP1 (pre-B-cell leukemia transcription factor-interacting protein 1) decreased during decidualization (5th day of culture) (FDR = 10%, p-value < 0.05). PSMC5 is a component of the 26S proteasome complex, which plays a critical role in protein degradation. FSCN1 is a key regulator of actin bundling and is involved in cell movement and invasion, while PBXIP1 plays important roles in cellular processes such as transcriptional regulation and apoptosis. In the RPL group, RPS25 (40S ribosomal protein S25) and ACADVL (very long-chain specific acyl-CoA dehydrogenase, mitochondrial) decreased between non-decidualized and decidualized samples (FDR = 10%, p-value < 0.05). ACADVL catalyses the first step of the fatty acid beta-oxidation pathway, which is critical for the decidualization process. In the group of fertile women, the proteins vimentin (VIM) and RPL23A (60S ribosomal protein L23a) exhibited decreased concentration (FDR = 10%, p-value < 0.05). After comparing expression ratios between decidualized and non-decidualized samples across all groups, six proteins with differential expression were identified: DUX4L2 (double homeobox protein 4-like protein 2), CNPY4 (protein canopy homologue 4), PDE7A (high affinity cAMP-specific 3′,5′-cyclic phosphodiesterase 7A), CTSK (cathepsin K), PCBP2 (poly(rC)-binding protein 2), and PSMD4 (26S proteasome non-ATPase regulatory subunit 4) (FDR = 10%,

p-value < 0.05). DUX4L2 is a member of the double homeobox (DUX) family of transcription factors. CNPY4 is a member of the Canopy (CNPY) family of proteins which plays a multifaceted role in maintaining cellular homeostasis by regulating protein folding, the ER stress response, and the secretion of proteins. PDE7A is an enzyme that participates in the regulation of intracellular levels of cyclic adenosine monophosphate (cAMP). CTSK is a cysteine protease enzyme which is involved in collagen degradation and PSMD4 is a subunit of the 19S regulatory particle of the 26S proteasome, which participates in the regulation of protein degradation. PCBP2 is a member of the heterogeneous nuclear ribonucleoprotein (hnRNP) family of RNA-binding proteins and has an important role in post-transcriptional regulation of gene expression. Serotransferrin also showed differential expression in the comparison between the RPL group and fertile women (FDR 3%, p-value < 0.01). Changes in the expression levels of serotransferrin, ANXA6, ACDVL, and VIM were further validated using the Western blot method [16].

In 2019, the research team of Bielfeld et al. conducted a proteomic analysis of endometrial tissue obtained through biopsy from patients with recurrent implantation failure (RIF) and from women with proven fertility. Using mass spectrometry, 2120 proteins were identified, three of which exhibited statistically significant changes in their quantity in the endometrial tissue of patients with RIF compared to fertile women. Specifically, the results showed an increase in the quantity of epiplakin-1 (EPPK1) and Bcl-2-associated transcription factor 1 (BCLAF1), and a decrease in the quantity of prothymosin-alpha (PTMA) in women with RIF. EPPK1 is a multifunctional protein crucial in maintaining the structural integrity of epithelial tissues, regulating cell adhesion and migration, and contributing to cytoskeletal dynamics. BCLAF1 plays important roles in various cellular processes, including apoptosis, transcriptional regulation, RNA splicing, and DNA damage response. PTMA is a ubiquitous polypeptide with both intracellular and extracellular functions. Intracellularly, it acts as an anti-apoptotic and proliferation mediator, while extracellularly, serves as a biologic response modifier, influencing immune responses and contributing to immune regulation. Additionally, an analysis of the endometrial tissue was performed following in vivo administration of a human chorionic gonadotropin (hCG) substitute. The endometrial administration of hCG helped increase the expression of intracellular proteins, HIF1 (Hypoxia-Inducible Factor 1) signaling, and chemokine production. Specifically, patients with RIF showed a 19% higher clinical pregnancy rate after endometrial hCG administration prior to embryo transfer (ET), compared to failed attempts in previous cycles. Based on these findings, the research team suggests that endometrial hCG administration before ET may improve chemical communication between the embryo and endometrium, enhance angiogenesis and immune response, thereby resulting in the increase in pregnancy rate in patients with RIF [17].

In the study conducted by Wang et al. and published in 2021, a screening was performed for endometrial proteins with differential expression during the window of implantation (WOI), using the iTRAQ labeling technique in combination with 2D LC-MS/MS, aiming to identify potential biomarkers for patients with recurrent implantation failure (RIF). The endometrial tissue samples were obtained by hysteroscopy during the phase of WOI, from September 2016 to December 2019, and simultaneously during this period, clinical data were collected. Patients were divided into two groups according to pregnancy outcomes: a group of women with reproductive failure (RIF) and a control group of women who achieved successful pregnancy. The results revealed 82 differentially expressed proteins in patients with RIF compared to the control group, including 55 proteins with increased expression (>1.50 fold, p-value < 0.05) and 27 proteins with decreased expression (<0.67 fold, p-value < 0.05). Bioinformatics analysis using the String analysis software highlighted interactions among these proteins, which were grouped into two categories: ribosomal proteins and homeostatic blood proteins. The most statistically significant enriched biological processes identified by Gene Ontology analysis included the downregulation of hydrolase activity, blood microparticles, and enzyme inhibition activity. Specifically, seven proteins (SPB6, APOA1, GMIP, THBG, CBG, ANT3, and FETUA) involved in hydrolase activity were identified, another seven proteins (VTDB, IGHG4, APOA1, A1AG2, FETUA, ANT3, and A1AG1) were found in the category of blood microparticles, and yet another seven proteins (ANT3, FETUA, CBG, ASPN, SPB6, THBG, and APOA1) were implicated in the inhibition of various enzymes. Additionally, verification was performed for the levels of antithrombin-III (ANT3), corticosteroid-binding globulin (CBG), and fetuin-A (FETUA) in the endometrium using the Western blot method, and significantly higher levels of CBG (1.39-fold, p-value = 0.003) and fetuin-A (1.47-fold, p-value = 0.002) were observed in patients with RIF. CBG is a glycoprotein whose main function is to bind glucocorticoids and progesterone in the bloodstream, thereby regulating their distribution and availability to target tissues throughout the body. FETUA is a multifunctional glycoprotein involved in various physiological processes including calcification inhibition, regulation of insulin sensitivity, modulation of inflammation, lipid metabolism, and bone mineralization. Based on the above results, the research team proposed corticosteroid-binding globulin (CBG) and fetuin-A as biomarkers for recurrent implantation failure [18].

The study by Fu et al. in 2022 demonstrated that aberrant expression of DNA topoisomerase-alpha (TOP2A), which is a critical enzyme involved in DNA replication, transcription, and repair, affects endometrial decidualization and alters the timing of the "window of implantation" thereby leading to implantation failure. The research team conducted proteomic analysis to assess differentially expressed proteins between endometrial tissue samples of patients with RIF and fertile women. The expression patterns of TOP2A in the pre-implantation endometrium of patients with RIF were determined using immunohistochemistry, Western blotting, and qRT-PCR. Furthermore, T-HESCs (Immortal human ESCs) were generated with TOP2A gene silencing (sh-TOP2A) using lentiviral vectors and the expression of TOP2A in T-HESCs was manipulated to investigate its role in the process of decidualization. The TOP2A-related changes in decidualization were examined using mRNA sequencing and subsequently validated by Western blotting and immunofluorescence. The results showed that TOP2A is widely expressed in both stromal and glandular epithelial cells of the endometrium, and its expression appeared to be significantly lower in the mid-secretory phase of the endometrium in women with RIF (p-value < 0.01). TOP2A expression was downregulated under stimulation by 8-bromo-cAMP and MPA [19].

In 2023, the research study by Yang et al. proposed that the levels of the proteins TPPP3 (tubulin polymerization-promoting protein family member 3), S100A13 (S100 Calcium Binding Protein A13), HSD17B2 (17b-hydroxysteroid dehydrogenase 2), and AZGP1 (alpha-2-glycoprotein 1, zinc binding) in the endometrium can be used as markers for endometrial receptivity and the diagnosis of women with recurrent implantation failure (RIF). TPPP3 is a member of the tubulin polymerization promoting protein family, involved in regulating microtubule dynamics within cells. S100A13 is a small calcium-binding protein belonging to the S100 family, which plays important roles in a series of cellular processes, such as calcium homeostasis, cell proliferation, apoptosis, and inflammation. HSD17B is an enzyme essential for the synthesis and metabolism of estrogens and androgens. AZGP1 is a secretory adipose factor which participates in metabolic processes such as lipolysis and glucose transport, acts as a tumor suppressor and may be involved in immune modulation. The research team compared endometrial tissues obtained from women with RIF to those from women with normal fertility, taken 7–9 days after the peak of luteinizing hormone (LH). Using the iTRAQ technique, 2063 proteins with differential expression were identified, which are involved in various biological processes such as protein translation, mitochondrial function, oxidoreductase activity, amino acid, and fatty acid metabolism. Ultimately, after bioinformatics analysis, the proteins TPPP3, S100A13, HSD17B2, and AZGP1 were identified as potential biomarkers of receptive endometrium and further validation was performed using Western blot and immunohistochemistry. Specifically, the iTRAQ analysis revealed that the expression of the proteins HSD17B2 and AZGP1 decreased in samples from patients with RIF compared to those of the control group, while the proteins TPPP3, APEX1, and S100A13 showed increased expression in the RIF group. The results from Western blot and immunohistochemistry showed that the levels of TPPP3,

HSD17B2, S100A13, and AZGP1 were significantly reduced in the endometrium of patients with RIF [20].

Another study published in 2023 by Zhao et al. compared the protein expression in endometrial tissues collected from women with recurrent implantation failure (RIF) and from women with recurrent implantation successes (RIS). The differential expression of proteins between individuals with RIF and those with RIS was identified using the iTRAQ and LC-MS/MS techniques. Overall, 35,071 peptides and 6290 proteins were identified in the samples of both comparison groups using the iTRAQ method. According to the criteria for defining differentially expressed proteins set by the research team (fold change > 1.3 or <0.77 and p-value < 0.05), 425 proteins with increased expression and 200 proteins with decreased expression were found in the RIF group compared to the RIS group. The bioinformatics analysis (GO enrichment and KEGG pathway analysis) revealed that these proteins were enriched in biological processes related to Wnt and TGF-β signaling, smooth muscle contraction, ubiquitin-mediated proteolysis, and tight junctions. To confirm the above results for the proteins that showed differential expression, validation was performed using qPCR and Western blotting. It was revealed that claudin-4, p38 kinase, AMP-activated protein kinase subunit beta (PRKAB), and NF-kB inhibitor subunit-beta (IKB-b) had increased expression, while myosin-2 and protein kinase G (PKG2) had significantly decreased expression in women with RIF [21]. Claudin-4 is a tight junction protein which plays a crucial role in maintaining the barrier function of tight junctions and regulates paracellular permeability. p38 kinase is a versatile signaling molecule which is involved in stress responses, inflammation, cell cycle regulation, apoptosis, differentiation, response to growth factors and tissue regeneration. PRKAB is a component of the AMPK complex, which acts as a cellular energy sensor and regulator of metabolic pathways, influencing cell growth and autophagy. IKB-b is a critical regulator of the NF-kB signaling pathway and its roles include regulating the inflammatory response, cell survival, development, and immune response. Myosin-2 is a versatile motor protein involved in muscle contraction, cell movement, cell adhesion and communication. PKG2 is involved in cGMP signaling pathways and plays roles in smooth muscle relaxation, cardiovascular function, platelet function, neuronal function, and the regulation of ion channels, cell cytoplasm and cytoskeleton array. However, contrary to the findings of this study, in the study by Pérez-Debén et al., where iTRAQ technology was also applied and a comparison was made between endometrial samples from fertile women, women with an intrauterine contraceptive device, and women with a history of recurrent implantation failure, no differences were found in the protein composition of the endometrium between patients with RIF and fertile women [22].

3.2. Comparison of Protein Expression between Endometrial Fluid Samples from Fertile Women and Women with Recurrent Implantation Failure

To investigate noninvasive methods for assessing endometrial receptivity, some studies have examined the different protein composition of endometrial fluid samples. In 2003, the team of Inagaki et al. used the method of zymography to compare the levels of interleukin-1beta (IL-1beta), tumor necrosis factor-alpha (TNF-alpha), interferon-gamma (IFN-gamma), leukemia inhibitory factor (LIF), interleukin-10 (IL-10), and the activity of matrix metalloproteinases 2 and 9 (MMP-2 and MMP-9) among samples of intrauterine fluid obtained from fertile women and patients with recurrent implantation failure (RIF). IL-1beta and TNF-alpha are pro-inflammatory cytokines that play a key role in the promotion of inflammation and immune responses. IFN-gamma is a potent cytokine which activates macrophages, enhances the activity of NK cells and cytotoxic T cells, and has antiviral effects. IL-10 is an anti-inflammatory cytokine that facilitates the regulation of the immune response and maintains immune balance, through suppression of pro-inflammatory cytokines and immune cells. MMP-2 and MMP-9, both members of the gelatinase subgroup of MMPs, are involved in tissue remodeling, ECM degradation, and various pathological processes. It was observed that the activity levels of MMP-2, MMP-9, and IL-1beta were increased in women RIF compared to fertile women, while the concentrations of IFN-gamma and IL-10 were significantly lower (p-value = 0.05). Regarding TNF-alpha, there was a trend towards increased expression in samples from women with RIF, but this difference was not statistically significant. Similarly, the expression of LIF did not show a statistically significant difference between the compared groups [23]. The higher levels of MMP-2 and MMP-9 in women with RIF were also confirmed by the study of Yoshii et al. in 2013 [24]. The research team indicated that this increase reflected an inflammatory state in the endometrium, and therefore, they proceeded with treatment using antibiotics and corticosteroids aiming to reduce inflammation in women with RIF. This treatment likely improved the endometrial environment by limiting the activity of matrix metalloproteinases (MMPs), and consequently led to significantly better pregnancy outcomes in the group of patients who underwent this therapy [24,25].

The study by Azkargorta et al., published in 2018, confirmed by large-scale proteomic techniques that the endometrial fluid exhibits a different protein composition between women who achieve successful embryo implantation in IVF cycles and those who experience implantation failure. The collection of endometrial fluid was performed immediately before embryo transfer. The results of the proteomic and bioinformatic analysis revealed that samples from women experiencing implantation failure exhibited significant dysregulation in processes controlling endometrial receptivity, such as antimicrobial response, cellular interaction, immune response and signaling during inflammation. Also, findings of this study indicate a scenario where the ability to respond to oxidative stress is compromised in non-receptive endometrial fluid aspirate (EFA). This is partly due to the potential inhibition of Nrf2, which is a key regulator of the oxidative stress response, as it is responsible for activating a range of antioxidant genes. Overall, eight proteins were identified with strong dysregulation: Mucin-16 (MUC16), Heat shock 70 kDa protein 4 (HSP74), Prostaglandin E synthase 3 (TEBP), Follistatin-related protein 3 (FSTL3), Glycogen phosphorylase (PYGB), Ubiquitin-like modifier-activating enzyme 1 (UBA1), Peptidyl-prolyl cis-trans isomerase A (PPIA), and 14-3-3 protein epsilon (1433E) ($q < 0.05$). One of them, glycogen phosphorylase B (PYGB), was selected for confirmatory analysis by Western blot, where its reduced expression in samples from women with RIF was verified (p-value < 0.05). PYGB is an enzyme that plays a key role in glycogen metabolism and dysregulation of PYGB can lead to glycogen storage diseases. MUC16 provides a protective, lubricating barrier against particles and infectious agents at mucosal surfaces, as well as suppresses the cytolytic responses of NK cells. HSP74 is a member of the HSP70 family, functioning as a molecular chaperone to assist in protein folding and refolding under stress conditions, while it also plays a crucial role in maintaining protein homeostasis. TEBP has anti-inflammatory and immunomodulatory effects. FSTL3 is a multifunctional protein involved in various biological processes, including cell development, inflammation regulation, and metabolism. UBA1 is an E1 enzyme in the ubiquitin-proteasome system (UPS), which is responsible for tagging proteins with ubiquitin for degradation. PPIA, also known as cyclophilin A, is an enzyme that catalyses protein folding, and plays a role in the regulation of the immune response and protein cycle. 1433E is a member of the 14-3-3 protein family, which binds to various target proteins to modulate their activity and is involved in the regulation of ion concentration, cell–cell adhesion and cellular signaling. Based on the results of this study, the research team supported that the analysis of endometrial fluid has the ability to detect the increased inflammatory status in non-receptive endometrial samples. Additionally, they proposed PYGB as a potential biomarker for predicting endometrial receptivity or the success of implantation [26].

The team of Kasvandik et al. in 2019, analyzed endometrial fluid samples (UF) obtained from the endometrium of early and mid-secretory phase of fertile women and women with RIF, to determine if the proteome of uterine fluid could be used to monitor the window of implantation (WOI). Using mass spectrometry, 367 proteins were identified, which underwent significant changes during the transition from the early to mid-secretory phase of the endometrium ($q \leq 0.05$, fold change (FC) range: -15.2 to $+60.9$). Subsequently,

45 of these proteins (with $|FC| \geq 5$, $q < 0.05$) were further analyzed by targeted MS, and 21 were found to exhibit similar levels between the early secretory phase group of fertile women and the mid-secretory phase group of women with RIF, indicating the temporal shift of the window of implantation in women with RIF. The panel of proteins PGR (progesterone receptor), NNMT (nicotinamide N-methyltransferase), SLC26A2 (Solute Carrier family 26 member 2), and LCN2 (lipocalin-2) showed high specificity (91.7%) and sensitivity (91.7%) in distinguishing samples from the mid-secretory phase from those of the early secretory phase. The same panel distinguished with high specificity (91.7%) and sensitivity (96.6%) the samples from the mid-secretory phase of the endometrium of fertile women from those of women with RIF. PGR is a nuclear receptor protein that mediates the biological effects of progesterone hormone. NNMT is an enzyme involved in the metabolism of nicotinamide, as well as in the regulation of cellular methylation and metabolism. SLC26A2 is a sulfate transporter protein involved in the transport of sulfate ions across cell membranes. LCN is an iron-trafficking protein participating in multiple processes such as apoptosis and innate immunity. Based on the above results, this study demonstrated that the proteins present in uterine fluid, obtained with minimal invasiveness, can be used to assess endometrial receptivity. Furthermore, women with RIF appear to have a differentiated protein profile during the mid-secretory phase of the endometrium, a factor that is highly likely to contribute to the low success rate of implantation [27].

Table 1 summarizes the proteins that showed differential expression in the endometrium of women with recurrent implantation failure (RIF) and is based on the results of all the studies mentioned in this review, both those that compared protein expression in endometrial biopsies and those that analyzed endometrial fluid samples.

Table 1. Summary of proteins with differential expression in the endometrium of women with recurrent implantation failure (RIF).

Protein	Basic Role/Function	Compared Groups	Specimen/Phase of the Cycle	Altered Expression in Women with RIF	Study
Apolipoprotein-A1 (apoA-I)	Lipid metabolism	RIF samples vs. Control	Endometrial biopsies/Follicular phase	Increased expression	Brosens et al. [12]
Interleukin-15 (IL-15)	NK cells proliferation	RIF samples vs. Control	Endometrial biopsies/Ovulation	Increased expression	Mariee et al. [13]
Leukemic inhibitory factor (LIF)	Immune tolerance between endometrial–blastocyst junction	RIF samples vs. Control	Endometrial biopsies/Ovulation	Decreased expression	Mariee et al. [13]
Phosphoglucomutase 1 (PGM1)	Carbohydrate metabolism	ERA-NR samples vs. ERA-R	Endometrial sample/Prereceptive	Decreased expression	Garrido-Gómez et al. [14]
Alpha-enolase (ENO1)	Carbohydrate metabolism	ERA-NR samples vs. ERA-R	Endometrial sample/Prereceptive	Increased expression	Garrido-Gómez et al. [14]
Sialic acid synthase (SIAS)	Carbohydrate metabolism	ERA-NR samples vs. ERA-R	Endometrial sample/Prereceptive	Decreased expression	Garrido-Gómez et al. [14]
Annexin-6 (ANXA6)	Mediates calcium-dependent secretion of exosomes during plasma membrane repair/Involvement in apoptosis mechanism	ERA-NR samples vs. ERA-R	Endometrial sample/Prereceptive	Increased expression	Garrido-Gómez et al. [14]
		RIF samples vs. Control	Cultured endometrial stromal cells/Secretory	Increased expression	Dhaenes et al. [16]
Progesterone receptor membrane component 1 (PGRMC1)	Progesterone binding/Heme homeostasis/Interaction with cytochromes P450 (CYPs)	ERA-NR samples vs. ERA-R	Endometrial sample/Prereceptive	Increased expression	Garrido-Gómez et al. [14]
Telomerase reverse transcriptase (TERT)	Creation of telomeres in DNA	RIF samples vs. Control	Endometrial biopsies/Implantation window	Increased expression	Long et al. [15]
Estrogen receptor alpha (ER alpha)	Estrogen binding/DNA binding/Transcription activation	RIF samples vs. Control	Endometrial biopsies/Implantation window	Decreased expression	Long et al. [15]

Table 1. *Cont.*

Protein	Basic Role/Function	Compared Groups	Specimen/Phase of the Cycle	Altered Expression in Women with RIF	Study
26S proteasome regulatory subunit 8 (PSMC5)	Protein degradation	RIF samples vs. Control	Cultured endometrial stromal cells/Secretory	Increased expression	Dhaenes et al. [16]
Fascin-1 (FSCN1)	Participation in the organization of the cellular cytoskeleton (formation of microfilaments)	RIF samples vs. Control	Cultured endometrial stromal cells/Secretory	Increased expression	Dhaenes et al. [16]
pre-B-cell leukaemia transcription factor-interacting protein 1 (PBXIP1)	Regulation of protein degradation and autophagy	RIF samples vs. Control	Cultured endometrial stromal cells/Secretory	Decreased expression	Dhaenes et al. [16]
double homeobox protein 4-like protein 2 (DUX4L2)	Regulation of gene expression	RIF non decidualized samples vs. RIF decidualized	Cultured endometrial stromal cells/Secretory	Decreased expression	Dhaenes et al. [16]
protein canopy homologue 4 (CNPY4)	Participation in cell adhesion and cell migration/Signaling/Maintenance of tissue homeostasis	RIF non decidualized samples vs. RIF decidualized	Cultured endometrial stromal cells/Secretory	Increased expression	Dhaenes et al. [16]
high affinity cAMP-specific 3′,5′-cyclic phosphodiesterase 7A (PDE7A)	Involved in the regulation of cyclic adenosine monophosphate (cAMP)	RIF non decidualized samples vs. RIF decidualized	Cultured endometrial stromal cells/Secretory	Decreased expression	Dhaenes et al. [16]
Cathepsin K (CTSK)	Involved in collagen degradation	RIF non decidualized samples vs. RIF decidualized	Cultured endometrial stromal cells/Secretory	Decreased expression	Dhaenes et al. [16]
poly(rC)-binding protein 2 (PCBP2)	Regulation of translation/Regulation of gene expression/Participation in intracellular signaling	RIF non decidualized samples vs. RIF decidualized	Cultured endometrial stromal cells/Secretory	Decreased expression	Dhaenes et al. [16]
26S proteasome non-ATPase regulatory subunit 4 (PSMD4)	Regulation of protein degradation	RIF non decidualized samples vs. RIF decidualized	Cultured endometrial stromal cells/Secretory	Decreased expression	Dhaenes et al. [16]
Epiplakin-1 (EPPK1)	Structural support of the epidermis/Immunological response to HPV infection	RIF samples vs. Control	Endometrial scratch biopsies/Luteal Phase	Increased expression	Bielfeld et al. [17]
Bcl-2-related transcription factor (BCLAF1)	Regulation of apoptosis/Regulation of gene transcription/Regulation of immune response	RIF samples vs. Control	Endometrial scratch biopsies/Luteal Phase	Increased expression	Bielfeld et al. [17]
Prothymosin-α (PTMA)	Intracellularly participates in the regulation of the cell cycle, transcription and apoptosis/Extracellularly acts as an immunomodulator	RIF samples vs. Control	Endometrial scratch biopsies/Luteal Phase	Decreased expression	Bielfeld et al. [17]
Corticosteroid-binding globulin (CBG)	Transport and regulation of corticosteroid hormone availability	RIF samples vs. Control	Endometrial biopsies	Increased expression	Wang et al. [18]
Fetuin-A (FETUA)	Involved in inflammatory response/Participation in calcium storage in tissues/Regulation of blood sugar	RIF samples vs. Control	Endometrial biopsies	Increased expression	Wang et al. [18]
DNA topoisomerase-alpha (TOP2A)	Involvement in DNA replication, splicing and repression	RIF samples vs. Control	Endometrial biopsies/Luteal Phase	Decreased expression	Fu et al. [19]
tubulin polymerization-promoting protein family member 3 (TPPP3)	Promotion of microtubule accumulation and maintenance of microtubule system stability	RIF samples vs. Control	Endometrial tissue/Luteal Phase	Decreased expression	Yang et al. [20]

Table 1. *Cont.*

Protein	Basic Role/Function	Compared Groups	Specimen/Phase of the Cycle	Altered Expression in Women with RIF	Study
S100 Calcium Binding Protein A13 (S100A13)	Calcium homeostasis/ Cell proliferation/ Apoptosis/Inflammation Response	RIF samples vs. Control	Endometrial tissue/Luteal Phase	Decreased expression	Yang et al. [20]
17b-hydroxysteroid dehydrogenase 2 (HSD17B2)	Synthesis and inactivation of estrogens and androgens	RIF samples vs. Control	Endometrial tissue/Luteal Phase	Decreased expression	Yang et al. [20]
alpha-2-glycoprotein 1, zinc binding (AZGP1)	Lipolysis/Glucose transport	RIF samples vs. Control	Endometrial tissue/Luteal Phase	Decreased expression	Yang et al. [20]
Claudin-4	Formation of tight junction between cells/Control of permeability of substances in epithelium	RIF samples vs. RIS samples	Endometrial biopsy/Luteal Phase	Increased expression	Zhao et al. [21]
Kinase p38	Involvement in stress and inflammatory response/Regulation of cell growth and apoptosis	RIF samples vs. RIS samples	Endometrial biopsy/Luteal Phase	Increased expression	Zhao et al. [21]
AMP-activated protein kinase subunit B (PRKAB)	Regulation of cellular energy balance	RIF samples vs. RIS samples	Endometrial biopsy/Luteal Phase	Increased expression	Zhao et al. [21]
Inhibitor of NF-kB subunit-b (IKB-b)	Regulation of inflammation and immune cellular response/Maintenance of cellular homeostasis	RIF samples vs. RIS samples	Endometrial biopsy/Luteal Phase	Increased expression	Zhao et al. [21]
Myosin-2	Formation of smooth muscle fiber arrays/Participation in movement and the mechanism of tightening the cell membrane	RIF samples vs. RIS samples	Endometrial biopsy/Luteal Phase	Decreased expression	Zhao et al. [21]
Protein Kinase G (PKG2)	Regulation of cell signaling/Regulation of the cell cytoplasm and cytoskeleton array	RIF samples vs. RIS samples	Endometrial biopsy/Luteal Phase	Decreased expression	Zhao et al. [21]
Matrix metalloproteinase-2 (MMP-2)	Degradation of collagen type IV/Participation in angiogenesis/Migration and spreading of cells	RIF samples vs. Control	Endometrial fluid/Luteal Phase	Increased expression	Inagaki et al. [23], Yoshii et al. [24]
Matrix metalloproteinase-9 (MMP-9)	Degradation of collagen and gelatin/Participation in tissue development and regeneration/Involvement in immune response	RIF samples vs. Control	Endometrial fluid/Luteal Phase	Increased expression	Inagaki et al. [23], Yoshii et al. [24]
Interleukin-1beta (IL-1beta)	Promotion of inflammatory and immune response	RIF samples vs. Control	Endometrial fluid/Luteal Phase	Increased expression	Inagaki et al. [23]
Interferon-gamma (IFN-gamma)	Regulation of lymphocyte activity/Control of inflammatory response	RIF samples vs. Control	Endometrial fluid/Luteal Phase	Decreased expression	Inagaki et al. [23]
Interleukin-10 (IL-10)	Suppression of the immune response/Anti-inflammatory action	RIF samples vs. Control	Endometrial fluid/Luteal Phase	Decreased expression	Inagaki et al. [23]
Glycogen phosphorylase B (PYGB)	Regulation of glycogen metabolism	RIF samples vs. Control	Endometrial fluid aspiration/Luteal Phase—Before Embryotransfer	Decreased expression	Azkargorta et al. [26]
Prostaglandin E synthase 3 (TEBP)	Anti-inflammatory and immunomodulatory effects	RIF samples vs. Control	Endometrial fluid aspiration/Luteal Phase—Before Embryotransfer	Decreased expression	Azkargorta et al. [26]
Heat shock 70 kDa protein 4 (HSP74)	Participation in cellular stress control mechanisms/Antigen presentation/Involvement in protein cycle regulation	RIF samples vs. Control	Endometrial fluid aspiration/Luteal Phase—Before Embryotransfer	Decreased expression	Azkargorta et al. [26]

Table 1. *Cont.*

Protein	Basic Role/Function	Compared Groups	Specimen/Phase of the Cycle	Altered Expression in Women with RIF	Study
Mucin-16	Regulation of immune responses	RIF samples vs. Control	Endometrial fluid aspiration/Luteal Phase—Before Embryotransfer	Increased expression	Azkargorta et al. [26]
Peptidyl-prolyl cis-trans isomerase A (PPIA)	Protein folding/Regulation of immune response and protein cycle	RIF samples vs. Control	Endometrial fluid aspiration/Luteal Phase—Before Embryotransfer	Decreased expression	Azkargorta et al. [26]
Follistatin-related protein 3 (FSTL3)	Participation in the differentiation of primitive hematopoietic cells/Regulation of metabolism/Possible influence on oocyte maturation	RIF samples vs. Control	Endometrial fluid aspiration/Luteal Phase—Before Embryotransfer	Increased expression	Azkargorta et al. [26]
14-3-3protein epsilon (1433E)	Regulation of ion concentration/Regulation of cell–cell adhesion/Regulation of cellular signaling	RIF samples vs. Control	Endometrial fluid aspiration/Luteal Phase—Before Embryotransfer	Decreased expression	Azkargorta et al. [26]
Ubiquitin-like modifier-activating enzyme 1 (UBA1)	Regulation of protein degradation	RIF samples vs. Control	Endometrial fluid aspiration/Luteal Phase—Before Embryotransfer	Decreased expression	Azkargorta et al. [26]
Progesterone receptor (PGR)	Regulation of menstrual cycle/Promotion of the secretory phase of the endometrium	RIF samples vs. Control	Endometrial fluid/Secretory Phase	Increased expression	Kasvandik et al. [27]
Nicotinamide N-methyltransferase (NNMT)	Methylation of nicotinamide/Regulation of metabolism/Epigenetic regulation/Participation in cell proliferation and differentiation/Participation in inflammatory response	RIF samples vs. Control	Endometrial fluid/Secretory Phase	Decreased expression	Kasvandik et al. [27]
Solute Carrier family 26 member 2 (SLC26A2)	Transport of ions and inorganic molecules/Regulation of ion balance	RIF samples vs. Control	Endometrial fluid/Secretory Phase	Decreased expression	Kasvandik et al. [27]
Lipocalin-2 (LCN2)	Antimicrobial action/Iron binding	RIF samples vs. Control	Endometrial fluid/Secretory Phase	Decreased expression	Kasvandik et al. [27]

RIF: recurrent implantation failure, ERA-NR: endometrial receptivity analysis—non-receptive, ERA-R: endometrial receptivity analysis—receptive, RIS: recurrent implantation successes.

4. Discussion

Recurrent implantation failure (RIF) undeniably constitutes a serious and multifaceted problem in assisted reproduction, for which significant research effort has been made in recent years by many scientific teams. The aim of the research studies that have been carried out to date, which, for the most part, included genetic and transcriptomic studies, has been to understand the causes and mechanisms that can lead to RIF, to develop specific tests for the early diagnosis of women prone to implantation failure and to find new therapeutic approaches.

Over the last two decades, many potential molecular markers and proteins associated with endometrial receptivity have been identified. Despite all efforts, current tests for endometrial receptivity prior to embryo transfer, which involve invasive biopsies and rely on endometrial transcriptome analysis, result in modest improvements in implantation outcomes. According to the results of a meta-analysis, the rates of ongoing pregnancy (OPR) and live births (LBR) were comparable between patients with RIF diagnosed after endometrial receptivity testing, with non-receptive endometrium, who underwent personalized embryo transfer (p-ET), and patients with receptive endometrium who underwent embryo transfer based on the standard protocol [28]. On the contrary, according to a recent multicenter cohort study in patients with a previous failed embryo transfer, the LBR and cumulative LBR were higher after embryo transfer based on the standard protocol compared to personalized embryo transfer (p-ET), which was performed after endometrial receptivity testing [29]. ESHRE supports that there is insufficient evidence to recommend the use of currently available endometrial receptivity tests in ART and states that more studies are needed to determine their value in managing patients with RIF [3]. Therefore, the field of human reproductive medicine needs more precise and quantitative, yet rapid and non-invasive assessments to further improve pregnancy rates.

Proteomics represents a modern, technology-driven science that studies proteins and their post-translational modifications and interactions, providing exceptionally high-precision qualitative and quantitative results. The proteome is more than the translated products of the genetic material, as proteins significantly differ in stability and rates of modification, have different spatiotemporal regulation, undergo epigenetic and post-translational modifications, and interact with other proteins to create structural and functional complexes [30]. Therefore, the proteomic profile is simultaneously multifaceted and dynamic, spatially and temporally, and proteomic analysis is capable of reflecting various phases of cell differentiation and states.

In transcriptomic studies, compelling evidence has shown that there are distinct transcriptional characteristics in the endometrium during various phases [31,32], and a recent test for endometrial receptivity (ERA) has been applied as a diagnostic tool in some assisted reproduction centers [33,34]. However, there are still some limitations in the depth of understanding of endometrial receptivity based on transcriptional results because not all RNA messages are translated into proteins, and post-transcriptional, translational, and post-translational regulations are extensively applied. The use of proteomic analysis in the investigation of endometrial receptivity is extremely useful and promising with the new innovative methods that it includes, as it can provide more information and contribute both in understanding the protein expression of the endometrium during the "window of implantation", as well as in finding reliable biomarkers for assessment of the receptivity of the endometrium, with the ultimate goal of timely and accurate therapeutic intervention in the cases of women with RIF.

Big data analysis and proteomics, the large-scale study of proteins, have become increasingly intertwined in modern biological research. One of the proteomic techniques that is widely used for protein identification and quantification is Mass spectrometry (MS). MS is a rapid and reliable method for proteomic analysis, especially when coupled with liquid chromatography (LC-MS/MS) for high-throughput applications. Additionally, with the appropriate setup, MS is able to provide simultaneous results for a large number and types of samples [35]. Multiplexed assays, such as immunoassays or protein arrays, can also be relatively fast depending on the specific technology and allow the simultaneous measurement of multiple proteins in a single sample, providing high throughput. They can also provide simultaneous results for a large number of samples, especially in the case of microarray-based methods and are preferred for targeted analysis of specific proteins or pathways [36].

In the present review, several important proteomic studies of the endometrium conducted over the last 20 years were discussed. Studies comparing endometrial tissues of fertile women with those of women with RIF mostly showed that there are proteins exhibiting differential expression between the compared groups during the receptive endometrial phase. Regarding studies focusing on protein expression in the endometrial fluid, they also demonstrate a differentiated proteomic profile during the mid-secretory phase of the endometrium. Overall, several proteins considered to be associated with endometrial receptivity have been identified in 14 of 15 studies that are concluded in this review, in both samples of endometrial tissue and endometrial fluid. However, the number and profile of proteins in different phases of the endometrium varied significantly among studies. These variations are most likely due to the different experimental conditions of studies. Nevertheless, it could be proposed that the proteins revealed to be important for endometrial receptivity and are common in the majority of studies may after further research serve as effective biomarkers. Such proteins are annexin-6 [14,16], progesterone receptor [14,27], MMP-2 and MMP-9 [23,24].

However, while many biomarkers have been proposed for endometrial receptivity, it is necessary for the optimal set of them to be selected and validated in multicenter, prospective, and reliable randomized trials to establish their clinical application in assisted reproduction. Additionally, due to the many discrepancies among studies, it is necessary to have common designs of proteomic and bioinformatic analysis experiments [11]. The publication by Altmäe et al. has proposed a guide for study design, sample collection and processing, data processing and analysis, as well as the validation of endometrial proteomic studies [37]. Furthermore, although many proteins with differential expression have been identified as correlated with endometrial receptivity through proteomics, achieving synchronization between the embryo and the endometrium is extremely important yet complex as a process. For this reason, the design of in vitro studies, which conduct simultaneous analysis of proteins produced by embryonic trophoblast cells and proteins produced by the endometrium, could be helpful.

5. Conclusions

In conclusion, the use of proteomics contributes towards understanding the protein expression of the endometrium in women with RIF and towards finding biomarkers of endometrial receptivity. To our knowledge this is the first review that aims to summarize the differentially expressed proteins in tissue and endometrial fluid in women with recurrent implantation failure. However, there is a need for a standardized model for designing proteomic and bioinformatics analysis experiments. Furthermore, a future goal is the more extensive analysis of proteins in endometrial fluid—which does not require invasive methods—and the implementation of new diagnostic tests using endometrial receptivity biomarkers in clinical practice, leading to personalized embryo transfer, after confirming the synchronization of embryo and endometrial development. It is also necessary to select the optimal set of proposed biomarkers and validate them in multicenter, prospective, and randomized controlled trials, to establish their application in clinical routine. The field of proteomics has strong potential to improve the embryo implantation rate after IVF in women with recurrent implantation failure (RIF), resulting in significantly increased pregnancy and birth rates.

Author Contributions: Conceptualization, A.P. and E.A.; methodology, D.M., P.P. and S.S.; validation, E.D., T.K. and C.S.; data curation, E.A.; writing—original draft preparation, A.P. and E.A.; writing—review and editing, P.M., S.T., E.D., D.M., T.K., A.Z. and P.D.; visualization, A.P.; supervision, C.S., P.P. and P.D.; project administration, S.S. All authors have read and agreed to the published version of the manuscript.

Funding: This research received no external funding.

Institutional Review Board Statement: Not applicable.

Informed Consent Statement: Not applicable.

Data Availability Statement: Not applicable.

Conflicts of Interest: The authors declare no conflicts of interest.

References

1. Busnelli, A.; Reschini, M.; Cardellicchio, L.; Vegetti, W.; Somigliana, E.; Vercellini, P. How common is real repeated implantation failure? An indirect estimate of the prevalence. *Reprod. Biomed. Online* **2020**, *40*, 91–97. [CrossRef] [PubMed]
2. Coughlan, C.; Ledger, W.; Wang, Q.; Liu, F.; Demirol, A.; Gurgan, T.; Cutting, R.; Ong, K.; Sallam, H.; Li, T.C. Recurrent implantation failure: Definition and management. *Reprod. Biomed. Online* **2014**, *28*, 14–38. [CrossRef]
3. Cimadomo, D.; de Los Santos, M.J.; Griesinger, G.; Lainas, G.; Le Clef, N.; McLernon, D.J.; Montjean, D.; Toth, B.; Vermeulen, N.; Macklon, N.; et al. ESHRE good practice recommendations on recurrent implantation failure. *Hum. Reprod. Open* **2023**, *2023*, hoad023. [CrossRef] [PubMed]

4. Vaduva, C.C.; Constantinescu, C.; Serbanescu, M.; Dara, L.; Oancea, M.D.; Carp-Veliscu, A. The association between endometrial polyps, chronic endometritis, and IVF outcomes. *Eur. Rev. Med. Pharmacol. Sci.* **2023**, *27*, 8895–8904. [CrossRef] [PubMed]
5. Buzzaccarini, G.; Vitagliano, A.; Andrisani, A.; Santarsiero, C.M.; Cicinelli, R.; Nardelli, C.; Ambrosini, G.; Cicinelli, E. Chronic endometritis and altered embryo implantation: A unified pathophysiological theory from a literature systematic review. *J. Assist. Reprod. Genet.* **2020**, *37*, 2897–2911. [CrossRef]
6. Panagopoulos, P.; Mavrogianni, D.; Christodoulaki, C.; Drakaki, E.; Chrelias, G.; Panagiotopoulos, D.; Potiris, A.; Drakakis, P.; Stavros, S. Effects of endocrine disrupting compounds on female fertility. *Best Pract. Res. Clin. Obstet. Gynaecol.* **2023**, *88*, 102347. [CrossRef]
7. Ma, J.; Gao, W.; Li, D. Recurrent implantation failure: A comprehensive summary from etiology to treatment. *Front. Endocrinol.* **2022**, *13*, 1061766. [CrossRef] [PubMed]
8. Potiris, A.; Perros, P.; Drakaki, E.; Mavrogianni, D.; Machairiotis, N.; Sfakianakis, A.; Karampitsakos, T.; Vrachnis, D.; Antonakopoulos, N.; Panagopoulos, P.; et al. Investigating the Association of Assisted Reproduction Techniques and Adverse Perinatal Outcomes. *J. Clin. Med.* **2024**, *13*, 328. [CrossRef]
9. Craciunas, L.; Gallos, I.; Chu, J.; Bourne, T.; Quenby, S.; Brosens, J.J.; Coomarasamy, A. Conventional and modern markers of endometrial receptivity: A systematic review and meta-analysis. *Hum. Reprod. Update* **2019**, *25*, 202–223. [CrossRef]
10. Aslam, B.; Basit, M.; Nisar, M.A.; Khurshid, M.; Rasool, M.H. Proteomics: Technologies and Their Applications. *J. Chromatogr. Sci.* **2017**, *55*, 182–196. [CrossRef]
11. Hernandez-Vargas, P.; Munoz, M.; Dominguez, F. Identifying biomarkers for predicting successful embryo implantation: Applying single to multi-OMICs to improve reproductive outcomes. *Hum. Reprod. Update* **2020**, *26*, 264–301. [CrossRef] [PubMed]
12. Brosens, J.J.; Hodgetts, A.; Feroze-Zaidi, F.; Sherwin, J.R.; Fusi, L.; Salker, M.S.; Higham, J.; Rose, G.L.; Kajihara, T.; Young, S.L.; et al. Proteomic analysis of endometrium from fertile and infertile patients suggests a role for apolipoprotein A-I in embryo implantation failure and endometriosis. *Mol. Hum. Reprod.* **2010**, *16*, 273–285. [CrossRef] [PubMed]
13. Mariee, N.; Li, T.C.; Laird, S.M. Expression of leukaemia inhibitory factor and interleukin 15 in endometrium of women with recurrent implantation failure after IVF; correlation with the number of endometrial natural killer cells. *Hum. Reprod.* **2012**, *27*, 1946–1954. [CrossRef] [PubMed]
14. Garrido-Gomez, T.; Quinonero, A.; Antunez, O.; Diaz-Gimeno, P.; Bellver, J.; Simon, C.; Dominguez, F. Deciphering the proteomic signature of human endometrial receptivity. *Hum. Reprod.* **2014**, *29*, 1957–1967. [CrossRef] [PubMed]
15. Long, N.; Liu, N.; Liu, X.L.; Li, J.; Cai, B.Y.; Cai, X. Endometrial expression of telomerase, progesterone, and estrogen receptors during the implantation window in patients with recurrent implantation failure. *Genet. Mol. Res.* **2016**, *15*, gmr.15027849. [CrossRef] [PubMed]
16. Dhaenens, L.; Lierman, S.; De Clerck, L.; Govaert, E.; Deforce, D.; Tilleman, K.; De Sutter, P. Endometrial stromal cell proteome mapping in repeated implantation failure and recurrent pregnancy loss cases and fertile women. *Reprod. Biomed. Online* **2019**, *38*, 442–454. [CrossRef]
17. Bielfeld, A.P.; Pour, S.J.; Poschmann, G.; Stuhler, K.; Krussel, J.S.; Baston-Bust, D.M. A Proteome Approach Reveals Differences between Fertile Women and Patients with Repeated Implantation Failure on Endometrial Level(-) Does hCG Render the Endometrium of RIF Patients? *Int. J. Mol. Sci.* **2019**, *20*, 425. [CrossRef] [PubMed]
18. Wang, C.; Feng, Y.; Zhou, W.J.; Cheng, Z.J.; Jiang, M.Y.; Zhou, Y.; Fei, X.Y. Screening and identification of endometrial proteins as novel potential biomarkers for repeated implantation failure. *PeerJ* **2021**, *9*, e11009. [CrossRef] [PubMed]
19. Fu, H.; Tan, W.; Chen, Z.; Ye, Z.; Duan, Y.; Huang, J.; Qi, H.; Liu, X. TOP2A deficit-induced abnormal decidualization leads to recurrent implantation failure via the NF-kappaB signaling pathway. *Reprod. Biol. Endocrinol.* **2022**, *20*, 142. [CrossRef] [PubMed]
20. Yang, J.; Wang, L.; Ma, J.; Diao, L.; Chen, J.; Cheng, Y.; Yang, J.; Li, L. Endometrial proteomic profile of patients with repeated implantation failure. *Front. Endocrinol.* **2023**, *14*, 1144393. [CrossRef]
21. Zhao, J.; Hao, J.; Xu, B.; Li, Y. Recurrent implantation failure versus recurrent implantation success: A preliminary study at proteomic level. *Gynecol. Endocrinol.* **2023**, *39*, 2217261. [CrossRef]
22. Perez-Deben, S.; Bellver, J.; Alama, P.; Salsano, S.; Quinonero, A.; Sebastian-Leon, P.; Diaz-Gimeno, P.; Dominguez, F. iTRAQ comparison of proteomic profiles of endometrial receptivity. *J. Proteom.* **2019**, *203*, 103381. [CrossRef] [PubMed]
23. Inagaki, N.; Stern, C.; McBain, J.; Lopata, A.; Kornman, L.; Wilkinson, D. Analysis of intra-uterine cytokine concentration and matrix-metalloproteinase activity in women with recurrent failed embryo transfer. *Hum. Reprod.* **2003**, *18*, 608–615. [CrossRef] [PubMed]
24. Yoshii, N.; Hamatani, T.; Inagaki, N.; Hosaka, T.; Inoue, O.; Yamada, M.; Machiya, R.; Yoshimura, Y.; Odawara, Y. Successful implantation after reducing matrix metalloproteinase activity in the uterine cavity. *Reprod. Biol. Endocrinol.* **2013**, *11*, 37. [CrossRef] [PubMed]
25. Benkhalifa, M.; Zayani, Y.; Bach, V.; Copin, H.; Feki, M.; Benkhalifa, M.; Allal-Elasmi, M. Does the dysregulation of matrix metalloproteinases contribute to recurrent implantation failure? *Expert. Rev. Proteom.* **2018**, *15*, 311–323. [CrossRef] [PubMed]
26. Azkargorta, M.; Escobes, I.; Iloro, I.; Osinalde, N.; Corral, B.; Ibanez-Perez, J.; Exposito, A.; Prieto, B.; Elortza, F.; Matorras, R. Differential proteomic analysis of endometrial fluid suggests increased inflammation and impaired glucose metabolism in non-implantative IVF cycles and pinpoints PYGB as a putative implantation marker. *Hum. Reprod.* **2018**, *33*, 1898–1906. [CrossRef] [PubMed]

27. Kasvandik, S.; Saarma, M.; Kaart, T.; Rooda, I.; Velthut-Meikas, A.; Ehrenberg, A.; Gemzell, K.; Lalitkumar, P.G.; Salumets, A.; Peters, M. Uterine Fluid Proteins for Minimally Invasive Assessment of Endometrial Receptivity. *J. Clin. Endocrinol. Metab.* **2020**, *105*, 219–230. [CrossRef]
28. Liu, Z.; Liu, X.; Wang, M.; Zhao, H.; He, S.; Lai, S.; Qu, Q.; Wang, X.; Zhao, D.; Bao, H. The Clinical Efficacy of Personalized Embryo Transfer Guided by the Endometrial Receptivity Array/Analysis on IVF/ICSI Outcomes: A Systematic Review and Meta-Analysis. *Front. Physiol.* **2022**, *13*, 841437. [CrossRef] [PubMed]
29. Cozzolino, M.; Diaz-Gimeno, P.; Pellicer, A.; Garrido, N. Use of the endometrial receptivity array to guide personalized embryo transfer after a failed transfer attempt was associated with a lower cumulative and per transfer live birth rate during donor and autologous cycles. *Fertil. Steril.* **2022**, *118*, 724–736. [CrossRef]
30. Ahrens, C.H.; Brunner, E.; Qeli, E.; Basler, K.; Aebersold, R. Generating and navigating proteome maps using mass spectrometry. *Nat. Rev. Mol. Cell Biol.* **2010**, *11*, 789–801. [CrossRef]
31. Riesewijk, A.; Martin, J.; van Os, R.; Horcajadas, J.A.; Polman, J.; Pellicer, A.; Mosselman, S.; Simon, C. Gene expression profiling of human endometrial receptivity on days LH+2 versus LH+7 by microarray technology. *Mol. Hum. Reprod.* **2003**, *9*, 253–264. [CrossRef] [PubMed]
32. Hu, S.; Yao, G.; Wang, Y.; Xu, H.; Ji, X.; He, Y.; Zhu, Q.; Chen, Z.; Sun, Y. Transcriptomic changes during the pre-receptive to receptive transition in human endometrium detected by RNA-Seq. *J. Clin. Endocrinol. Metab.* **2014**, *99*, E2744–E2753. [CrossRef] [PubMed]
33. Hromadova, L.; Tokareva, I.; Vesela, K.; Travnik, P.; Vesely, J. Endometrial Receptivity Analysis—A tool to increase an implantation rate in assisted reproduction. *Ces. Gynekol.* **2019**, *84*, 177–183.
34. Diaz-Gimeno, P.; Ruiz-Alonso, M.; Blesa, D.; Bosch, N.; Martinez-Conejero, J.A.; Alama, P.; Garrido, N.; Pellicer, A.; Simon, C. The accuracy and reproducibility of the endometrial receptivity array is superior to histology as a diagnostic method for endometrial receptivity. *Fertil. Steril.* **2013**, *99*, 508–517. [CrossRef]
35. Aebersold, R.; Mann, M. Mass-spectrometric exploration of proteome structure and function. *Nature* **2016**, *537*, 347–355. [CrossRef] [PubMed]
36. Chen, J.; Schwarz, E. Opportunities and Challenges of Multiplex Assays: A Machine Learning Perspective. *Methods Mol. Biol.* **2017**, *1546*, 115–122. [CrossRef]
37. Altmae, S.; Esteban, F.J.; Stavreus-Evers, A.; Simon, C.; Giudice, L.; Lessey, B.A.; Horcajadas, J.A.; Macklon, N.S.; D'Hooghe, T.; Campoy, C.; et al. Guidelines for the design, analysis and interpretation of 'omics' data: Focus on human endometrium. *Hum. Reprod. Update* **2014**, *20*, 12–28. [CrossRef]

Journal of
Clinical Medicine

MDPI

Review

Comprehensive Review of In Vitro Human Follicle Development for Fertility Restoration: Recent Achievements, Current Challenges, and Future Optimization Strategies

Francisco Vitale [1] and Marie-Madeleine Dolmans [1,2,*]

1 Gynecology Research Unit, Institut de Recherche Expérimentale et Clinique, Université Catholique de Louvain, Avenue Mounier 52, 1200 Brussels, Belgium; francisco.vitale@uclouvain.be

2 Gynecology Department, Cliniques Universitaires Saint-Luc, 1200 Brussels, Belgium

* Correspondence: marie-madeleine.dolmans@uclouvain.be; Tel.: +32-2-764-5237

Abstract: Ovarian tissue cryopreservation (OTC) and subsequent transplantation (OTT) is a fertility preservation technique widely offered to prepubertal girls and young fertile women who need to undergo oncological treatment but are at a high risk of infertility. However, OTT is not considered safe in patients with certain diseases like leukemia, Burkitt's lymphoma, and ovarian cancer because of the associated risk of malignant cell reintroduction. In vitro follicle development has therefore emerged as a promising means of obtaining mature metaphase II (MII) oocytes from the primordial follicle (PMF) pool contained within cryopreserved ovarian tissue, without the need for transplantation. Despite its significant potential, this novel approach remains highly challenging, as it requires replication of the intricate process of intraovarian folliculogenesis. Recent advances in multi-step in vitro culture (IVC) systems, tailored to the specific needs of each follicle stage, have demonstrated the feasibility of generating mature oocytes (MII) from early-stage human follicles. While significant progress has been made, there is still room for improvement in terms of efficiency and productivity, and a long way to go before this IVC approach can be implemented in a clinical setting. This comprehensive review outlines the most significant improvements in recent years, current limitations, and future optimization strategies.

Keywords: folliculogenesis; follicle activation; human ovarian tissue; bovine ovarian tissue; in vitro culture; in vitro growth; in vitro maturation

1. Introduction

Young fertile cancer patients undergoing treatment like chemotherapy or radiotherapy face the threat of iatrogenic fertility impairment due to the gonadotoxicity of these interventions [1–4]. Among fertility preservation techniques developed to address this issue, ovarian tissue cryopreservation (OTC) with subsequent transplantation (OTT) is the only available option for prepubertal girls and patients who cannot postpone their treatment [5,6]. However, auto-transplantation carries the potential risk of reintroducing neoplastic cells, especially in the case of blood-borne malignancies like leukemia and non-Hodgkin's lymphoma, as well as ovarian cancer [7–9].

In recent years, in vitro follicle development has emerged as a promising means of obtaining mature metaphase II (MII) oocytes from the primordial follicle (PMF) pool contained within cryopreserved ovarian cortex, without the need for OTT [10,11]. Indeed, PMFs are a key target for fertility restoration, as they are the most abundant follicle population and can tolerate freezing and thawing procedures [12,13].

Achieving complete in vitro folliculogenesis involves initial activation of quiescent PMFs, further growth and progression through the different stages of development, and then final oocyte maturation prior to in vitro fertilization (IVF). While encouraging, this novel approach remains extremely challenging, since not all signaling mechanisms involved in follicle development are yet fully understood [11,14]. Although it was possible to generate newborns from completely in vitro-derived ovarian follicles in mice well over two decades ago [15], replicating this technique in larger mammals and humans has proven much more problematic. Bovines share greater similarities to humans in terms of reproductive cycles and ovarian follicle kinetics, being a mono-ovular species, in contrast to pigs and mice, which are poly-ovular. Numerous studies were therefore conducted using bovine ovarian tissue as a better model for research into human follicle development.

A few decades ago, insights obtained from ultrasound techniques in cattle paved the way for a deeper understanding of follicle kinetics in humans [16]. Both species' ovarian cycles exhibit follicle waves characterized by synchronized growth of follicle cohorts, with one eventually emerging as dominant while others regress. During ovulation in both species, LH levels increase, triggering ovulation of the dominant follicle. This shared pattern highlights fundamental parallels in the mechanisms underlying follicle wave generation, dominant follicle selection, and the ultimate release of a single egg in both humans and bovines, making the bovine model an ideal framework for extrapolating results to human clinical applications.

We searched the PubMed database (https://pubmed.ncbi.nlm.nih.gov/, accessed on 1 August 2023) for English-language articles relevant to the subject, published up to June 2023. The search specifically targeted in vitro folliculogenesis studies using the following keywords: 'in vitro culture' AND 'ovarian tissue' AND 'ovarian follicles'. A total of 809 articles initially matched these criteria. After identifying original studies that used human or bovine ovarian tissue and were methodologically adequate, the authors selected and reviewed 43 articles. The present review summarizes key advances in in vitro follicle development in humans and bovines in recent years, the main challenges that remain, and strategies to optimize outcomes.

2. Different In Vitro Culture Systems

Since the successful creation of mouse embryos from a complete in vitro follicle development system was first reported [15], various research groups have attempted to devise different in vitro culture (IVC) strategies to mimic the same process in humans. Two principal but opposing approaches have been described: isolated PMF culture versus in situ culture of PMFs within ovarian cortex.

Early attempts to culture isolated PMFs failed to induce growth [17,18] and it became clear that preserving interactions between PMFs and neighboring stromal cells in cortical tissue is crucial to their survival and initial growth [19–21]. This approach typically involves IVC of thin cortical fragments (no more than 1 mm thick) [10]. Physical factors, including tissue surface area and stiffness, can also compromise in vitro cell behavior. The ovarian cortex must therefore be fragmented and any excess medulla removed to optimize the balance between cultured cells and nutrients. Indeed, disproportion between the tissue surface and medium volume could lead to nutrient insufficiency and tissue necrosis, especially during prolonged IVC [22].

Telfer and colleagues recently developed human MII oocytes from PMFs within ovarian tissue using a multi-step IVC procedure [10] (Figure 1). The first step involved activation and early growth of PMFs. Secondary follicles (100–150 μm) were then isolated and individually cultured in V-shaped wells to reach the antral stage, forming cumulus-oocyte complexes (COCs). The final step was maturation of the remaining COCs to the preovulatory stage, enabling collection of mature MII oocytes.

While this approach served to demonstrate the feasibility of the technique, it also revealed its limited effectiveness, yielding only 9 MII oocytes from 160 initial ovarian tissue fragments. Further refinement of the technique is clearly essential before its implementation in clinical practice.

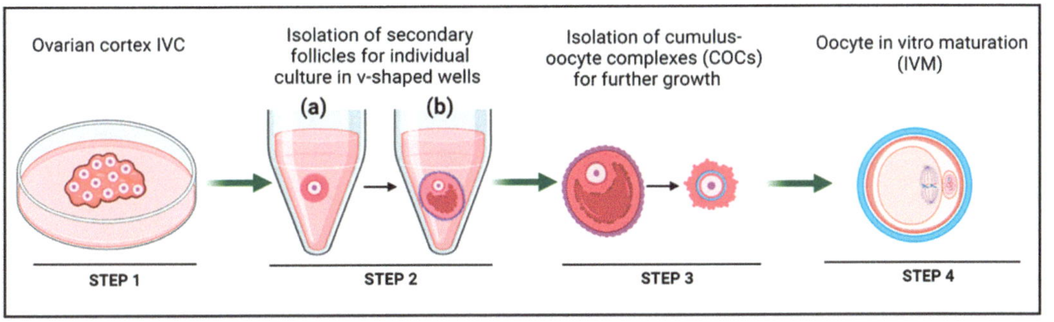

Figure 1. Illustrative representation of the multi-step IVC system supporting in vitro follicle development from PMFs contained within the ovarian cortex to mature MII oocytes, as described by McLaughlin et al., 2018 [10]. Step 1: PMF activation. Step 2: Isolation of secondary follicles (a) and subsequent individual culture in V-shaped wells until the antral follicle stage (b). Step 3: Mechanical dissection of COCs. Step 4: Oocyte IVM until reaching the MII stage. Created with BioRender.com, accessed on 1 January 2024.

3. Follicle Activation: From PMFs to Secondary Follicles

Table 1 summarizes different IVC systems, culture periods, medium components, biomaterials, and isolation methods from publications reporting transition of PMFs to secondary follicles in humans and bovines.

3.1. Culture Medium Composition for the First Step

Culture medium composition is pivotal to maintaining viability, growth, and proliferation of cells in an IVC system. The most commonly used basal media for this phase of human ovarian tissue IVC are alpha minimal essential medium (αMEM) [17,19,20,23–32] and McCoy's 5a [21,33–39]. Waymouth's medium [40–46] is the most widely used medium for bovine ovarian tissue culture (Table 1). In recent years, there has been a consensus on supplements that should be added to the basal culture medium to support follicle survival and growth. Glucose and amino acids like L-glutamine are usually used as energy sources. Insulin, transferrin, and selenium (ITS) are added to increase uptake of soluble metabolic precursors. Antibiotics such as penicillin and streptomycin are given to prevent microorganism growth. In addition, soluble antioxidants like ascorbic acid are frequently added to culture medium, having been shown to reduce cell apoptosis and increase follicle integrity [47–49]. Follicle-stimulating hormone (FSH) and activin A are often included thanks to their effect on granulosa cell (GC) proliferation [10,21]. Medium supplements may also contain serum, such as fetal bovine serum, or serum substitutes, like human serum albumin commonly used as protein complements.

It is essential to replace culture medium after a fixed amount of time in order to prevent nutrient depletion and ensure elimination of toxic waste products, like ammonia and lactic acid. In studies involving IVC for more than four days, standard practice is to replace half of the culture medium every other day [10,21,38,50–53].

Table 1. Publications reporting transition of PMFs to secondary follicles in humans and bovines (step 1).

Publication.	Source	Type of Culture	Culture Period	Culture Medium	Culture System	Biomaterial	Isolation Method
Hovatta et al., 1997 [19]	Human	Ovarian tissue	21 days	αMEM	2D	Extracellular matrix	N/A
Wright et al., 1999 [20]	Human	Ovarian tissue	15 days	αMEM	2D	Matrigel	N/A

Table 1. *Cont.*

Publication.	Source	Type of Culture	Culture Period	Culture Medium	Culture System	Biomaterial	Isolation Method
Abir et al., 1999 [17]	Human	Isolated follicles	1 day	αMEM	3D	Collagen gel	Enzymatic
Hreinsson et al., 2002 [24]	Human	Ovarian tissue	14 days	αMEM	2D	Extracellular matrix	N/A
Scott et al., 2004 [25]	Human	Ovarian tissue	7 days	αMEM	N/A	No	N/A
Amorim et al., 2009 [26]	Human	Isolated follicles	7 days	αMEM	3D	Alginate	Enzymatic
Kedem et al., 2011 [54]	Human	Ovarian tissue	14 days	αMEM	3D	Alginate	N/A
Camboni et al., 2013 [27]	Human	Isolated follicles	7 days	αMEM	3D	Alginate	Enzymatic
Lerer-Serfaty et al., 2013 [28]	Human	Ovarian tissue	12 days	αMEM	3D	PEG-fibrinogen	N/A
Wang et al., 2014 [55]	Human	Isolated follicles	8 days	αMEM	3D	Alginate	Enzymatic + mechanical
Laronda et al., 2014 [29]	Human	Isolated follicles	3 days	αMEM	3D	Alginate	Enzymatic
Yin et al., 2016 [56]	Human	Isolated follicles	30 days	αMEM	3D	Alginate	Enzymatic
Hosseini et al., 2017 [30]	Human	Isolated follicles	10 days	αMEM	3D	Alginate	Enzymatic
Hosseini et al., 2019 [57]	Human	Ovarian tissue	8 days	αMEM	N/A	No	N/A
Ghezelayagh et al., 2020 [31]	Human	Ovarian tissue	7 days	αMEM	3D	Agar scaffold	N/A
Ghezelayagh et al., 2021 [32]	Human	Ovarian tissue	7 days	αMEM	3D	Matrigel	N/A
Telfer et al., 2008 [21]	Human	Ovarian tissue	10 days	McCoy's 5a	N/A	No	Mechanical
Khosravi et al., 2013 [35]	Human	Ovarian tissue	7 days	McCoy's 5a	N/A	No	N/A
McLaughlin et al., 2011 [33]	Human	Ovarian tissue	6 days	McCoy's 5a	N/A	No	N/A
McLaughlin et al., 2014 [34]	Human	Ovarian tissue	6 days	McCoy's 5a	N/A	No	Mechanical
Asadi et al., 2017 [36]	Human	Ovarian tissue	6 days	McCoy's 5a	N/A	No	N/A
Grosbois et al., 2018 [37]	Human	Ovarian tissue	6 days	McCoy's 5a	N/A	No	N/A
Hossay et al., 2023 [38]	Human	Ovarian tissue	6 days	McCoy's 5a	N/A	No	N/A
Subiran Adrados et al., 2023 [39]	Human	Isolated follicles	8 days	McCoy's 5a	3D	Alginate	Enzymatic + mechanical
Dadashzadeh et al., 2023 [58]	Human	Isolated follicles	7 days	DMEM/F12	3D	PEG hydrogels	Enzymatic
Wandji et al., 1996 [40]	Bovine	Ovarian tissue	7 days	Waymouth	N/A	No	N/A
Fortune et al., 1998 [41]	Bovine	Ovarian tissue	7 days	Waymouth	N/A	No	N/A
Gigli et al., 2006 [42]	Bovine	Ovarian tissue	7 days	Waymouth	N/A	No	N/A
Yang and Fortune, 2006 [43]	Bovine	Ovarian tissue	10 days	Waymouth	N/A	No	N/A
Yang and Fortune, 2007 [44]	Bovine	Ovarian tissue	10 days	Waymouth	N/A	No	N/A
Yang and Fortune, 2008 [45]	Bovine	Ovarian tissue	10 days	Waymouth	N/A	No	N/A
Yang et al., 2017 [46]	Bovine	Ovarian tissue	12 days	Waymouth	N/A	No	N/A

N/A: not applicable.

3.2. Molecular Signaling Pathways

Follicle activation is the first step in folliculogenesis and appears to be the key feature of in vitro follicle development. Due to an absence of gonadotropin receptors within PMFs and their limited irrigation supply, PMF activation is most likely gonadotropin-independent, with reliance on paracrine signaling both within follicles and throughout the local intraovarian environment [59]. While still not fully understood, regulation of PMF activation looks to involve intricate coordination between stimulating and inhibiting signals.

3.2.1. Oocyte-GC Crosstalk

Cell communication pathways between the oocyte and GCs are critical features in PMF activation. Previous studies suggest that growth differentiation factor 9 (GDF9) and bone morphogenetic protein 15 (BMP15), two members of the transforming growth factor beta (TGFβ) superfamily specifically secreted by oocytes, may be involved in initiating follicle growth and subsequent stage transition [60,61]. It has been documented that after follicle activation, the recruited oocyte initiates GDF9 and BMP15 secretion, directly impacting both GC proliferation and expansion, and thereby promoting follicle transition [62,63]. Indeed, addition of human recombinant GDF9 and BMP15 to human ovarian tissue IVC has been found to promote increased activation of PMFs and higher estradiol secretion [54]. On the other hand, GDF9 knockout mice showed significant impairment of follicle development, which hampers progression beyond the primary stage [64], while BMP15 knockout mice exhibited subfertility, with lower ovulation and fertilization rates [65].

Another hormone regulating follicle activation is anti-Müllerian hormone (AMH) [66], also a member of the TGFβ superfamily. AMH is secreted by GCs from the primary follicle stage onwards and peaks during the secondary and small antral follicle stages [67]. AMH from growing follicles has an inhibitory effect on follicle activation in neighboring quiescent PMFs [68], designed to maintain a balanced and coordinated process of follicle recruitment and development. Certainly, studies in AMH-knockout mice revealed increased numbers of antral follicles, coupled with a decrease in the PMF count [69]. It has also been demonstrated that supplementing human [70] and bovine [46] ovarian tissue IVC with AMH curbs follicle activation.

3.2.2. Hippo Signaling

Among the different molecular pathways, Hippo signaling appears to play a key role in PMF activation (Figure 2). This pathway regulates organ size, tissue homeostasis, and cell differentiation [71]. The Hippo pathway functions through downstream effectors, namely transcriptional coactivator yes-associated protein (YAP) and transcriptional coactivator PDZ-binding motif (TAZ) [72,73]. While active, this kinase-regulated suppressive pathway eventually causes phosphorylation of the YAP/TAZ complex, resulting in its retention and degradation within the cytoplasm, and thereby preventing its nuclear localization and activation of transcription factors. Conversely, during ovarian tissue fragmentation, transformation of globular actin into filamentous actin disrupts this signaling pathway, leading to accumulation of unphosphorylated YAP/TAZ in the nucleus, which subsequently enhances cell proliferation-related gene expression [72,74–76]. Lunding and colleagues demonstrated that fragmentation of human ovaries boosted actin polymerization, causing inhibition of the Hippo pathway by dephosphorylation and nuclear translocation of YAP, and ultimately leading to follicle and oocyte growth [77]. Likewise, immunostaining techniques (targeting YAP) on human ovarian tissue have revealed that in vitro tissue fragmentation activates PMFs through the Hippo pathway [78]. Grosbois and colleagues were even able to prove that after IVC, follicles situated closer to the fragmentation site were more developed than those localized deeper in cortical tissue [37].

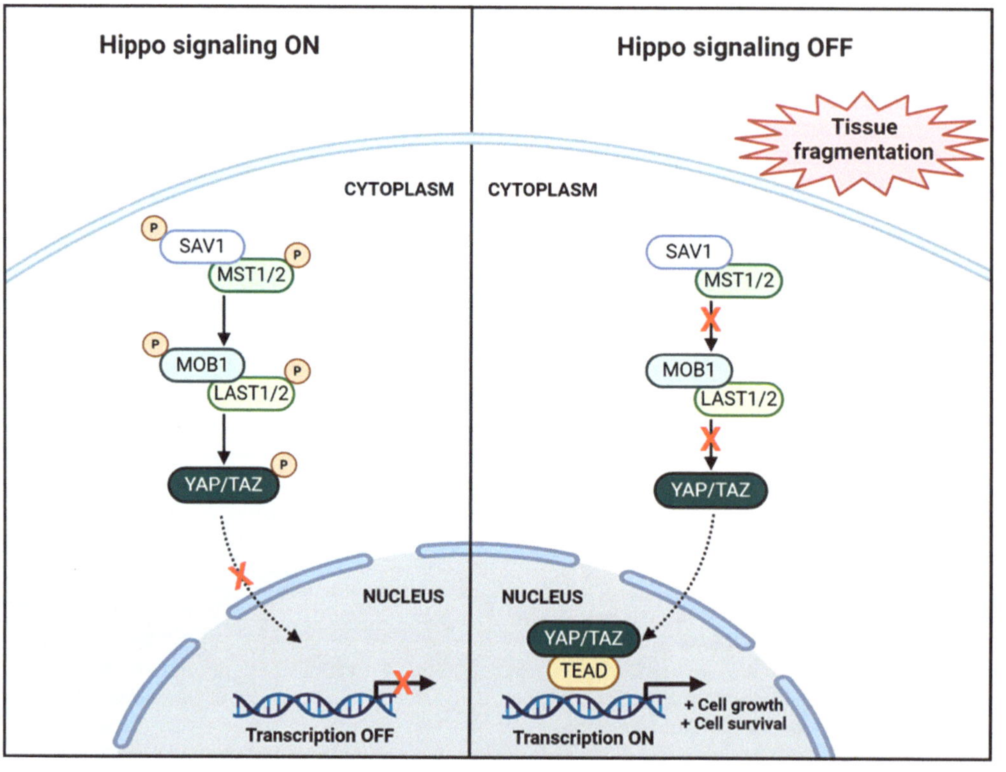

Figure 2. When the Hippo pathway is active (**left**), SAV1 and MST1/2 complex phosphorylates LATS1/2 and MOB1. Activated LATS1/2 subsequently phosphorylates the YAP/TAZ complex, resulting in cytoplasmic retention and no DNA transcription. Conversely, when the Hippo pathway is disrupted (**right**) during ovarian tissue fragmentation, dephosphorylated YAP1/TAZ translocates to the nucleus to bind with TEAD, leading to transcriptional activation of genes associated with cell growth and survival. Created with BioRender.com. Abbreviations: LATS1/2 (large tumor suppressor kinase 1/2); MOB1 (Mps one binder 1); MST1/2 (mammalian Ste20-like serine/threonine kinases 1/2); P (phosphorylated); SAV1 (protein salvador homolog 1; TEAD (TEA domain family members).

3.2.3. PI3K/AKT Pathway

The phosphoinositide 3-kinase (PI3K)-protein kinase B (AKT) signaling pathway has also been implicated in PMF activation [34,50] (Figure 3). The PI3K/AKT pathway is activated by various growth factors. Platelet-derived growth factor (PDGF) and basic fibroblast growth factor (bFGF) are among those able to trigger oocyte activation by boosting oocyte-GC crosstalk through c-kit/kit ligand signaling [59,79,80]. Upon binding of the c-kit receptor to the oocyte membrane, increased kit ligand expression and secretion from GCs activate the PI3K/AKT pathway [81,82]. Other growth factors such as vascular endothelial growth factor (VEGF), epidermal growth factor (EGF), and hormones like insulin are able to directly stimulate the PI3K/AKT pathway upon binding to tyrosine-kinase receptors [59,79,83]. After receptor activation, phosphatidylinositol-4,5-bisphosphate (PIP2) phosphorylates into phosphatidylinositol 3,4,5-triphosphate (PIP3). AKT is then phosphorylated and translocated to the nucleus, where it in turn phosphorylates the transcriptional factor forkhead box O (FOXO), resulting in its export into the cytoplasm. After translocation, inactive FOXO ceases its inhibitory influence over follicle growth [84,85]. Mammalian target of rapamycin complex (mTORC), another AKT downstream effector, is also involved in early-stage follicle activation and development. When active, mTORC regulates protein synthesis and cell growth through ribosomal biogenesis, enhancing follicle activation [86]. Conversely, phosphatase and tensin homolog (PTEN) has a negative impact on PI3K/AKT signaling, counteracting conversion of PIP2 into PIP3 [75]. Past research has demonstrated upregulation of the PI3K/AKT and mTORC pathways and a decrease in PTEN signaling upon analysis of oocyte transcriptomic profiles during primordial-to-primary follicle transition in human ovarian follicles [87].

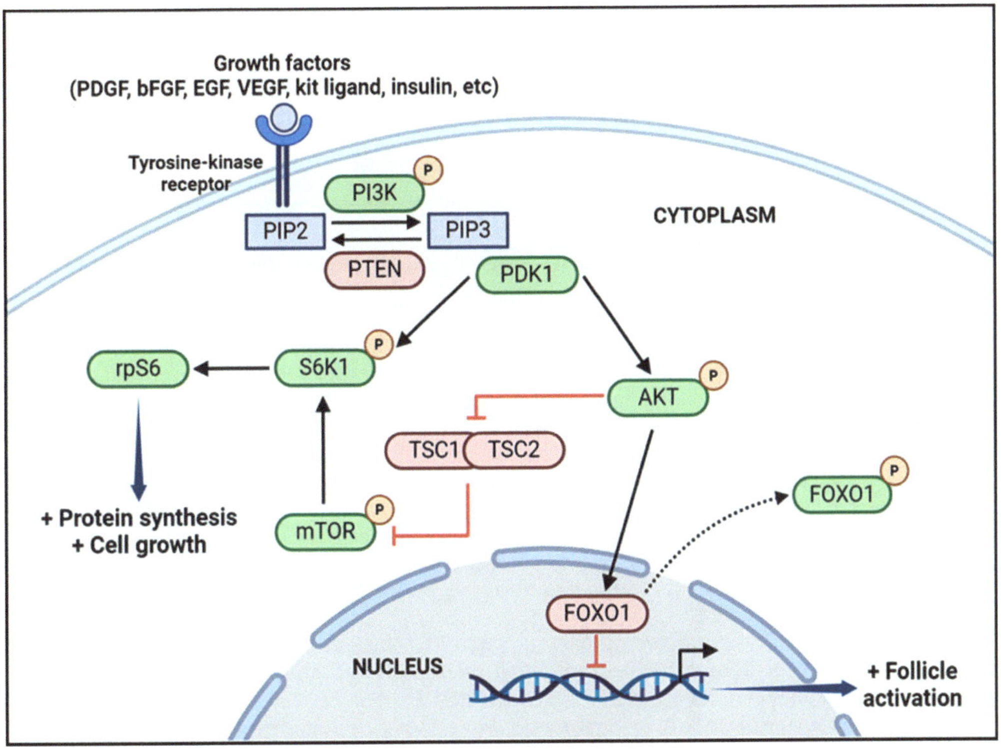

Figure 3. The PI3K/AKT pathway is activated following binding of several growth factors to tyrosine-kinase receptors on cell membranes. This interaction leads to PIP2 transformation into PIP3. AKT is then phosphorylated and translocated to the nucleus where it phosphorylates FOXO1, resulting in its export into the cytoplasm. After translocation, inactive FOXO1 ceases its inhibitory effect over transcriptional factors, enhancing follicle activation and growth. mTOR, another AKT downstream effector regulates protein synthesis and cell growth through ribosomal biosynthesis, also promoting follicle activation. PTEN, on the other hand, counteracts the conversion of PIP2 into PIP3, inhibiting the pathway. Activators are represented in green and inhibitors in red. Created with BioRender.com. Abbreviations: AKT (protein kinase B); bFGF (basic fibroblast growth factor); EGF (epidermal growth factor); FOXO1 (forkhead box O1); mTOR (mammalian target of rapamycin); P (phosphorylated); PDGF (platelet-derived growth factor); PDK1 (phosphoinositide-dependent kinase-1); PI3K (phosphatidylinositol 3-kinase); PIP2 (phosphatidylinositol 4,5-bisphosphate); PIP3 (phosphatidylinositol 3,4,5-trisphosphate); PTEN (phosphatase and tensin homolog); rpS6 (ribosomal protein S6); S6K1 (S6 kinase 1); TSC1 and TSC2 (tuberous sclerosis complex 1 and 2); VEGF (vascular endothelial growth factor).

3.3. Spontaneous In Vitro Follicle Activation: Friend or Foe?

In vivo, PMF quiescence is maintained by an intricate balance between stimulatory and inhibitory autocrine and paracrine cues within the intraovarian setting. However, follicle activation occurs spontaneously in vitro after a few days in both humans [10,21,38,50] and bovines [40,41]. This might be due to disruption of follicle activation-suppressing mechanisms after the cortical fragment is extracted from its natural environment [88]. Such uncontrolled in vitro activation stands in sharp contrast to the natural physiological process, where PMFs are gradually recruited in regulated waves. Indeed, this highly coordinated development is estimated to take at least 80 days in vivo [89], raising questions about the quality and genomic integrity of in vitro-derived follicles that reach the same growth stage in around 10 days. Previous studies [10,21] have in fact found that despite rapid in vitro activation, only a limited number of PMFs are capable of progressing to the next stage of follicle growth, while the majority face follicle death or development arrest. Not all activated follicles manage to grow and develop to further stages [10], but whether this developmental defect lies in the initial uncontrolled activation or happens at some later stage cannot yet be determined.

In recent years, numerous investigations have sought to increase follicle activation using pharmacological agents to enhance ovarian tissue IVC. Short-term in vitro exposure to low doses of PTEN inhibitors like bisperoxovanadium(pic) [bpV(pic)] or bisperoxovanadium(HOpic) [bpV(HOpic)] was found to improve human PMF activation and growth in vitro [34,90] and promote estradiol secretion [90]. Creating a favorable environment for follicle growth could certainly be beneficial in clinical settings. Kawamura and colleagues reported human pregnancies after grafting ovarian cortex previously exposed to a PTEN inhibitor to patients with premature ovarian failure [72,91,92]. However, iatrogenically forcing follicle activation may not be harmless to follicle health. Apart from its function in follicle activation, PTEN also plays a role in maintaining genomic stability [93,94]. Indeed, studies have demonstrated that PTEN inhibition causes greater follicle DNA damage, impairs DNA repair mechanisms [95] and increases histomorphological follicle abnormalities, such as loss of GC-oocyte contacts, steroidogenesis defects, and poor survival of growing follicles [28,34,37].

Conversely, other researchers have hypothesized that an ideal IVC system should limit extensive follicle activation to mimic the natural intraovarian environment. Pharmacological inhibition of mTORC, a downstream effector of the PI3K/AKT pathway, has been used to attenuate follicle in vitro activation. Exposure to rapamycin, an mTORC1 inhibitor, resulted in high rates of oocyte loss and an 'empty follicle' pattern in ovarian tissue culture [33]. Surprisingly, better outcomes were observed with everolimus (EVE), an analog of rapamycin. EVE has been reported to have a protective effect on maintaining PMF dormancy and avoiding IVC-induced spontaneous activation [37]. Furthermore, adding AMH to ovarian tissue IVC could be a valuable approach to control follicle activation. Recombinant AMH exposure was also shown to prevent PMF activation in cultured ovarian tissue both in humans [70] and bovines [46].

Regulation of in vitro activation by ovarian tissue IVC offers a promising avenue for fertility treatments but raises concerns about follicle health and genetic integrity. While the results may look encouraging, it is essential to remain cautious regarding potential impairments to follicle health, quality, and genetic and epigenetic integrity. Long-term impacts of genetic instability on oocytes and subsequent offspring remain uncertain. Indeed, these new reproductive techniques still have a long way to go before they can be safely employed in a clinical setting [96].

3.4. Mimicking the In Vivo Environment: The Key to Success

Physical and biological parameters like base media and additives, nutrients, temperature, oxygen (O_2) tension, and light exposure should be meticulously analyzed to determine the optimal IVC strategy. Ultimately, the IVC system that most closely mimics the intraovarian physiological environment is one that causes the least cell distress and yields the best viability.

Optimal temperatures for IVC can vary from species to species depending on normal body temperatures, like 37 °C for human tissue and 38.5–39 °C for bovine tissue. Determining species-specific temperature requirements is crucial to successful IVC.

In recent years, cell-based co-culture systems have attracted attention for their potential to replicate the intraovarian microenvironment [97,98]. It appears that 'feeder cells', such as different types of mesenchymal stem cells (MSCs), exert their influence on neighboring cells due to their capacity to release a secretome containing cytokines, chemokines, and growth factors. Among these cells, bone marrow-derived (BM)-MSCs were found to enhance follicle growth and decrease follicle apoptosis in a human ovarian tissue co-culture model [57]. It has also been very recently demonstrated that addition of adipose tissue-derived stem cell (ASC)-conditioned medium, which includes the secretome, to bovine ovarian tissue IVC significantly boosts follicle viability, development, and estradiol secretion [99]. Indeed, MSC derivatives like conditioned medium could emerge as powerful optimization tools, as they reduce the risk of cell differentiation and nutrient competition within shared culture media. They also provide a more secure option, given its ease of collection, storage, and standardization, thereby ensuring consistent and reproducible outcomes.

Oxygen tension is another crucial environmental factor affecting IVC follicle outcomes. Optimal O_2 tension is difficult to determine in culture. It is estimated that quiescent PMFs reside within the ovarian cortex at physiological O_2 tension levels ranging between 2% and 8% [100,101]. Elevated O_2 tension causes accumulation of reactive oxygen species (ROS), eventually leading to oxidative stress damage and cell dysfunction. Consequently, culturing PMFs at O_2 tension beyond physiological levels may result in increased follicle distress and reduced viability. In line with these data, a study reported that human ovarian tissue cultured at 5% O_2 tension yielded lower follicle apoptosis rates, mainly by generating less oxidative stress damage and fewer DNA double-strand breaks [51] than culture at 20% O_2 tension. It was also reported that hypoxia induces a dormant state in oocytes through FOXO3, a downstream effector of the PI3K/AKT signaling pathway [102]. Atmospheric O_2 tension could therefore be another factor contributing to large-scale spontaneous human follicle activation invariably observed in vitro.

Conversely, there is no clear directive on O_2 tension in bovine ovarian tissue IVC. Jorssen and colleagues found no significant differences in follicle viability or growth between 5% and 20% O_2 tension [103]. Although the role of O_2 tension has not yet been fully elucidated, it is clear that it varies according to follicle stage. Low O_2 tension is most critical during the early stages of IVC, while higher tension may be required during later stages to support normal development of GCs and steroidogenesis [42]. This mirrors in vivo follicle dynamics, where PMFs migrate from the avascular periphery towards the highly irrigated medulla as they grow.

Finally, it is worth noting that low in vitro survival and growing follicle rates are likely due to suboptimal culture medium composition. Determining which culture supplements should be added to enhance IVC outcomes is extremely challenging, as factors, proteins, and signaling pathways involved in follicle activation, growth, and maturation are still largely unknown. This lack of understanding of the complex processes of folliculogenesis is undoubtedly a significant limitation to achieving favorable in vitro follicle outcomes.

4. Follicle In Vitro Growth (IVG): From Secondary to Antral Follicles

Table 2 summarizes different IVC systems, culture periods, medium components, biomaterials, and isolation methods from publications reporting transition of secondary follicles to antral follicles in humans and bovines.

Table 2. Publications reporting transition of secondary to antral follicles in humans and bovines (step 2).

Publication	Source	Culture Period	Culture Medium	Culture System	Biomaterial	Isolation Method
Roy et al., 1993 [104]	Human	5 days	D-MEM	2D	Agar	Enzymatic
Abir et al., 1997 [23]	Human	28 days	αMEM	2D	Extracellular matrix	Mechanical
Xu et al., 2009 [105]	Human	30 days	αMEM	3D	Alginate	Enzymatic + mechanical
Xia et al., 2015 [106]	Human	8 days	αMEM	3D	Alginate	Enzymatic + mechanical
Xiao et al., 2015 [107]	Human	40 days	αMEM	3D	Alginate	Mechanical
Yin et al., 2016 [56]	Human	30 days	αMEM	3D	Alginate	Enzymatic
Telfer et al., 2008 [21]	Human	10 days	McCoy's 5a	V-shaped microwell	No	Mechanical
McLaughlin et al., 2014 [34]	Human	6 days	McCoy's 5a	V-shaped microwell	No	Mechanical
McLaughlin et al., 2018 [10]	Human	23 days	McCoy's 5a	V-shaped microwell	No	Mechanical
Xu et al., 2021 [108]	Human	42 days	αMEM	N/A	No	Mechanical
Subiran Adrados et al., 2023 [39]	Human	8 days	McCoy's 5a	3D	Alginate	Enzymatic + mechanical
Thomas et al., 2007 [109]	Bovine	6 days	McCoy's 5a	V-shaped microwell	No	Mechanical
McLaughlin and Telfer, 2010 [110]	Bovine	15 days	McCoy's 5a	V-shaped microwell	No	Mechanical
Rossetto et al., 2013 [52]	Bovine	16 days	α-MEM, McCoy's 5a and TCM-199	V-shaped microwell	No	Mechanical
Paulino et al., 2018 [53]	Bovine	18 days	TCM-199	Droplets culture	No	Mechanical

N/A: not applicable.

4.1. Isolation Techniques

After reaching the secondary follicle stage consisting of a multilayer of GCs, follicles cannot survive within the cortical environment, so isolation from surrounding ovarian cells is a prerequisite for further in vitro development. This is not surprising as, during intraovarian development, follicles migrate from the rigid cortex towards the less dense medulla. Secondary follicle isolation can be performed either enzymatically [56,58,104,111], mechanically by microdissection [10,21,23,34,52,53,107,109,110], or a combination of both [39,105,106] (Table 2). The microdissection approach, using fine-gauge needles, has been established as the most appropriate, as it maintains an intact follicle basement membrane, thereby preserving oocyte-GC communications [10,21].

4.2. Secondary Follicle Culture Systems and Medium Composition

The physical setting of isolated follicles is hugely important at this stage. In the past, follicle IVG studies only took a few days, and 2D culture systems enabling follicles to attach to a flat surface appeared to function adequately [104]. However, with establishment of long-term IVC techniques, the 2D method exhibited significant limitations, such as loss of cell-to-cell communication and follicle growth arrest [112]. Researchers, therefore, shifted to 3D culture systems using biomaterials to encapsulate follicles to better mimic the intraovarian environment (Table 2). Among these bio-matrices, natural compounds like alginate and Matrigel (a commercialized solubilized basal membrane matrix) were found to support IVG of isolated human secondary follicles [56,105]. Moreover, synthetic components such as polyethylene glycol (PEG)-ylated fibrin hydrogels were successfully utilized to promote human secondary follicle development in vitro [58]. Other approaches using decellularized ovarian tissue [113] and 3D microporous scaffolds [114] were also shown to support follicle IVG. However, IVG can in fact be performed without any extracellular matrix or scaffold at all [10]. In the multi-step IVC system, isolated secondary follicles can be cultured individually in V-shaped well culture dishes without any added biomaterial until the antral stage [10]. Numerous studies on isolated bovine follicles have consistently demonstrated that V-shaped microwell plates facilitate follicle growth and proliferation [52,109,110], although the droplet culture approach has also been successfully applied [53].

Medium composition is also crucial to IVG. The most commonly used media in human IVG systems are αMEM [23,56,105,107,108], McCoy's 5a [10,21,34,39], Dulbecco's MEM (DMEM) [104], or mixed media (DMEM+F12) [58], while McCoys' 5a [109,110] and TCM-199 [53] are typically utilized in bovines (Table 2).

Addition of activin A and low-dose FSH at this stage has been found to impart a stabilizing influence on intercellular connections, improve the quality of oocytes and promote antrum formation in both humans [10,21,107] and bovines [115]. In this context, it has been reported that FSH receptors (FSHRs) are mainly present during growth stages [116] and, upon binding to FSH, they initiate intracellular mechanisms involved in GC proliferation [117]. Activin has also been shown to act in coordination with FSH, preserving the integrity of intercellular connections within follicles [118]. In oocytes, activin is involved in modulation of nuclear gene transcription, promoting maturation [119,120]. Isolated follicle growth and survival can also be enhanced with other culture additives such as bFGF [55], antioxidants like ascorbic acid that mitigate oxidative stress damage [21,47], and platelet-rich plasma or human platelet lysate containing high concentrations of growth factors [30,39]. While various research groups have tested different additives, further studies are needed to determine their effectiveness. It is crucial to establish clear guidelines on exactly which supplements should be added to standard IVC growth medium.

4.3. Antrum Formation

This step involves enlargement of the oocyte, further replication and expansion of GCs, and formation of a central fluid-filled cavity known as the antrum. As preantral follicles develop, areas of fluid initially accumulate between GCs, eventually leading to the creation of a large central antrum. This central fluid-filled space serves as a reservoir for various substances and plays a crucial role in providing essential support and nourishment to the oocyte as it continues to mature. Based on in vivo migration of growing follicles from the cortex to the medulla during physiological development, it is thought that antrum formation and expansion might be influenced by biomechanical environmental factors. Follicles in collagen-dense ovarian cortex are less likely to grow, while those in the medulla benefit from a biomechanical environment that supports further development and antrum formation [121]. Xiao and colleagues found that while human follicles encapsulated in alginate could grow to a diameter of 110 μm after 30 days, oocytes within these follicles were unable to progress to the MII stage, instead remaining at the germinal vesicle (GV) stage or deteriorating, most probably due to limitations imposed by the physical surroundings. However, when antral follicles were removed from the alginate hydrogel and further cultured in low-attachment plates using a dynamic two-step system, they were able to reach the MII stage [107]. Indeed, these findings emphasize the importance of providing a dynamic in vitro environment for follicle development.

5. Oocyte In Vitro Maturation (IVM): The Final Step

This technique has advanced significantly over the last 30 years [122–124]. It involves oocyte maturation to achieve meiosis resumption, chromatin condensation, development of the meiotic spindle, and expulsion of the initial polar body, reaching the mature stage of MII oocyte [125] (Figure 4A). This technique can be performed either on (i) immature oocytes obtained from oocyte pick-up or (ii) oocytes from in vitro-derived follicles. The former technique entails puncturing small and mid-antral follicles before they reach periovulatory size ranges (between 6–12 mm) without previous hormone stimulation, and final oocyte maturation is achieved in vitro [123]. In this review, our focus is on the latter option, where IVM is performed on completely in vitro-derived follicles. Table 3 summarizes different IVC systems, culture periods, medium components, and use of biomaterials from publications reporting oocyte IVM from in vitro-derived follicles.

Table 3. Publications reporting the generation of mature oocytes MII from in vitro-derived human follicles.

Publication	Source	Type of Culture	Culture Period	Culture Medium	Culture System	Biomaterial
Xiao et al., 2015 [107]	Human	Isolated follicles	40 days	αMEM	3D	Alginate
McLaughlin et al., 2018 [10]	Human	Ovarian tissue	23 days	McCoy's 5a	N/A	No
Xu et al., 2021 [108]	Human	Ovarian tissue	42 days	αMEM	N/A	No

N/A: not applicable.

IVM from In Vitro-Derived Follicles

Achieving successful IVM from in vitro-derived follicles poses considerable technical challenges. Oocyte competence is gained progressively throughout follicle development and involves gradual accumulation of RNA molecules and proteins throughout oocyte growth, which will constitute the oocyte genome [79]. Previous research in mammals has shown that the oocyte genome may be strongly influenced by the environment [126], so follicle IVC will clearly have an impact on oocyte RNA and protein regulation. Environmental epigenomic modifications mainly include DNA methylation, chromatin reorganization, and histone modifications [127], all of which contribute to proper segregation of chromosomes during meiosis.

To date, only three research groups have documented successful maturation of oocytes from cultured human follicles (Table 3), albeit invariably showing suboptimal oocyte developmental competence. Unlike animal models where fertilization rates can be measured, the only viable options to assess human oocyte developmental competence are morphological parameters like establishment of the meiotic spindle, chromosomal alignment, polar body formation, and cytoplasmic ultrastructure, obviously due to ethical concerns (Figure 4A–D).

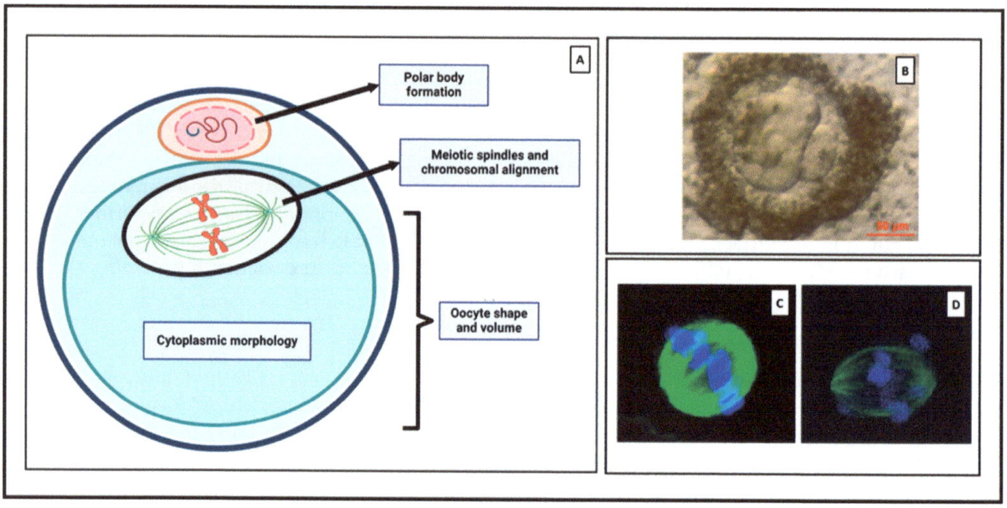

Figure 4. (**A**) Schematic representation of morphological parameters used to assess oocyte competence. Created with BioRender.com. (**B**) Bright field image showing a MII oocyte with and enlarged abnormal polar body. Reproduced with permission from [10]. Confocal images displaying (**C**) equatorially aligned chromosomes (blue) and meiotic spindles (green), and (**D**) chromosomal misalignment. Reproduced with permission from [128].

Xiao and colleagues reported the generation of MII oocytes from mechanically isolated secondary follicles, with a typical meiosis spindle configuration. However, polar body fragmentation was observed [107], which denotes low oocyte quality for potential IVF. Likewise, McLaughlin's team achieved MII oocyte production from early-stage follicles cultured in a multi-step IVC system, but this approach exhibited limited effectiveness, yielding only 9 MII oocytes from 160 ovarian tissue fragments. Furthermore, these oocytes displayed abnormally large polar bodies [10]. Similarly, Xu's team demonstrated development of MII oocytes from early-stage follicles cultured in situ within cortical fragments in a more recent study. By the end, 3 out of 14 MII oocytes showed normal spindle configuration, adequate polar body size, and typical intracellular ultrastructure [108]. All in all, these results highlight the challenges associated with achieving optimal oocyte competence using in vitro folliculogenesis systems.

6. Future Directions

Creating a successful and efficient long-term IVC system for human follicles is a demanding pursuit. Researchers have recently been exploring ways of generating dynamic microfluidic culture systems in assisted reproduction devices, such as reproductive organs-on-a-chip [129], in vitro spermatogenesis [130], and testis culture [131]. The dynamic microfluidic approach aims to establish a constant flow of culture medium around tissue, closely mimicking the physiological ovarian microenvironment by facilitating continuous exchange of metabolites and cell waste. This innovative technique might have the potential to overcome limitations associated with static IVC approaches, hopefully improving follicle survival and development. Moreover, employing a dynamic O_2 tension IVC system could be advantageous. As previously mentioned, quiescent PMFs initially reside in the avascular cortical region and gradually migrate to the highly irrigated medulla, as they progress through developmental stages [89]. This increasing O_2 gradient is crucial to GC proliferation, steroidogenesis, and oocyte maturation during follicle growth [132]. Indeed, applying dynamic O_2 tension throughout IVC could positively impact follicle quality and competence, as it mimics O_2 gradients experienced during physiological ovarian follicle development.

Another avenue for advancement involves implementation of ovarian organoids. This concept refers to in vitro generation of miniature histological structures resembling ovarian source tissue [133]. Such a 3D approach could be used not only as an alternative for fertility restoration purposes, but also as a novel opportunity to investigate disease mechanisms, the impact of gonadotoxic agents, and potential therapeutic strategies. Li and colleagues recently developed an ovarian organoid using mouse female germline stem cells, resulting in differentiated heterogenic tissue containing germ cells and somatic cells like GCs and theca cells [134]. This model demonstrated reproductive functions, including oocyte and offspring production, and endocrine activity, with secretion of progesterone and estradiol. Use of ovarian organoids in humans certainly holds great promise as a brand-new approach to fertility restoration, offering the potential for improved outcomes and broader applications in the field of reproductive medicine.

To validate such innovative strategies for human tissue in clinical practice, it is imperative to follow a structured approach. The European Society of Human Reproduction and Embryology (ESHRE) task force on ethics and law outlines a comprehensive research pathway to evaluate the efficacy and safety of new assisted reproductive technologies, including four key steps: (i) conducting animal studies; (ii) undertaking preclinical embryo research; (iii) performing clinical trials on human subjects; and (iv) conducting follow-up studies to monitor long-term outcomes [135]. Research in animals has already been developed according to these principles, but perhaps the most challenging step is human embryo research, because of ethical regulations that restrict this practice in many European countries. That said, it is also very important to stress that regulatory considerations, including obtaining ethical approval and compliance with medical device regulations from institutional boards, are crucial throughout the entire validation process. This systematic approach should be adhered to, so that approval for these innovative techniques can be granted before their integration into clinical settings.

7. Patient Perspectives

A diagnosis of cancer represents a profound challenge for young women, triggering both the psychological shock of the diagnosis itself and the potential repercussion on fertility due to gonadotoxic treatments [136]. Concerns about fertility can indeed dash their hopes of a family, causing considerable emotional distress. Moreover, facing the complex landscape of treatment decisions and medical interventions associated with cancer therapy can be hugely overwhelming. Among oncological patients, those with pathologies that contraindicate OTT are most acutely affected by this uncertainty. For this category of patients, we may advocate OTC for fertility preservation in very young girls, in the hope of continued (albeit slow and difficult) progress in the field in the future.

8. Conclusions

In vitro follicle development has shown significant potential as a novel method for fertility restoration in young cancer patients with OTT contraindications. Despite ongoing challenges associated with the in vitro technique, some studies have demonstrated the ability to generate mature human MII oocytes from early-stage follicles. Indeed, there is a widely accepted consensus on the benefits of culturing PMFs in situ within ovarian cortex to achieve follicle activation, along with mechanical microdissection of secondary follicles for further growth. In addition, IVC medium composition has been standardized over the years, albeit with slight variations between species, the most common being αMEM and McCoy's 5a for humans and Waymouth and TCM-199 for bovines.

New strategies, such as dynamic microfluidic culture systems and dynamic O_2 tension IVC systems, aim to better replicate the physiological ovarian microenvironment, potentially enhancing follicle survival and development rates. The use of ovarian organoids offers exciting prospects for both fertility restoration and investigation of disease mechanisms and therapeutic strategies.

Further optimization and refinement could ultimately make in vitro follicle development a safe, accessible, and cost-effective option for fertility restoration in a clinical setting, providing a valuable alternative for subjects who cannot undergo OTT.

Author Contributions: Writing—original draft preparation, F.V. and M.-M.D.; writing—review and editing, F.V. and M.-M.D. All authors have read and agreed to the published version of the manuscript.

Funding: This study was supported by grants from the Fonds National de la Recherche Scientifique de Belgique (FNRS-PDR T.0064.22, CDR J.0063.20 and grant 5/4/150/5 awarded to M.-M.D.).

Data Availability Statement: No new data were created or analyzed in this study. Data sharing is not applicable to this article.

Acknowledgments: The authors thank Mira Hryniuk, for reviewing the English language of the article.

Conflicts of Interest: The authors declare no conflicts of interest.

References

1. Meirow, D. The Effects of Radiotherapy and Chemotherapy on Female Reproduction. *Hum. Reprod. Update* **2001**, *7*, 535–543. [CrossRef]
2. Schmidt, K.; Larsen, E.; Andersen, C.; Andersen, A. Risk of Ovarian Failure and Fertility Preserving Methods in Girls and Adolescents with a Malignant Disease: Fertility Preserving Methods in Girls with Cancer. *BJOG Int. J. Obstet. Gynaecol.* **2010**, *117*, 163–174. [CrossRef] [PubMed]
3. Donnez, J.; Dolmans, M.-M. Fertility Preservation in Women. *N. Engl. J. Med.* **2017**, *377*, 1657–1665. [CrossRef] [PubMed]
4. Wallace, W.H.B.; Kelsey, T.W.; Anderson, R.A. Fertility Preservation in Pre-Pubertal Girls with Cancer: The Role of Ovarian Tissue Cryopreservation. *Fertil. Steril.* **2016**, *105*, 6–12. [CrossRef] [PubMed]
5. Dolmans, M.-M.; von Wolff, M.; Poirot, C.; Diaz-Garcia, C.; Cacciottola, L.; Boissel, N.; Liebenthron, J.; Pellicer, A.; Donnez, J.; Andersen, C.Y. Transplantation of Cryopreserved Ovarian Tissue in a Series of 285 Women: A Review of Five Leading European Centers. *Fertil. Steril.* **2021**, *115*, 1102–1115. [CrossRef] [PubMed]

6. Dolmans, M.-M.; Hossay, C.; Nguyen, T.Y.T.; Poirot, C. Fertility Preservation: How to Preserve Ovarian Function in Children, Adolescents and Adults. *J. Clin. Med.* **2021**, *10*, 5247. [CrossRef]
7. Dolmans, M.-M.; Marinescu, C.; Saussoy, P.; Van Langendonckt, A.; Amorim, C.; Donnez, J. Reimplantation of Cryopreserved Ovarian Tissue from Patients with Acute Lymphoblastic Leukemia Is Potentially Unsafe. *Blood* **2010**, *116*, 2908–2914. [CrossRef] [PubMed]
8. Dolmans, M.-M.; Luyckx, V.; Donnez, J.; Andersen, C.Y.; Greve, T. Risk of Transferring Malignant Cells with Transplanted Frozen-Thawed Ovarian Tissue. *Fertil. Steril.* **2013**, *99*, 1514–1522. [CrossRef]
9. Rosendahl, M.; Andersen, M.T.; Ralfkiær, E.; Kjeldsen, L.; Andersen, M.K.; Andersen, C.Y. Evidence of Residual Disease in Cryopreserved Ovarian Cortex from Female Patients with Leukemia. *Fertil. Steril.* **2010**, *94*, 2186–2190. [CrossRef]
10. McLaughlin, M.; Albertini, D.F.; Wallace, W.H.B.; Anderson, R.A.; Telfer, E.E. Metaphase II Oocytes from Human Unilaminar Follicles Grown in a Multi-Step Culture System. *Mol. Hum. Reprod.* **2018**, *24*, 135–142. [CrossRef]
11. Telfer, E.E.; Andersen, C.Y. In Vitro Growth and Maturation of Primordial Follicles and Immature Oocytes. *Fertil. Steril.* **2021**, *115*, 1116–1125. [CrossRef]
12. Shaw, J.M.; Oranratnachai, A.; Trounson, A.O. Fundamental Cryobiology of Mammalian Oocytes and Ovarian Tissue. *Theriogenology* **2000**, *53*, 59–72. [CrossRef]
13. Amorim, C.A.; Dolmans, M.-M.; David, A.; Jaeger, J.; Vanacker, J.; Camboni, A.; Donnez, J.; Van Langendonckt, A. Vitrification and Xenografting of Human Ovarian Tissue. *Fertil. Steril.* **2012**, *98*, 1291–1298.e2. [CrossRef] [PubMed]
14. Oktem, O.; Urman, B. Understanding Follicle Growth in Vivo. *Hum. Reprod.* **2010**, *25*, 2944–2954. [CrossRef] [PubMed]
15. Eppig, J.J. Development in Vitro of Mouse Oocytes from Primordial Follicles. *Biol. Reprod.* **1996**, *54*, 197–207. [CrossRef] [PubMed]
16. Adams, G.P.; Pierson, R.A. Bovine Model for Study of Ovarian Follicular Dynamics in Humans. *Theriogenology* **1995**, *43*, 113–120. [CrossRef]
17. Abir, R. Pilot Study of Isolated Early Human Follicles Cultured in Collagen Gels for 24 Hours. *Hum. Reprod.* **1999**, *14*, 1299–1301. [CrossRef]
18. Hovatta, O.; Wright, C.; Krausz, T.; Hardy, K.; Winston, R.M.L. Human Primordial, Primary and Secondary Ovarian Follicles in Long-Term Culture: Effect of Partial Isolation. *Hum. Reprod.* **1999**, *14*, 2519–2524. [CrossRef] [PubMed]
19. Hovatta, O.; Silye, R.; Abir, R.; Krausz, T.; Winston, R.M. Extracellular Matrix Improves Survival of Both Stored and Fresh Human Primordial and Primary Ovarian Follicles in Long-Term Culture. *Hum. Reprod.* **1997**, *12*, 1032–1036. [CrossRef] [PubMed]
20. Wright, C.S.; Hovatta, O.; Margara, R.; Trew, G.; Winston, R.M.; Franks, S.; Hardy, K. Effects of Follicle-Stimulating Hormone and Serum Substitution on the in-Vitro Growth of Human Ovarian Follicles. *Hum. Reprod.* **1999**, *14*, 1555–1562. [CrossRef] [PubMed]
21. Telfer, E.E.; McLaughlin, M.; Ding, C.; Thong, K.J. A Two-Step Serum-Free Culture System Supports Development of Human Oocytes from Primordial Follicles in the Presence of Activin. *Hum. Reprod.* **2008**, *23*, 1151–1158. [CrossRef]
22. Smitz, J.; Dolmans, M.M.; Donnez, J.; Fortune, J.E.; Hovatta, O.; Jewgenow, K.; Picton, H.M.; Plancha, C.; Shea, L.D.; Stouffer, R.L.; et al. Current Achievements and Future Research Directions in Ovarian Tissue Culture, in Vitro Follicle Development and Transplantation: Implications for Fertility Preservation. *Hum. Reprod. Update* **2010**, *16*, 395–414. [CrossRef]
23. Abir, R.; Franks, S.; Mobberley, M.A.; Moore, P.A.; Margara, R.A.; Winston, R.M. Mechanical Isolation and in Vitro Growth of Preantral and Small Antral Human Follicles. *Fertil. Steril.* **1997**, *68*, 682–688. [CrossRef]
24. Hreinsson, J.G.; Scott, J.E.; Rasmussen, C.; Swahn, M.L.; Hsueh, A.J.W.; Hovatta, O. Growth Differentiation Factor-9 Promotes the Growth, Development, and Survival of Human Ovarian Follicles in Organ Culture. *J. Clin. Endocrinol. Metab.* **2002**, *87*, 316–321. [CrossRef]
25. Scott, J.E.; Carlsson, I.B.; Bavister, B.D.; Hovatta, O. Human Ovarian Tissue Cultures: Extracellular Matrix Composition, Coating Density and Tissue Dimensions. *Reprod. Biomed. Online* **2004**, *9*, 287–293. [CrossRef]
26. Amorim, C.A.; Van Langendonckt, A.; David, A.; Dolmans, M.-M.; Donnez, J. Survival of Human Pre-Antral Follicles after Cryopreservation of Ovarian Tissue, Follicular Isolation and in Vitro Culture in a Calcium Alginate Matrix. *Hum. Reprod.* **2009**, *24*, 92–99. [CrossRef]
27. Camboni, A.; Van Langendonckt, A.; Donnez, J.; Vanacker, J.; Dolmans, M.M.; Amorim, C.A. Alginate Beads as a Tool to Handle, Cryopreserve and Culture Isolated Human Primordial/Primary Follicles. *Cryobiology* **2013**, *67*, 64–69. [CrossRef]
28. Lerer-Serfaty, G.; Samara, N.; Fisch, B.; Shachar, M.; Kossover, O.; Seliktar, D.; Ben-Haroush, A.; Abir, R. Attempted Application of Bioengineered/Biosynthetic Supporting Matrices with Phosphatidylinositol-Trisphosphate-Enhancing Substances to Organ Culture of Human Primordial Follicles. *J. Assist. Reprod. Genet.* **2013**, *30*, 1279–1288. [CrossRef] [PubMed]
29. Laronda, M.M.; Duncan, F.E.; Hornick, J.E.; Xu, M.; Pahnke, J.E.; Whelan, K.A.; Shea, L.D.; Woodruff, T.K. Alginate Encapsulation Supports the Growth and Differentiation of Human Primordial Follicles within Ovarian Cortical Tissue. *J. Assist. Reprod. Genet.* **2014**, *31*, 1013–1028. [CrossRef]
30. Hosseini, L.; Shirazi, A.; Naderi, M.M.; Shams-Esfandabadi, N.; Borjian Boroujeni, S.; Sarvari, A.; Sadeghnia, S.; Behzadi, B.; Akhondi, M.M. Platelet-Rich Plasma Promotes the Development of Isolated Human Primordial and Primary Follicles to the Preantral Stage. *Reprod. Biomed. Online* **2017**, *35*, 343–350. [CrossRef]
31. Ghezelayagh, Z.; Abtahi, N.S.; Rezazadeh Valojerdi, M.; Mehdizadeh, A.; Ebrahimi, B. The Combination of Basic Fibroblast Growth Factor and Kit Ligand Promotes the Proliferation, Activity and Steroidogenesis of Granulosa Cells during Human Ovarian Cortical Culture. *Cryobiology* **2020**, *96*, 30–36. [CrossRef] [PubMed]

32. Ghezelayagh, Z.; Abtahi, N.S.; Khodaverdi, S.; Rezazadeh Valojerdi, M.; Mehdizadeh, A.; Ebrahimi, B. The Effect of Agar Substrate on Growth and Development of Cryopreserved-Thawed Human Ovarian Cortical Follicles in Organ Culture. *Eur. J. Obs. Gynecol. Reprod. Biol.* **2021**, *258*, 139–145. [CrossRef] [PubMed]
33. McLaughlin, M.; Patrizio, P.; Kayisli, U.; Luk, J.; Thomson, T.C.; Anderson, R.A.; Telfer, E.E.; Johnson, J. MTOR Kinase Inhibition Results in Oocyte Loss Characterized by Empty Follicles in Human Ovarian Cortical Strips Cultured in Vitro. *Fertil. Steril.* **2011**, *96*, 1154–1159.e1. [CrossRef]
34. McLaughlin, M.; Kinnell, H.L.; Anderson, R.A.; Telfer, E.E. Inhibition of Phosphatase and Tensin Homologue (PTEN) in Human Ovary in Vitro Results in Increased Activation of Primordial Follicles but Compromises Development of Growing Follicles. *Mol. Hum. Reprod.* **2014**, *20*, 736–744. [CrossRef] [PubMed]
35. Khosravi, F.; Reid, R.L.; Moini, A.; Abolhassani, F.; Valojerdi, M.R.; Kan, F.W.K. In Vitro Development of Human Primordial Follicles to Preantral Stage after Vitrification. *J. Assist. Reprod. Genet.* **2013**, *30*, 1397–1406. [CrossRef]
36. Asadi, E.; Najafi, A.; Moeini, A.; Pirjani, R.; Hassanzadeh, G.; Mikaeili, S.; Salehi, E.; Adutwum, E.; Soleimani, M.; Khosravi, F.; et al. Ovarian Tissue Culture in the Presence of VEGF and Fetuin Stimulates Follicle Growth and Steroidogenesis. *J. Endocrinol.* **2017**, *232*, 205–219. [CrossRef]
37. Grosbois, J.; Demeestere, I. Dynamics of PI3K and Hippo Signaling Pathways during in Vitro Human Follicle Activation. *Hum. Reprod.* **2018**, *33*, 1705–1714. [CrossRef]
38. Hossay, C.; Tramacere, F.; Cacciottola, L.; Camboni, A.; Squifflet, J.-L.; Donnez, J.; Dolmans, M.-M. Follicle Outcomes in Human Ovarian Tissue: Effect of Freezing, Culture, and Grafting. *Fertil. Steril.* **2023**, *119*, 135–145. [CrossRef]
39. Subiran Adrados, C.; Cadenas, J.; Zheng, M.; Lund, S.; Larsen, E.C.; Tanvig, M.H.; Greve, V.H.; Blanche, P.; Andersen, C.Y.; Kristensen, S.G. Human Platelet Lysate Improves the Growth and Survival of Cultured Human Pre-Antral Follicles. *Reprod. Biomed. Online* **2023**, *47*, 103256. [CrossRef]
40. Wandji, S.-A.; Sršeň, V.; Voss, A.K.; Eppig, J.J.; Fortune, J.E. Initiation in Vitro of Growth of Bovine Primordial Follicles1. *Biol. Reprod.* **1996**, *55*, 942–948. [CrossRef]
41. Fortune, J.E.; Kito, S.; Wandji, S.-A.; Sršeň, V. Activation of Bovine and Baboon Primordial Follicles in Vitro. *Theriogenology* **1998**, *49*, 441–449. [CrossRef] [PubMed]
42. Gigli, I.; Byrd, D.D.; Fortune, J.E. Effects of Oxygen Tension and Supplements to the Culture Medium on Activation and Development of Bovine Follicles in Vitro. *Theriogenology* **2006**, *66*, 344–353. [CrossRef] [PubMed]
43. Yang, M.Y.; Fortune, J.E. Testosterone Stimulates the Primary to Secondary Follicle Transition in Bovine Follicles in Vitro1. *Biol. Reprod.* **2006**, *75*, 924–932. [CrossRef]
44. Yang, M.Y.; Fortune, J.E. Vascular Endothelial Growth Factor Stimulates the Primary to Secondary Follicle Transition in Bovine Follicles in Vitro. *Mol. Reprod. Dev.* **2007**, *74*, 1095–1104. [CrossRef] [PubMed]
45. Yang, M.Y.; Fortune, J.E. The Capacity of Primordial Follicles in Fetal Bovine Ovaries to Initiate Growth In Vitro Develops During Mid-Gestation and Is Associated with Meiotic Arrest of Oocytes1. *Biol. Reprod.* **2008**, *78*, 1153–1161. [CrossRef] [PubMed]
46. Yang, M.Y.; Cushman, R.A.; Fortune, J.E. Anti-Müllerian Hormone Inhibits Activation and Growth of Bovine Ovarian Follicles in Vitro and Is Localized to Growing Follicles. *Mol. Hum. Reprod.* **2017**, *23*, 282–291. [CrossRef]
47. Thomas, F.; Leask, R.; Srsen, V.; Riley, S.; Spears, N.; Telfer, E. Effect of Ascorbic Acid on Health and Morphology of Bovine Preantral Follicles during Long-Term Culture. *Reproduction* **2001**, *122*, 487–495. [CrossRef]
48. Andrade, E.R.; van den Hurk, R.; Lisboa, L.A.; Hertel, M.F.; Melo-Sterza, F.A.; Moreno, K.; Bracarense, A.P.F.R.L.; Landim-Alvarenga, F.C.; Seneda, M.M.; Alfieri, A.A. Effects of Ascorbic Acid on in Vitro Culture of Bovine Preantral Follicles. *Zygote* **2012**, *20*, 379–388. [CrossRef]
49. Tagler, D.; Makanji, Y.; Tu, T.; Bernabé, B.P.; Lee, R.; Zhu, J.; Kniazeva, E.; Hornick, J.E.; Woodruff, T.K.; Shea, L.D. Promoting Extracellular Matrix Remodeling via Ascorbic Acid Enhances the Survival of Primary Ovarian Follicles Encapsulated in Alginate Hydrogels. *Biotechnol. Bioeng.* **2014**, *111*, 1417–1429. [CrossRef]
50. Terren, C.; Nisolle, M.; Munaut, C. Pharmacological Inhibition of the PI3K/PTEN/Akt and MTOR Signalling Pathways Limits Follicle Activation Induced by Ovarian Cryopreservation and in Vitro Culture. *J. Ovarian Res.* **2021**, *14*, 95. [CrossRef]
51. Vitale, F.; Cacciottola, L.; Yu, F.S.; Barretta, M.; Hossay, C.; Donnez, J.; Dolmans, M.M. Importance of Oxygen Tension in Human Ovarian Tissue *in Vitro* Culture. *Hum. Reprod.* **2023**, *38*, 1538–1546. [CrossRef] [PubMed]
52. Rossetto, R.; Saraiva, M.V.A.; dos Santos, R.R.; da Silva, C.M.G.; Faustino, L.R.; Chaves, R.N.; Brito, I.R.; Rodrigues, G.Q.; Lima, I.M.T.; Donato, M.A.M.; et al. Effect of Medium Composition on the in Vitro Culture of Bovine Pre-Antral Follicles: Morphology and Viability Do Not Guarantee Functionality. *Zygote* **2013**, *21*, 125–128. [CrossRef] [PubMed]
53. Paulino, L.R.F.M.; Cunha, E.V.; Barbalho Silva, A.W.; Souza, G.B.; Lopes, E.P.F.; Donato, M.A.M.; Peixoto, C.A.; Matos-Brito, B.G.; van den Hurk, R.; Silva, J.R.V. Effects of Tumour Necrosis Factor-alpha and Interleukin-1 Beta on in Vitro Development of Bovine Secondary Follicles. *Reprod. Domest. Anim.* **2018**, *53*, 997–1005. [CrossRef] [PubMed]
54. Kedem, A.; Fisch, B.; Garor, R.; Ben-Zaken, A.; Gizunterman, T.; Felz, C.; Ben-Haroush, A.; Kravarusic, D.; Abir, R. Growth Differentiating Factor 9 (GDF9) and Bone Morphogenetic Protein 15 Both Activate Development of Human Primordial Follicles in Vitro, with Seemingly More Beneficial Effects of GDF9. *J. Clin. Endocrinol. Metab.* **2011**, *96*, E1246–E1254. [CrossRef]
55. Wang, T.; Yan, L.; Yan, J.; Lu, C.; Xia, X.; Yin, T.; Zhu, X.; Gao, J.; Ding, T.; Hu, W.; et al. Basic Fibroblast Growth Factor Promotes the Development of Human Ovarian Early Follicles during Growth in Vitro. *Hum. Reprod.* **2014**, *29*, 568–576. [CrossRef]

56. Yin, H.; Kristensen, S.G.; Jiang, H.; Rasmussen, A.; Andersen, C.Y. Survival and Growth of Isolated Pre-Antral Follicles from Human Ovarian Medulla Tissue during Long-Term 3D Culture. *Hum. Reprod.* **2016**, *31*, 1531–1539. [CrossRef]
57. Hosseini, M.; Salehpour, S.; Ghaffari Novin, M.; Shams Mofarahe, Z.; Abdollahifar, M.-A.; Piryaei, A. Improvement of in Situ Follicular Activation and Early Development in Cryopreserved Human Ovarian Cortical Tissue by Co-Culturing with Mesenchymal Stem Cells. *Cells Tissues Organs* **2019**, *208*, 48–58. [CrossRef]
58. Dadashzadeh, A.; Moghassemi, S.; Peaucelle, A.; Lucci, C.M.; Amorim, C.A. Mind the Mechanical Strength: Tailoring a 3D Matrix to Encapsulate Isolated Human Preantral Follicles. *Hum. Reprod. Open* **2023**, *2023*, hoad004. [CrossRef]
59. Hsueh, A.J.W.; Kawamura, K.; Cheng, Y.; Fauser, B.C.J.M. Intraovarian Control of Early Folliculogenesis. *Endocr. Rev.* **2015**, *36*, 1–24. [CrossRef] [PubMed]
60. Margulis, S.; Abir, R.; Felz, C.; Nitke, S.; Krissi, H.; Fisch, B. Bone Morphogenetic Protein 15 Expression in Human Ovaries from Fetuses, Girls, and Women. *Fertil. Steril.* **2009**, *92*, 1666–1673. [CrossRef] [PubMed]
61. Oron, G.; Fisch, B.; Ao, A.; Zhang, X.Y.; Farhi, J.; Haroush, A.B.; Kesseler-Icekson, G.; Abir, R. Expression of Growth-Differentiating Factor 9 and Its Type 1 Receptor in Human Ovaries. *Reprod. BioMedicine Online* **2010**, *21*, 109–117. [CrossRef]
62. Hussein, T.S.; Thompson, J.G.; Gilchrist, R.B. Oocyte-Secreted Factors Enhance Oocyte Developmental Competence. *Dev. Biol.* **2006**, *296*, 514–521. [CrossRef]
63. Gilchrist, R.B.; Lane, M.; Thompson, J.G. Oocyte-Secreted Factors: Regulators of Cumulus Cell Function and Oocyte Quality. *Hum. Reprod. Update* **2008**, *14*, 159–177. [CrossRef] [PubMed]
64. Dong, J.; Albertini, D.F.; Nishimori, K.; Kumar, T.R.; Lu, N.; Matzuk, M.M. Growth Differentiation Factor-9 Is Required during Early Ovarian Folliculogenesis. *Nature* **1996**, *383*, 531–535. [CrossRef] [PubMed]
65. Yan, C.; Wang, P.; DeMayo, J.; DeMayo, F.J.; Elvin, J.A.; Carino, C.; Prasad, S.V.; Skinner, S.S.; Dunbar, B.S.; Dube, J.L.; et al. Synergistic Roles of Bone Morphogenetic Protein 15 and Growth Differentiation Factor 9 in Ovarian Function. *Mol. Endocrinol.* **2001**, *15*, 854–866. [CrossRef] [PubMed]
66. Farhat, S.A.; Jabbari, F.; Jabbari, P.; Rezaei, N. Targeting Signaling Pathways Involved in Primordial Follicle Growth or Dormancy: Potential Application in Prevention of Follicular Loss and Infertility. *Expert. Opin. Biol. Ther.* **2022**, *22*, 871–881. [CrossRef] [PubMed]
67. Weenen, C.; Laven, J.S.E.; Von Bergh, A.R.M.; Cranfield, M.; Groome, N.P.; Visser, J.A.; Kramer, P.; Fauser, B.C.J.M.; Themmen, A.P.N. Anti-Müllerian Hormone Expression Pattern in the Human Ovary: Potential Implications for Initial and Cyclic Follicle Recruitment. *Mol. Hum. Reprod.* **2004**, *10*, 77–83. [CrossRef] [PubMed]
68. Meinsohn, M.-C.; Saatcioglu, H.D.; Wei, L.; Li, Y.; Horn, H.; Chauvin, M.; Kano, M.; Nguyen, N.M.P.; Nagykery, N.; Kashiwagi, A.; et al. Single-Cell Sequencing Reveals Suppressive Transcriptional Programs Regulated by MIS/AMH in Neonatal Ovaries. *Proc. Natl. Acad. Sci. USA* **2021**, *118*, e2100920118. [CrossRef] [PubMed]
69. Durlinger, A.L.; Kramer, P.; Karels, B.; de Jong, F.H.; Uilenbroek, J.T.; Grootegoed, J.A.; Themmen, A.P. Control of Primordial Follicle Recruitment by Anti-Müllerian Hormone in the Mouse Ovary. *Endocrinology* **1999**, *140*, 5789–5796. [CrossRef]
70. Carlsson, I.B.; Scott, J.E.; Visser, J.A.; Ritvos, O.; Themmen, A.P.N.; Hovatta, O. Anti-Müllerian Hormone Inhibits Initiation of Growth of Human Primordial Ovarian Follicles in Vitro. *Hum. Reprod.* **2006**, *21*, 2223–2227. [CrossRef]
71. Pan, D. Hippo Signaling in Organ Size Control. *Genes. Dev.* **2007**, *21*, 886–897. [CrossRef]
72. Kawamura, K.; Cheng, Y.; Suzuki, N.; Deguchi, M.; Sato, Y.; Takae, S.; Ho, C.; Kawamura, N.; Tamura, M.; Hashimoto, S.; et al. Hippo Signaling Disruption and Akt Stimulation of Ovarian Follicles for Infertility Treatment. *Proc. Natl. Acad. Sci. USA* **2013**, *110*, 17474–17479. [CrossRef] [PubMed]
73. Lv, X.; He, C.; Huang, C.; Wang, H.; Hua, G.; Wang, Z.; Zhou, J.; Chen, X.; Ma, B.; Timm, B.K.; et al. Timely Expression and Activation of YAP1 in Granulosa Cells Is Essential for Ovarian Follicle Development. *FASEB J.* **2019**, *33*, 10049–10064. [CrossRef] [PubMed]
74. Plewes, M.R.; Hou, X.; Zhang, P.; Liang, A.; Hua, G.; Wood, J.R.; Cupp, A.S.; Lv, X.; Wang, C.; Davis, J.S. Yes-Associated Protein 1 Is Required for Proliferation and Function of Bovine Granulosa Cells in Vitro†. *Biol. Reprod.* **2019**, *101*, 1001–1017. [CrossRef] [PubMed]
75. Masciangelo, R.; Hossay, C.; Chiti, M.C.; Manavella, D.D.; Amorim, C.A.; Donnez, J.; Dolmans, M.-M. Role of the PI3K and Hippo Pathways in Follicle Activation after Grafting of Human Ovarian Tissue. *J. Assist. Reprod. Genet.* **2020**, *37*, 101–108. [CrossRef] [PubMed]
76. Barretta, M.; Cacciottola, L.; Hossay, C.; Donnez, J.; Dolmans, M.-M. Impact of Human Ovarian Tissue Manipulation on Follicles: Evidence of a Potential First Wave of Follicle Activation during Fertility Preservation Procedures. *J. Assist. Reprod. Genet.* **2023**, *40*, 2769–2776. [CrossRef]
77. Lunding, S.A.; Andersen, A.N.; Hardardottir, L.; Olesen, H.Ø.; Kristensen, S.G.; Andersen, C.Y.; Pors, S.E. Hippo Signaling, Actin Polymerization, and Follicle Activation in Fragmented Human Ovarian Cortex. *Mol. Reprod. Devel.* **2020**, *87*, 711–719. [CrossRef]
78. De Roo, C.; Lierman, S.; Tilleman, K.; De Sutter, P. In-Vitro Fragmentation of Ovarian Tissue Activates Primordial Follicles through the Hippo Pathway. *Hum. Reprod. Open* **2020**, *2020*, hoaa048. [CrossRef]
79. Zuccotti, M.; Merico, V.; Cecconi, S.; Redi, C.A.; Garagna, S. What Does It Take to Make a Developmentally Competent Mammalian Egg? *Hum. Reprod. Update* **2011**, *17*, 525–540. [CrossRef]
80. Adhikari, D.; Liu, K. Molecular Mechanisms Underlying the Activation of Mammalian Primordial Follicles. *Endocr. Rev.* **2009**, *30*, 438–464. [CrossRef] [PubMed]

81. Zhang, H.; Liu, K. Cellular and Molecular Regulation of the Activation of Mammalian Primordial Follicles: Somatic Cells Initiate Follicle Activation in Adulthood. *Hum. Reprod. Update* **2015**, *21*, 779–786. [CrossRef]
82. Reddy, P.; Zheng, W.; Liu, K. Mechanisms Maintaining the Dormancy and Survival of Mammalian Primordial Follicles. *Trends Endocrinol. Metab.* **2010**, *21*, 96–103. [CrossRef] [PubMed]
83. Gougeon, A. Human Ovarian Follicular Development: From Activation of Resting Follicles to Preovulatory Maturation. *Ann. D'endocrinologie* **2010**, *71*, 132–143. [CrossRef] [PubMed]
84. Castrillon, D.H.; Miao, L.; Kollipara, R.; Horner, J.W.; DePinho, R.A. Suppression of Ovarian Follicle Activation in Mice by the Transcription Factor Foxo3a. *Science* **2003**, *301*, 215–218. [CrossRef] [PubMed]
85. Albamonte, M.I.; Calabró, L.Y.; Albamonte, M.S.; Zuccardi, L.; Stella, I.; Halperin, J.; Vitullo, A.D. PTEN and FOXO3 Expression in the Prenatal and Postnatal Human Ovary. *J. Assist. Reprod. Genet.* **2020**, *37*, 1613–1622. [CrossRef]
86. Tong, Y.; Li, F.; Lu, Y.; Cao, Y.; Gao, J.; Liu, J. Rapamycin-Sensitive MTORC1 Signaling Is Involved in Physiological Primordial Follicle Activation in Mouse Ovary: Primordial Follicle Activation Entails mTORC1. *Mol. Reprod. Dev.* **2013**, *80*, 1018–1034. [CrossRef]
87. Ernst, E.H.; Grøndahl, M.L.; Grund, S.; Hardy, K.; Heuck, A.; Sunde, L.; Franks, S.; Andersen, C.Y.; Villesen, P.; Lykke-Hartmann, K. Dormancy and Activation of Human Oocytes from Primordial and Primary Follicles: Molecular Clues to Oocyte Regulation. *Hum. Reprod.* **2017**, *32*, 1684–1700. [CrossRef]
88. Nagamatsu, G.; Shimamoto, S.; Hamazaki, N.; Nishimura, Y.; Hayashi, K. Mechanical Stress Accompanied with Nuclear Rotation Is Involved in the Dormant State of Mouse Oocytes. *Sci. Adv.* **2019**, *5*, eaav9960. [CrossRef] [PubMed]
89. Gougeon, A. Dynamics of Follicular Growth in the Human: A Model from Preliminary Results. *Hum. Reprod.* **1986**, *1*, 81–87. [CrossRef]
90. Novella-Maestre, E.; Herraiz, S.; Rodríguez-Iglesias, B.; Díaz-García, C.; Pellicer, A. Short-Term PTEN Inhibition Improves In Vitro Activation of Primordial Follicles, Preserves Follicular Viability, and Restores AMH Levels in Cryopreserved Ovarian Tissue from Cancer Patients. *PLoS ONE* **2015**, *10*, e0127786. [CrossRef]
91. Li, J.; Kawamura, K.; Cheng, Y.; Liu, S.; Klein, C.; Liu, S.; Duan, E.-K.; Hsueh, A.J.W. Activation of Dormant Ovarian Follicles to Generate Mature Eggs. *Proc. Natl. Acad. Sci. USA* **2010**, *107*, 10280–10284. [CrossRef] [PubMed]
92. Suzuki, N.; Yoshioka, N.; Takae, S.; Sugishita, Y.; Tamura, M.; Hashimoto, S.; Morimoto, Y.; Kawamura, K. Successful Fertility Preservation Following Ovarian Tissue Vitrification in Patients with Primary Ovarian Insufficiency. *Hum. Reprod.* **2015**, *30*, 608–615. [CrossRef]
93. Shen, W.H.; Balajee, A.S.; Wang, J.; Wu, H.; Eng, C.; Pandolfi, P.P.; Yin, Y. Essential Role for Nuclear PTEN in Maintaining Chromosomal Integrity. *Cell* **2007**, *128*, 157–170. [CrossRef]
94. Jagarlamudi, K.; Liu, L.; Adhikari, D.; Reddy, P.; Idahl, A.; Ottander, U.; Lundin, E.; Liu, K. Oocyte-Specific Deletion of Pten in Mice Reveals a Stage-Specific Function of PTEN/PI3K Signaling in Oocytes in Controlling Follicular Activation. *PLoS ONE* **2009**, *4*, e6186. [CrossRef]
95. Maidarti, M.; Clarkson, Y.L.; McLaughlin, M.; Anderson, R.A.; Telfer, E.E. Inhibition of PTEN Activates Bovine Non-Growing Follicles *in Vitro* but Increases DNA Damage and Reduces DNA Repair Response. *Hum. Reprod.* **2019**, *34*, 297–307. [CrossRef] [PubMed]
96. Griesinger, G.; Fauser, B.C.J.M. Drug-Free in-Vitro Activation of Ovarian Cortex; Can It Really Activate the 'Ovarian Gold Reserve'? *Reprod. BioMedicine Online* **2020**, *40*, 187–189. [CrossRef]
97. Tingen, C.M.; Kiesewetter, S.E.; Jozefik, J.; Thomas, C.; Tagler, D.; Shea, L.; Woodruff, T.K. A Macrophage and Theca Cell-Enriched Stromal Cell Population Influences Growth and Survival of Immature Murine Follicles in Vitro. *Reproduction* **2011**, *141*, 809–820. [CrossRef] [PubMed]
98. Tagler, D.; Tu, T.; Smith, R.M.; Anderson, N.R.; Tingen, C.M.; Woodruff, T.K.; Shea, L.D. Embryonic Fibroblasts Enable the Culture of Primary Ovarian Follicles Within Alginate Hydrogels. *Tissue Eng. Part. A* **2012**, *18*, 1229–1238. [CrossRef] [PubMed]
99. Vitale, F.; Cacciottola, L.; Camboni, A.; Donnez, J.; Dolmans, M.M. Assessing the Effect of Adipose Tissue-Derived Stem Cell-Conditioned Medium on Follicles and Stromal Cells in Bovine Ovarian Tissue Culture. *RBM Online*, 2024; *accepted, in press*.
100. Redding, G.P.; Bronlund, J.E.; Hart, A.L. Mathematical Modelling of Oxygen Transport-Limited Follicle Growth. *Reproduction* **2007**, *133*, 1095–1106. [CrossRef]
101. Redding, G.P.; Bronlund, J.E.; Hart, A.L. Theoretical Investigation into the Dissolved Oxygen Levels in Follicular Fluid of the Developing Human Follicle Using Mathematical Modelling. *Reprod. Fertil. Dev.* **2008**, *20*, 408. [CrossRef]
102. Shimamoto, S.; Nishimura, Y.; Nagamatsu, G.; Hamada, N.; Kita, H.; Hikabe, O.; Hamazaki, N.; Hayashi, K. Hypoxia Induces the Dormant State in Oocytes through Expression of *Foxo3*. *Proc. Natl. Acad. Sci. USA* **2019**, *116*, 12321–12326. [CrossRef]
103. Jorssen, E.P.A.; Langbeen, A.; Fransen, E.; Martinez, E.L.; Leroy, J.L.M.R.; Bols, P.E.J. Monitoring Preantral Follicle Survival and Growth in Bovine Ovarian Biopsies by Repeated Use of Neutral Red and Cultured in Vitro under Low and High Oxygen Tension. *Theriogenology* **2014**, *82*, 387–395. [CrossRef]
104. Roy, S.K.; Treacy, B.J. Isolation and Long-Term Culture of Human Preantral Follicles. *Fertil. Steril.* **1993**, *59*, 783–790. [CrossRef] [PubMed]
105. Xu, M.; Barrett, S.L.; West-Farrell, E.; Kondapalli, L.A.; Kiesewetter, S.E.; Shea, L.D.; Woodruff, T.K. In Vitro Grown Human Ovarian Follicles from Cancer Patients Support Oocyte Growth. *Hum. Reprod.* **2009**, *24*, 2531–2540. [CrossRef] [PubMed]

106. Xia, X.; Wang, T.; Yin, T.; Yan, L.; Yan, J.; Lu, C.; Liang, Z.; Li, M.; Zhang, Y.; Jin, H.; et al. Mesenchymal Stem Cells Facilitate In Vitro Development of Human Preantral Follicle. *Reprod. Sci.* **2015**, *22*, 1367–1376. [CrossRef] [PubMed]
107. Xiao, S.; Zhang, J.; Romero, M.M.; Smith, K.N.; Shea, L.D.; Woodruff, T.K. In Vitro Follicle Growth Supports Human Oocyte Meiotic Maturation. *Sci. Rep.* **2015**, *5*, 17323. [CrossRef] [PubMed]
108. Xu, F.; Lawson, M.S.; Bean, Y.; Ting, A.Y.; Pejovic, T.; De Geest, K.; Moffitt, M.; Mitalipov, S.M.; Xu, J. Matrix-Free 3D Culture Supports Human Follicular Development from the Unilaminar to the Antral Stage in Vitro Yielding Morphologically Normal Metaphase II Oocytes. *Hum. Reprod.* **2021**, *36*, 1326–1338. [CrossRef] [PubMed]
109. Thomas, F.H.; Campbell, B.K.; Armstrong, D.G.; Telfer, E.E. Effects of IGF-I Bioavailability on Bovine Preantral Follicular Development in Vitro. *Reproduction* **2007**, *133*, 1121–1128. [CrossRef]
110. McLaughlin, M.; Telfer, E.E. Oocyte Development in Bovine Primordial Follicles Is Promoted by Activin and FSH within a Two-Step Serum-Free Culture System. *Reproduction* **2010**, *139*, 971–978. [CrossRef] [PubMed]
111. Dolmans, M.-M.; Michaux, N.; Camboni, A.; Martinez-Madrid, B.; Van Langendonckt, A.; Annarita Nottola, S.; Donnez, J. Evaluation of Liberase, a Purified Enzyme Blend, for the Isolation of Human Primordial and Primary Ovarian Follicles. *Hum. Reprod.* **2006**, *21*, 413–420. [CrossRef] [PubMed]
112. Green, L.J.; Shikanov, A. In Vitro Culture Methods of Preantral Follicles. *Theriogenology* **2016**, *86*, 229–238. [CrossRef]
113. Pors, S.E.; Ramløse, M.; Nikiforov, D.; Lundsgaard, K.; Cheng, J.; Andersen, C.Y.; Kristensen, S.G. Initial Steps in Reconstruction of the Human Ovary: Survival of Pre-Antral Stage Follicles in a Decellularized Human Ovarian Scaffold. *Hum. Reprod.* **2019**, *34*, 1523–1535. [CrossRef]
114. Laronda, M.M.; Rutz, A.L.; Xiao, S.; Whelan, K.A.; Duncan, F.E.; Roth, E.W.; Woodruff, T.K.; Shah, R.N. A Bioprosthetic Ovary Created Using 3D Printed Microporous Scaffolds Restores Ovarian Function in Sterilized Mice. *Nat. Commun.* **2017**, *8*, 15261. [CrossRef] [PubMed]
115. McLaughlin, M.; Bromfield, J.J.; Albertini, D.F.; Telfer, E.E. Activin Promotes Follicular Integrity and Oogenesis in Cultured Pre-Antral Bovine Follicles. *Mol. Hum. Reprod.* **2010**, *16*, 644–653. [CrossRef] [PubMed]
116. Bhartiya, D.; Patel, H. An Overview of FSH-FSHR Biology and Explaining the Existing Conundrums. *J. Ovarian Res.* **2021**, *14*, 144. [CrossRef]
117. Navalakhe, R.M.; Jagtap, D.D.; Nayak, S.U.; Nandedkar, T.D.; Mahale, S.D. Effect of FSH Receptor-Binding Inhibitor-8 on FSH-Mediated Granulosa Cell Signaling and Proliferation. *Chem. Biol. Drug Des.* **2013**, *82*, 178–188. [CrossRef]
118. Tian, S.; Zhang, H.; Chang, H.-M.; Klausen, C.; Huang, H.-F.; Jin, M.; Leung, P.C.K. Activin A Promotes Hyaluronan Production and Upregulates Versican Expression in Human Granulosa Cells†. *Biol. Reprod.* **2022**, *107*, 458–473. [CrossRef] [PubMed]
119. Wijayarathna, R.; de Kretser, D.M. Activins in Reproductive Biology and Beyond. *Hum. Reprod. Update* **2016**, *22*, 342–357. [CrossRef]
120. Cadenas, J.; Poulsen, L.C.; Nikiforov, D.; Grøndahl, M.L.; Kumar, A.; Bahnu, K.; Englund, A.L.M.; Malm, J.; Marko-Varga, G.; Pla, I.; et al. Regulation of Human Oocyte Maturation in Vivo during the Final Maturation of Follicles. *Hum. Reprod.* **2023**, *38*, 686–700. [CrossRef] [PubMed]
121. Woodruff, T.K.; Shea, L.D. A New Hypothesis Regarding Ovarian Follicle Development: Ovarian Rigidity as a Regulator of Selection and Health. *J. Assist. Reprod. Genet.* **2011**, *28*, 3–6. [CrossRef] [PubMed]
122. Edwards, R.G. Maturation in Vitro of Mouse, Sheep, Cow, Pig, Rhesus Monkey and Human Ovarian Oocytes. *Nature* **1965**, *208*, 349–351. [CrossRef] [PubMed]
123. De Vos, M.; Grynberg, M.; Ho, T.M.; Yuan, Y.; Albertini, D.F.; Gilchrist, R.B. Perspectives on the Development and Future of Oocyte IVM in Clinical Practice. *J. Assist. Reprod. Genet.* **2021**, *38*, 1265–1280. [CrossRef] [PubMed]
124. Gilchrist, R.B.; Smitz, J. Oocyte in Vitro Maturation: Physiological Basis and Application to Clinical Practice. *Fertil. Steril.* **2023**, *119*, 524–539. [CrossRef] [PubMed]
125. Keefe, D.; Kumar, M.; Kalmbach, K. Oocyte Competency Is the Key to Embryo Potential. *Fertil. Steril.* **2015**, *103*, 317–322. [CrossRef] [PubMed]
126. Osman, E.; Franasiak, J.; Scott, R. Oocyte and Embryo Manipulation and Epigenetics. *Semin. Reprod. Med.* **2018**, *36*, e1–e9. [CrossRef] [PubMed]
127. Laprise, S.L. Implications of Epigenetics and Genomic Imprinting in Assisted Reproductive Technologies. *Mol. Reprod. Dev.* **2009**, *76*, 1006–1018. [CrossRef]
128. Coticchio, G.; Sciajno, R.; Hutt, K.; Bromfield, J.; Borini, A.; Albertini, D.F. Comparative Analysis of the Metaphase II Spindle of Human Oocytes through Polarized Light and High-Performance Confocal Microscopy. *Fertil. Steril.* **2010**, *93*, 2056–2064. [CrossRef]
129. Nagashima, J.B.; El Assal, R.; Songsasen, N.; Demirci, U. Evaluation of an Ovary-on-a-Chip in Large Mammalian Models: Species Specificity and Influence of Follicle Isolation Status. *J. Tissue Eng. Regen. Med.* **2018**, *12*, e1926–e1935. [CrossRef]
130. Önen, S.; Atik, A.C.; Gizer, M.; Köse, S.; Yaman, Ö.; Külah, H.; Korkusuz, P. A Pumpless Monolayer Microfluidic Device Based on Mesenchymal Stem Cell-Conditioned Medium Promotes Neonatal Mouse in Vitro Spermatogenesis. *Stem Cell Res. Ther.* **2023**, *14*, 127. [CrossRef]
131. Sharma, S.; Venzac, B.; Burgers, T.; Le Gac, S.; Schlatt, S. Microfluidics in Male Reproduction: Is Ex Vivo Culture of Primate Testis Tissue a Future Strategy for ART or Toxicology Research? *Mol. Hum. Reprod.* **2020**, *26*, 179–192. [CrossRef]

132. Van Blerkom, J. Intrafollicular Influences on Human Oocyte Developmental Competence: Perifollicular Vascularity, Oocyte Metabolism and Mitochondrial Function. *Hum. Reprod.* **2000**, *15* (Suppl. S2), 173–188. [CrossRef] [PubMed]
133. Lancaster, M.A.; Knoblich, J.A. Organogenesis in a Dish: Modeling Development and Disease Using Organoid Technologies. *Science* **2014**, *345*, 1247125. [CrossRef] [PubMed]
134. Li, X.; Zheng, M.; Xu, B.; Li, D.; Shen, Y.; Nie, Y.; Ma, L.; Wu, J. Generation of Offspring-Producing 3D Ovarian Organoids Derived from Female Germline Stem Cells and Their Application in Toxicological Detection. *Biomaterials* **2021**, *279*, 121213. [CrossRef] [PubMed]
135. ESHRE Task Force on Ethics and Law including; Pennings, G.; de Wert, G.; Shenfield, F.; Cohen, J.; Tarlatzis, B.; Devroey, P. ESHRE Task Force on Ethics and Law 13: The Welfare of the Child in Medically Assisted Reproduction. *Hum. Reprod.* **2007**, *22*, 2585–2588. [CrossRef] [PubMed]
136. Crawshaw, M. Psychosocial Oncofertility Issues Faced by Adolescents and Young Adults over Their Lifetime: A Review of the Research. *Hum. Fertil.* **2013**, *16*, 59–63. [CrossRef]

MDPI AG
Grosspeteranlage 5
4052 Basel
Switzerland
Tel.: +41 61 683 77 34

Journal of Clinical Medicine Editorial Office
E-mail: jcm@mdpi.com
www.mdpi.com/journal/jcm

www.ingramcontent.com/pod-product-compliance
Lightning Source LLC
Chambersburg PA
CBHW041357210926
51850CB00013B/3106
9783725843657